Ahlin/White/Tsamtsouris/Saadia

Maxillofacial Orthopedics: A Clinical Approach for the Growing Child

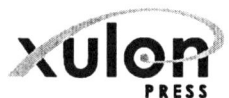

Copyright © 2004 by Ahlin/White/Tsamtsouris/Saadia

Maxillofacial Orthopedics:
A Clinical Approach for the Growing Child
by Ahlin/White/Tsamtsouris/Saadia

Printed in the United States of America

ISBN 1-591609-40-2

All rights reserved. No part of this publication may be reproduced or transmitted in any form or by any means without written permission of the publisher.

Xulon Press
www.XulonPress.com

Xulon Press books are available in bookstores everywhere, and on the Web at www.XulonPress.com.

Dedication

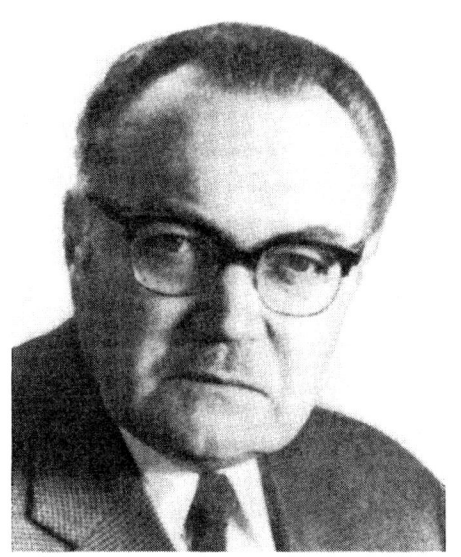

Prof. Wilhelm Balters

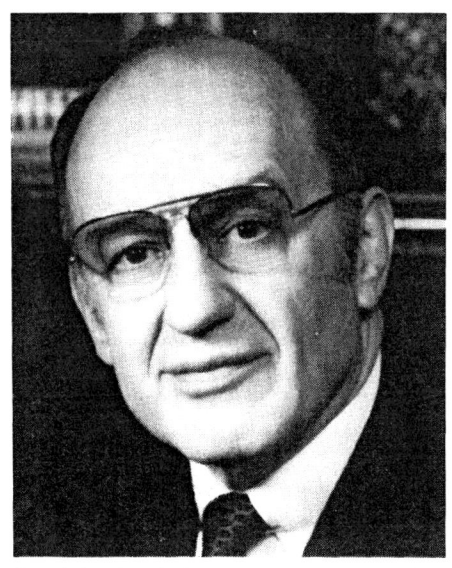

Dr. John W. Witzig

This work is dedicated to two clinicians who had much influence in recent developments of the treatment of malocclusion in America: Professor Wilhelm Balters (1893–1973) and Dr. John W. Witzig.

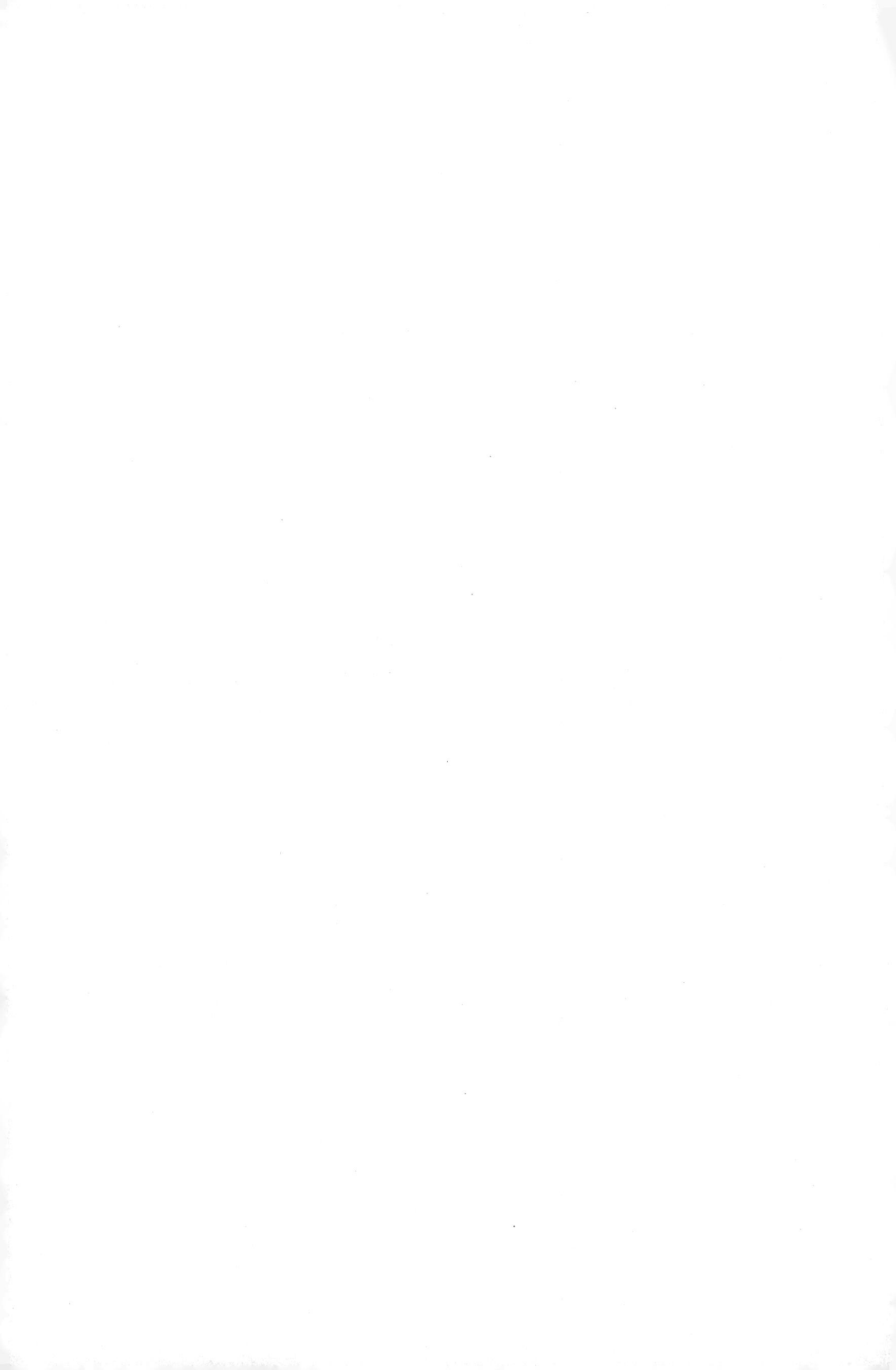

Contents

Part 1 Historical and Scientific Background

Chapter 1	Historical Development of Maxillofacial Orthopedic Technique	15
Chapter 2	Biological Shaping of the Craniofacial Complex	29
Chapter 3	Craniofacial Response to Maxillofacial Orthopedic Therapy	73

Part 2 Evaluation

Chapter 4	Examination and Diagnosis for Malocclusion	83
Chapter 5	Postural and Nutritional Considerations	117
Chapter 6	Treatment Planning	139

Part 3 Treatment

Chapter 7	Class I Malocclusion	155
Chapter 8	Class II Malocclusion	177
Chapter 9	Class III Malocclusion	203
Chapter 10	Treatment of Craniomandibular Disorders With Maxillofacial Orthopedic Appliances	217

Contents

Part 4 Special Considerations

Chapter 11	Extraction for Treatment of Malocclusion	265
Chapter 12	Special Problems in Treatment of Malocclusion	283
Chapter 13	Critical Errors in Diagnosis and Treatment of Malocclusion	301
Chapter 14	The Future	317
Index		320

Foreword

There is strong worldwide demand on the part of health-oriented consumers and clinicians for high-quality treatment for malocclusion in the growing child. Many types of malocclusion can be prevented with early treatment and guidance of the developing occlusion.

Preventing or intercepting malocclusion at the earliest possible time has always been one of my primary goals. Treatment must be effective but not damaging to the teeth or periodontal tissues. Therapy that is biologically oriented can be used for all types of malocclusion without danger to the surrounding tissues.

Early in my professional career I saw that excellent results could be obtained with treatment based on the biological principles of maxillofacial orthopedic techniques. In a search for efficient and effective treatment, I visited and was inspired by Dr. A. M. Schwarz in Vienna, Austria. Professor Schwarz had devoted his life to realizing the fullest treatment potential from removable appliances.

Heightened interest in maxillofacial orthopedic appliances has made essential the publication of a reliable, readable textbook outlining the logical, sequential technique that effective treatment requires. *Maxillofacial Orthopedics* presents a practical, time-saving approach to the treatment of malocclusion and temporomandibular joint disorder. It has been written to help practitioners treat their patients more intelligently and efficiently. Clinicians who utilize the techniques described in this book will be drawing on superior knowledge of prevention, interception, and treatment of malocclusion and disorders of the craniomandibular articulation.

In January 1973, I introduced the bionator appliance (developed by Professor Balters of Bonn, West Germany) in the United States. In order to shorten the treatment time, reduce the expense of another appliance, and give superior results, I later modified the bionator appliance into the orthopedic corrector appliance. The appliances presented here are used to achieve the most efficient changes in anteroposterior, transverse, and vertical skeletal relationships. Today the clinician using a combination of removable orthopedic and fixed appliances can achieve end results for his or her patients that are far superior to those obtained using one appliance system alone.

This text will give doctors a better perspective into the philosophy and use of maxillofacial orthopedic appliances. Incorporated into a treatment plan, these appliances will give orthopedic and orthodontic results difficult to attain with other forms of treatment.

This book will serve as a guide to help further progress in treating malocclusion; it will be instrumental in producing increased quality of final results. The role of maxillofacial orthopedic techniques is well-established in the literature. These appliances should be part of the armamentarium of every practitioner treating malocclusion and temporomandibular joint disorder.

It is my belief that the application of maxillofacial orthopedic techniques for the growing child with a malocclusion will guide and stimulate the proper craniofacial development.

John W. Witzig, D.D.S.

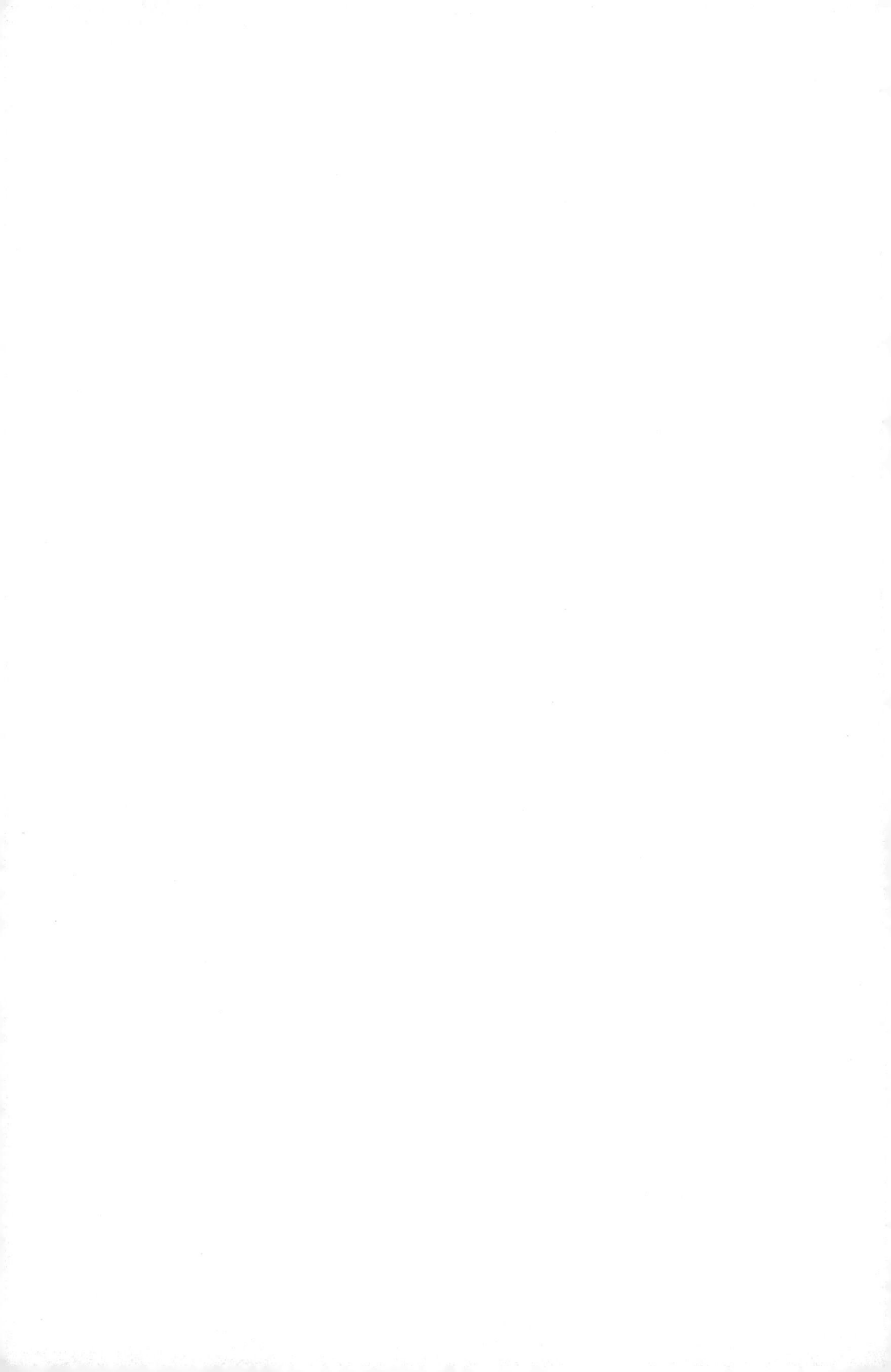

Preface

Maxillofacial Orthopedics is for the clinician. It is not the purpose of this text to provide a simplified approach to orthodontic treatment so that those who are untrained may attempt shortcuts to complete care. It is written by clinicians whose primary concern is the development of a healthy, functional, esthetic, and stable occlusion with minimal occlusal and craniomandibular discrepancies.

Each chapter contains several investigators' efforts to formulate an in-depth, readable guide of specific problems of and solutions to malocclusion. An orthopedic view of correction of malocclusion will aid the clinician in arriving at the best treatment alternative for each individual.

Correction of malocclusions can be time-consuming. Several examples of what orthopedic appliances can and cannot accomplish will direct the clinician to the best course of treatment. In most cases of malocclusion, the least complex solution will be the treatment of choice for the growing child.

This book emphasizes an orthopedic approach for treatment of malocclusion. It should be stressed, however, that early correction of many types of malocclusion may require additional techniques such as fixed multibonded appliances and nonfunctional removable appliances.

In the past, care for malocclusion in the United States has been accomplished primarily with fixed multibanded techniques. Although the treatment rendered has been excellent, there has been a growing need for a more complete orthodontic armamentarium. Functional orthopedic techniques first became popular in Europe in the early 1950s. Their excellent results in treatment have gained notice in America over the past 10 years. The growth in popularity of maxillofacial orthopedic continuing education courses attests to a real desire on the part of orthodontists, pedodontists, periodontists, prosthodontists, oral surgeons, and generalists to find better methods for treating their patients.

Ninety-five percent of the population could benefit by some form of treatment for malocclusion. It will take a concerted team effort by generalists and specialists to provide this care in the next century.

Generalists in the 1980s will be treating fewer restorative and prosthetic patients and more periodontic and orthodontic patients than ever before. There are two highly commendable reasons for this shift. First, the numbers of carious lesions have been dramatically reduced by the growth of community water fluoridation, topically applied fluorides, occlusal sealants, and a critical view of refined sugars in the diet. Second, and even more important, the clinician is more conscious of treating the entire dental-alveolar-facial complex. One can no longer consider treatment of an isolated tooth without an awareness of total health. Moreover, treatment for malocclusion cannot proceed without regard for facial esthetics, temporomandibular joint function, and periodontal health. We can little afford to take a chance on achieving less than optimal treatment results.

Prevention has always been easier and less expensive than treatment. The central theme of this book is dedicated to a discussion of prevention and early treatment of malocclusion.

Facial esthetics are very important. The basic treatment objective is to achieve harmonious facial esthetics with well-balanced dental, muscular, and skeletal components. The clinician is obliged to learn more about the psychological and psychosocial implications of unattractive faces, and do something about them. General body posture is also important. Poor posture may be exacerbated by a craniomandibular disorder. A consideration of condylar position, the orthostatic position of the head, and the relationship to the cervical spine is important for excellent overall treatment results.

The chapters develop logically with the more common types of malocclusion receiving the most emphasis. The first three chapters are devoted to the history of maxillofacial orthopedics and the physiology and biological shaping of the craniofacial complex. The next three chapters are devoted to patient evaluation, diagnosis, and treatment planning. Orthopedic appliance treatment of the Angle classifications of malocclusion is presented as well as orthopedic appliance treatment of temporomandibular joint (capsular) disorder. Dental extraction for treatment of malocclusion is discussed in depth. Special problems and critical errors in treating malocclusion are also evaluated. Each section represents a cross-fertilization of ideas from several pedodontists, orthodontists, and generalists.

Dentistry is a medical speciality. If we are to provide a leadership role in the 21st century, many dental subspecialties must be integrated into a cohesive multiphasic health treatment delivery system for the total care of the individual. *Maxillofacial Orthopedics* is dedicated to one of the first clinicians to consider the whole patient in his treatment of malocclusion, and to another whose work in disseminating these treatment ideas has made more complete care available to children with malocclusion.

Professor Wilhelm Balters (1893–1973) was a man ahead of his time. He looked at malocclusion as part of a larger problem of abnormal muscular and breathing functions, faulty posture, and deviant craniofacial spatial relationships. His treatment for malocclusion was based on the use of the bionator appliance he developed and used in conjunction with postural exercises and controlled nutrition. While at first many of Professor Balter's concepts were dismissed as unrealistic, by the early 1980s clinicians around the world were following many of his ideas with excellent results.

Dr. John W. Witzig is known best for his contributions to dental education and for his modification of the sagittal and bionator appliances. The techniques that Dr. Witzig recommends for treatment of craniomandibular disorders and correction of malocclusion are noninvasive, biologically and physiologically sound, and easily tolerated by the patient.

Acknowledgments

It is difficult to cite all those who were instrumental in bringing this project to fruition. Dr. John Witzig provided new ideas, inspiration, enthusiasm, and several patients' histories. Dr. Ira Yerkes provided excellent suggestions for treating patients with pain associated with the temporomandibular joint. Drs. Lawrence Funt, Brendon Stack, Bruce Kinnie, William Farrar, William McCarty, Harvey Peck, Sheldon Peck, Donald Tuverson, Lee Graber, T. M. Graber, William Solberg, and Glenn Clark were most generous in allowing different aspects of their work to be reproduced in this text.

Our thanks to Dr. James Dunning, professor emeritus from the Harvard School of Dental Medicine, for his critique and comments on Chapter 14, and to Dr. and Mrs. Hoffmann-Axthelm of Freiberg, West Germany, who provided material on the life of Dr. Balters.

The staffs of the National Library of Medicine and the Library of the National Institutes of Health, and the dental staff at the National Naval Medical Center, were most generous with their time. Dr. G. P. F. Schmuth, professor and chairman of the University of Bonn's Department of Orthodontics, was most helpful in his critique of Chapter 1. Dr. George Eversaul gave freely of his time and suggestions for the chapters on nutrition and treatment of craniomandibular disorders. Dr. Richard Valachovic, director of Clinics, Harvard School of Dental Medicine, was helpful in his critique of Chapters 4 and 5. Dr. Wilma A. Simões of São Paulo, Brazil, and Dr. Kazuhiko Ogiwara, associate professor, Pediatric Division, Nippon Dental University, Tokyo, Japan, were very supportive in sending translations of reprinted publications from their countries.

The staffs at the Tufts and Harvard medical libraries gave generously of their time and provided computer access when it was needed. June Harrington of the Countway Library deserves special thanks for her kindness.

An acknowledgment of thanks and deep appreciation for an overworked but tireless staff is needed: Ms. Dawn Brawley, Ms. Debora Siciliano, Mrs. Tami Lowe, Mrs. Laurie Feener, and Mrs. Helen Madison all helped keep our office functioning smoothly during the two years of preparation of the final draft. Particular gratitude is due to Mrs. Linda Buddenhagen for her long hours of typing and suggestions for the manuscript. My thanks to Ms. Nancy Weems for her help in gathering much of the research material for Chapters 10 through 12.

Many of the excellent photographs of appliances are due to the kindness of Mr. Jack Skay and his staff at Dyna-Flex Laboratories in St. Louis, Missouri. The expertise of Ms. Marlene Wolfe was invaluable in selecting, drawing, and editing the medical illustrations. Mr. Alex Grey has drawn very exacting and educationally rewarding illustrations of the temporomandibular joint musculature and types of malocclusion.

It was very rewarding to see our colleagues, friends, patients, staff, and families provide continual support and understanding. Their team effort made this project possible.

Part 1　　Historical and Scientific Background

Chapter 1

Historical Development of Maxillofacial Orthopedic Technique

Clinical need

Maxillofacial orthopedic appliances have developed as a result of clinical necessity. Clinicians who treat craniofacial growth problems in children have found that a fixed, multibanded technique has not always been entirely reliable for solving all growth discrepancies and resulting malocclusions. Although a fixed appliance regime has proven excellent for full three-axis control of individual tooth movement, a method of guiding maxillomandibular osseous growth was needed.

Early development

Several concepts and inventions from past centuries have been refined, modified, and discarded in a search for the most efficient methods of correcting malocclusion. One of the first "regulating" appliances was introduced in France by Fauchard in 1726. The principle function of this appliance was to expand the dental arch to form an "ideal" arch.[1] The English surgeon, John Hunter, had published *The Natural History of Human Teeth* in 1771.[2] His work gives the first accurate analysis of mandibular growth. A later book, *A Practical Treatise on the Diseases of the Teeth*,[3] developed many of the early principles for treatment of malocclusion.

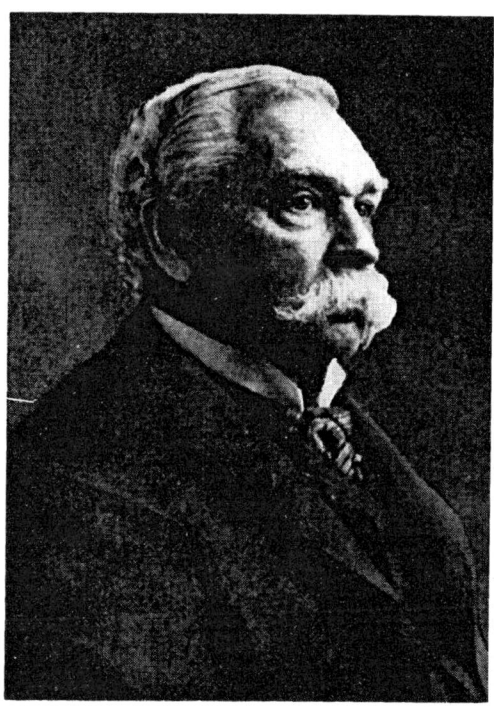

Fig. 1-1 Norman William Kingsley (1829–1913). (Reprinted from *History of Dentistry* [Quintessence Publishing Co., 1981] with permission of Dr. Hoffmann-Axthelm.)

Norman William Kingsley (Fig. 1-1) is often considered the "father of orthodontics" in American literature.[4] His life spanned 84 years. Born in Stockholm, New York, October 26, 1829, he received his first dental education from his uncle. His early

Historical Development of Maxillofacial Orthopedic Technique

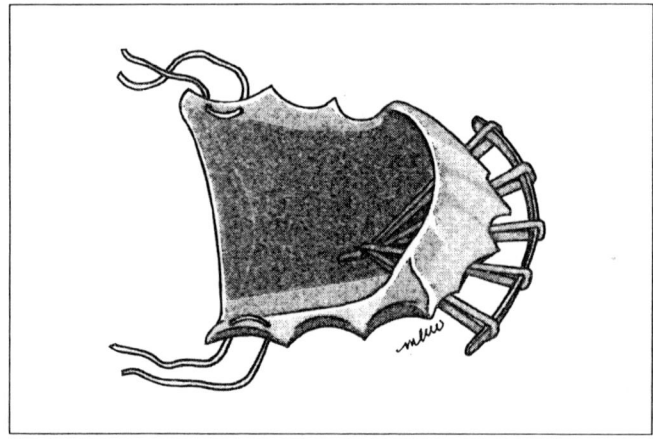

Fig. 1-2 Kingsley's 1880 bite plane for "jumping the bite." (Reprinted from *History of Dentistry* [Quintessence Publishing Co., 1981] with permission of Dr. Hoffmann-Axthelm.)

essays proposed *jumping the bite* by the abrupt repositioning of the mandible from a distal bite to a more forward or normal position. The concepts presented were similar to methods utilized in orthopedic appliances developed later by Robin,[5] and Andresen and Häupl.[6] In 1880[7] Dr. Kingsley had published the design of the appliance used for treating retrognathia by repositioning the mandible forward (Fig. 1-2). Dr. Kingsley also introduced extraoral occipital anchorage for treatment of maxillary anterior protrusion. The concept of extraoral anchorage is still widely used for limiting and correcting maxillary skeletal protrusion.

Influence of E. H. Angle

The importance of a thorough knowledge of growth and development combined with clinical skill was stressed in 1900 in the introduction to the sixth edition of the textbook by Dr. Angle:[1]

It is not enough to simply move into correct alignment irregular teeth. We should have a proper conception of the influence of the malocclusion in arresting or modifying the development of the alveolus, jaws, and muscles, and in shaping the contour of the face. We must consider the numerous possible changes which may follow the movement of teeth into correct positions, with the restoration of the natural functions of the occlusal planes, and the assistance the changes will lend to Nature. . . . It is now well known that the structural changes which follow the correction of malocclusion are often pronounced. In many cases there can be no intelligent diagnosis or plan of treatment unless the change probabilities be fully considered. (pp. 3–4)

Dr. Angle's words were truly prophetic. Although his life was devoted to teaching, research, and the development of a system of correcting malocclusion using regulating appliances, he never relied on any particular mechanical device. In his introduction Dr. Angle also comments:

In reality the regulating appliances are only secondary to many more important considerations. They are only a means to an end, and are no more to the orthodontist than are the colors to the artist, whose success depends on the breadth of his knowledge, the purity of his conception, and his skill in their use.[1] (p. 4)

The genius and creativity of Dr. Angle (Fig. 1-3) have had a worldwide effect on clinicians who study and treat malocclusion. His efforts have placed orthodontics on a firm scientific foundation. His introduction of tubes in 1886 simplified the means of attachment between the cemented bands and the fixed appliance. In 1887, he began utilizing German silver, which greatly simplified the manufacturing of the "regulating" appliances he was developing. In 1899, he published his "Classification of Malocclusion,"[8] which classified occlusal discrepancies based on the occlusal relation of the maxillary and mandibular first molars. Throughout his life, he rejected the extraction of any teeth. In 1928, two years before his death, he developed the edgewise arch as a device to move teeth without causing tipping movement.

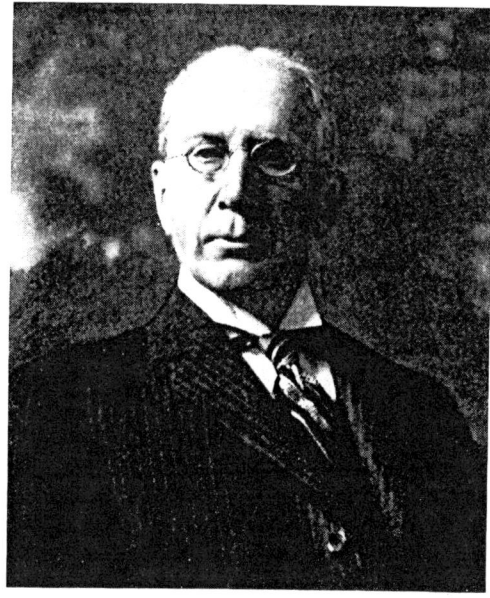

Fig. 1-3 Edward Hartley Angle (1855–1930). (Reprinted from *History of Dentistry* [Quintessence Publishing Co., 1981] with permission of Dr. Hoffmann-Axthelm.)

The European Orthodontic Society

The European Orthodontic Society was founded on September 27, 1907. William G. Law, an American practicing in Berlin, was a founding member of the society and president from 1907 through 1909.[9] However, the force behind the foundation of the European Orthodontic Society was very much due to the influence of Dr. Angle. Dr. Law had taken the Angle Course in 1903; five of the 10 founding members of the Society had either taken the Angle Course or had close association with Dr. Angle.[10] The Society grew slowly in the early years and tried to meet annually. World War I intervened from 1915 to 1921, and World War II began shortly after the society met in Bonn in 1939. The next (24th) meeting of the society was held in Brussels in October 1947. This site was chosen because Brussels was spared the food rationing that was common in other European countries at the time.[10]

Many eminent members of the European Orthodontic Society were involved in the development of maxillofacial orthopedic appliance technique. Expansion screw plates were introduced in the early part of the 1900s. Babcock[11] developed an expansion plate in 1911. Nord[12] discussed screw plates at the 1929 meeting of the society. By 1938, Schwarz[13] had published a textbook demonstrating the design and technical use of more refined appliances. The expansion appliances were highly effective when used in conjunction with the functional appliances that were then being developed.

The influence of Dr. P. Robin on maxillofacial orthopedic technique

The earliest literary references to orthopedic appliances include Kingsley 1880,[7] Robin 1902,[5] and Andresen and Häupl 1936.[6] Certainly, other eminent clinicians and researchers contributed greatly to the literature, but the activator, as currently modified, evolved primarily from the work of Kingsley, Robin, and Andresen and Häupl. Although the appliance created by Kingsley in the late 1870s was designed to reposition the mandible forward, it was Dr. Pierre Robin that combined the repositioned mandible with bimaxillary expansion in a single appliance. In 1902, Dr. Robin presented a paper to the French Society of Stomatology that described the "monobloc" appliance. The paper, entitled "A New Appliance for the Straightening of Teeth,"[5] discussed a method for correction of malocclusion by expansion of the osseous facial structures and repositioning of the mandible using a loose-fitting appliance. The appliance was later discussed by Watry[14] as a device "not meant to be an implement for the straightening of teeth but a passive guide aiming to achieve correction by natural means."

Maxillofacial orthopedic techniques were again discussed in a thesis by Fauconnier presented in 1915 to the Medical Faculty of Paris for partial fulfillment of a degree in medicine.

In 1918, Mershon modified some of the Angle techniques and introduced the lingual arch.[15] Kantorowicz and one of his students, Korkhaus, studied the etiology of malocclusion at the dental school in Bonn.[16] Some of the principles they developed differed from the purely morphological system initiated by Angle. A diagnostic system based on genetic and etiologic considerations was suggested.[17] Many of the ideas in the Kantorowicz-Korkhaus study of diagnostic principles were influential in the biogenetic classification of malocclusion developed by Dr. A. M. Schwarz.[18,19] Understanding the etiology of malocclusion helped develop an awareness of preventive and interceptive procedures for treatment.

From the early 1920s the influence of Dr. George Crozat and Dr. Albert Wiebrecht has been felt in the development of maxillofacial orthopedic techniques. These colleagues furthered the development of a gnathological approach to the correction of malocclusion by encouraging the development of full dental arches and the avoidance of premolar extraction. The Crozat appliance is still in use today.

Between 1924 and 1936, Dr. F. M. Watry gave several presentations based on theories initiated by Dr. Robin. Watry, however, had been influenced by the work of Alfred P. Rogers and the development of facial muscles.[20,21] Although Watry recommended the monoblock appliance, it was to be used as an exercise appliance to reeducate the facial musculature.[22]

The Andresen-Häupl activator

Dr. Viggo Andresen developed a functional appliance as early as 1908 and in 1910 discussed the use of this appliance in the literature.[23] Although first developed as a temporary retaining appliance, Andresen noticed favorable improvement of the occlusion in his patients when they returned from their summer vacations. The work of Drs. Kingsley, Farrar, and Robin helped influence the development of the Andresen activator appliance. The "retainer" device, developed by the American clinician C. A. Hawley also gave form and impetus to the development of the activator appliance. By modifying the appliance developed by Kingsley, which repositioned the mandible forward, and utilizing the loose-fitting monoblock technique of Robin, Andresen was

The Andresen-Häupl Activator

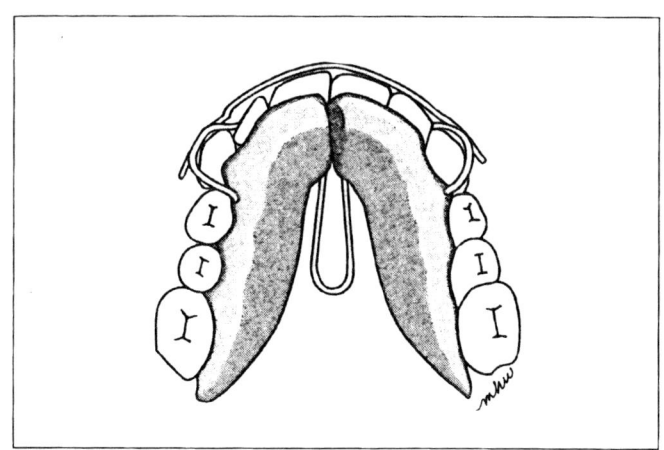

Fig. 1-4 The Andresen activator appliance (1936).

able to develop the precursor to many later variations of the maxillomandibular orthopedic appliance.

By 1927, Dr. Andresen was professor and director of the orthodontic department of the dental school in Oslo. A colleague, Dr. Karl Häupl, was instrumental in developing with Andresen a technique for correcting malocclusion called "functional jaw orthopedics." Between 1910 and 1942 Professor Andresen had published more than 40 journal articles dedicated to the correction of malocclusion. Many of these publications delineate the Norwegian System of functional orthopedic correction.[24-29] This system was discussed by Dr. Oscar Hoffer in 1947 as preferable to other methods because "it works with physiological forces without damaging the tissues."[30]

Although neither Dr. Andresen nor Dr. Häupl were orthodontic specialists (Andresen was a general dentist and Häupl a researcher in periodontology), both pursued the idea of simplifying mechanical therapy by utilizing muscle activation. The Andresen-Häupl activator was designed to increase the availability of treatment for patients. However, Andresen felt that utilization of standardized analysis did not account for the wide biological variation common among any group of patients.[31]

Andresen had read and been influenced by the work of Dr. Farrar. The appliance (Fig. 1-4) was to be a passive appliance which would place intermittent pressure on the facial structures and be controlled by the facial and tongue muscles of the patient. Each appliance was designed to correct malocclusion by altering mandibular position and altering the patient's chewing pattern. The loose-fitting appliance caused the muscles of mastication to become active in order to hold the appliance in the correct position in the mouth. This muscle activator was designed for night use only.[32,33]

The Andresen-Häupl activator appliance was to utilize the functional adaptation of a new mandibular position in order to reposition the teeth and change the direction of osseous growth. Much of this theory was based on earlier work by Roux[34] and Wolff,[35] which advocated that a change in function would bring about a change in bone structure. The appliance was to reflexively evoke contraction of the muscles of mastication by increasing the interocclusal molar distance 2 to 4 mm while worn only at night. Dr. A. M. Schwarz, however, felt that the principle orthodontic force produced by the activator would come with continued wear and active biting on the appliance.[36] The idea of increasing wear-

19

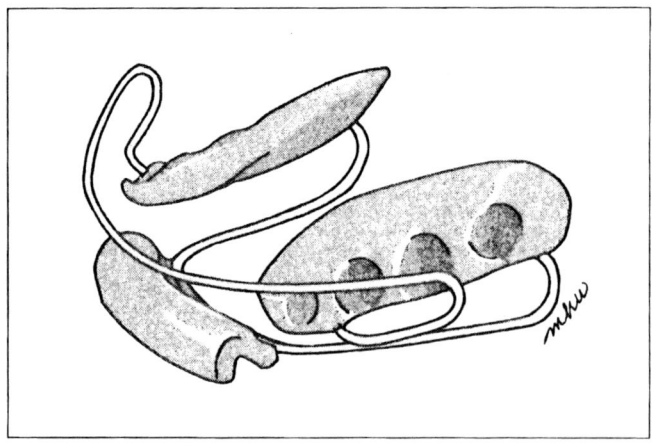

Fig. 1-5 Bimler: 1948 primary appliance with redoubling U-loop.

ing time for the activator and increasing the interocclusal and forward displacement of the mandible has been studied by several authors. Harvold, Selmer-Olsen, Herren, and Ahlgren have developed much of the current philosophy.

Harvold[37] advocated an increased interocclusal distance in order to activate the principle masticatory muscles. (Selmer-Olsen[38] had earlier expressed a similar mandibular position in 1937.) In 1959, Herren[39] discussed the mode of action of the activator and suggested that the intermittent stimulating forces of the appliance on the dental tissues offered protection against traumatic effects on the periodontium. Ahlgren studied the electromyographic response to activator treatment in 1960 and found no increase in muscular activity during sleep with nighttime-only activator treatment.[40] In order to improve clinical response from activator treatment, Ahlgren suggested taking the construction bite below and forward of the mandibular postural rest position suggested by Andresen. In addition, daytime wear was found to increase the effectiveness of treatment.

As interest in and understanding of activator appliance treatment increased, it became necessary to find appliances that could be worn with comfort for all or most of the day. The most widely used appliances, in order of development, are the *Bimler oral adaptor*,[41] the *kinetor* by Stockfisch,[42] the *functional regulator* by Fränkel,[43] and the *bionator* developed by Balters.[44] All of these adaptations of and improvements to the Andresen activator appliance came after World War II.

At the 1939 European Orthodontic Society meeting in Bonn, the primary topic for discussion was functional therapy. At this meeting, Dr. Watry paid homage to Dr. Pierre Robin, the man considered by many to have laid the foundation for the evolution and development of maxillofacial orthopedics.

Post–World War II

The onset of World War II did much to interrupt the flow of scientific thinking and the development of maxillofacial orthopedic technique. Many of the best European scientists were channeled away from medical and dental research; steel and other appliance materials were diverted toward the war effort.

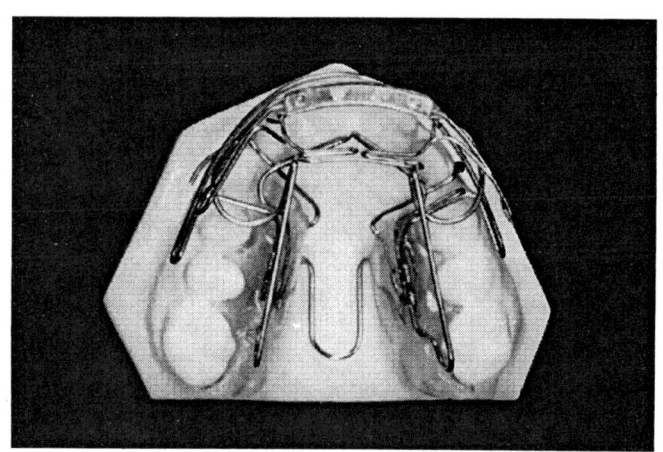

Fig. 1-6 The Bimler appliance (1980). (Courtesy of Dyna-Flex Orthodontic Laboratories, St. Louis, Mo.)

It was not until 1949 that the Bimler appliance, or "oral adaptor," was developed and introduced in Germany by Dr. H. P. Bimler.[41] The appliance was designed to be worn day and night except while eating or participating in active sports. The early appliance was very basic in design (Fig. 1-5). It was developed utilizing a combination of European functional technique and American wire construction, as follows:[45] Two acrylic pads on the palate and lingual surfaces of the maxillary posterior teeth were joined to an acrylic cap over the mandibular incisors by a maxillary labial arch wire and a mandibular lingual arch wire. Later evolutionary developments in the "oral adaptor" were variations of this first appliance (Fig. 1-6).

Many of the concepts and techniques of maxillofacial orthopedic appliances that were developed up until the early 1950s have been detailed in *Textbook of Functional Jaw Orthopaedics* by Professors K. Häupl, W. Grossman, and P. Clarkson.[46] The written text details the development of the human dentition, the etiology of malocclusion, and diagnosis and treatment planning with functional orthopedic appliances. The later chapters discuss treatment methods, "systematic" extractions, tissue changes during treatment, and surgical orthodontics. The functional appliance used for treatment is the activator developed by Andresen and Häupl. The clasped, removable appliances detailed are those of Nord and Schwarz. (Nord had introduced the expansion plate in Heidelberg at the 1934 Congress of the European Orthodontic Society.) Schwarz described "active" expansion appliances in the first edition of *Gebissregelung mit Platten* in 1938. Many later orthopedic appliances incorporated active expansion and functional modalities into the same appliance.

The *kinetor appliance* was developed by Dr. Hugo Stockfisch in the 1950s and 1960s.[42] The appliance utilizes a combination of functional and active-screw forces. The maxillary and mandibular acrylic parts of the kinetor act as lateral active expansion appliances (Fig. 1-7). The two acrylic parts are positioned and held together by wire vestibular loops that help reverse the inward pressure of the buccinator muscle and widen the dental arches. Small rubber tubes placed between the occlusal surfaces of the teeth help give the appliance a three-dimensional quality: *(1)* horizontal or transverse—from the active screws, *(2)* vertical—from the chewing action on the

Historical Development of Maxillofacial Orthopedic Technique

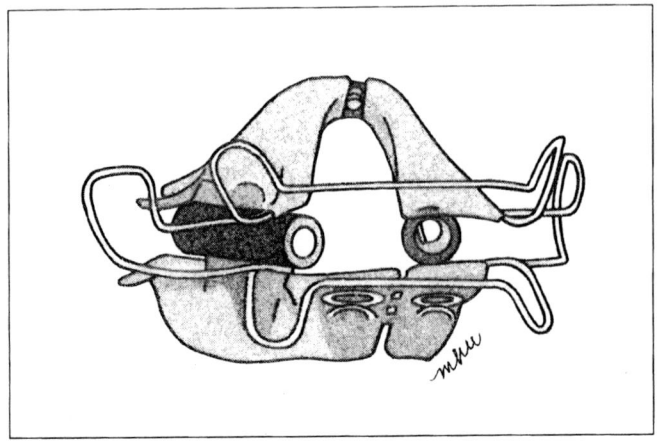

Fig. 1-7 The kinetor appliance (1951).

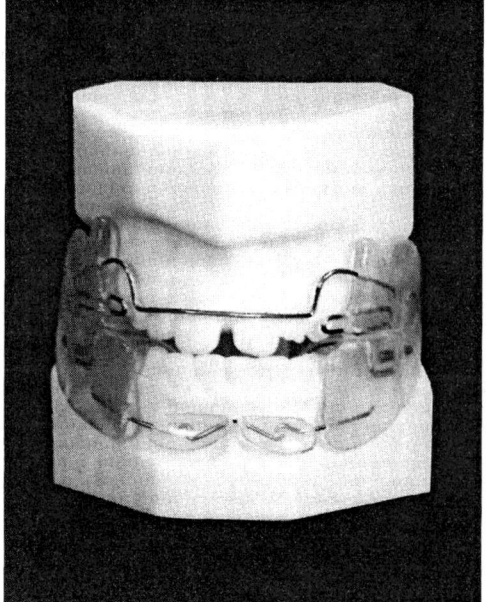

Fig. 1-8 The FR appliance (1980). (Courtesy of Dyna-Flex Orthodontic Laboratories, St. Louis, Mo.)

rubber tubes, and (3) sagittal—from mandibular repositioning.

By combining functional and active forces with vestibular interruption of pressure from the buccinator muscle, Dr. Stockfisch has developed an effective method for treating most (including Class III) cases of malocclusion.[47] The kinetor is an important appliance because it illustrates concepts that have influenced further development of maxillofacial orthopedic techniques.

Recent developments

The *function regulator,* or *FR appliance,* developed by Dr. Rolf Fränkel in the 1950s and 1960s, represents the incorporation of vestibular shields for the interruption of buccinator muscle pressure. By preventing the buccinator and orbicularis oris muscles from exerting pressure on the developing maxillofacial area, the osseous structures can be guided to new functional growth relationships. Instead of utilizing pressure from an expansion screw or coffin spring to widen the dental arches, crowding is minimized by withholding muscle force from the dentition and osseous structures. In addition to withholding muscle pressure, the lip pads and cheek shields also exert a direct mechanical influence by extending and gently stretching the soft tissue.[48] The most advantageous treatment time for using the FR appliance is during dental eruption. The

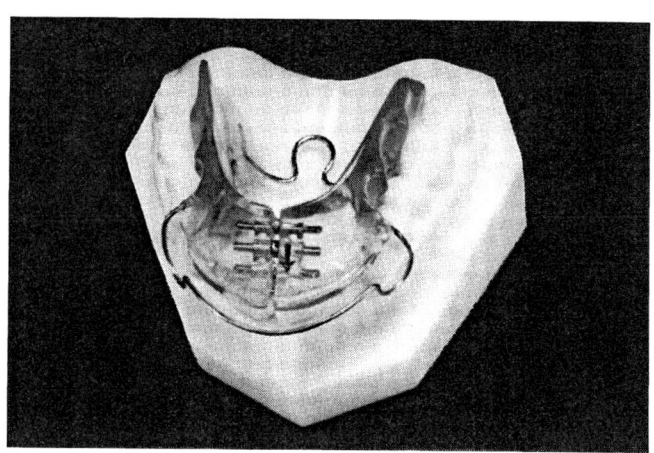

Fig. 1-9 Bionator appliance with midline screw, viewed from below (1980). (Courtesy of DynaFlex Orthodontic Laboratories, St. Louis, Mo.)

vestibular shields and pads take advantage of the soft tissue environment to produce a guidance effect on the eruptive path of the teeth (Fig. 1-8).[49]

The concept of bringing about dentoalveolar growth changes indirectly via intervention of the external muscular environment is gaining worldwide acceptance. Dr. Fränkel has developed an appliance that does not directly "straighten teeth," but guides dentoalveolar osseous growth. The successful results of treatment depend (as with all removable orthopedic appliances) on full patient cooperation. The appliance may seem awkward initially, but continued use brings good patient acceptance.

Patient acceptance is essential when the appliance is removable. The development of the functional orthopedic appliance variations of the Andresen activator were designed with the intent that the patient could speak more easily while wearing the appliance. With a comfortable appliance for talking, the patient would accept wearing the appliance during the day. Witt[50] found that daytime wear of the bionator appliance encouraged forward repositioning of the mandible. The work of Petrovic et al.[51] has shown a high level of mitotic activity in condylar prechondroblasts in animals while awake, but not during sleep.

The influence of Dr. W. Balters

The *bionator appliance,* developed by Balters in the late 1950s and 1960s, is a variation of the Andresen-Häupl activator but with much less bulk (Fig. 1-9). Since Balters considered space for the tongue essential, the bionator appliance was designed to allow maximum tongue movement and comfort in daytime wear. The lips are encouraged to attain closure while the incisors are brought to an edge-to-edge relationship. Balters has developed an appliance that stimulates the oral and masticatory musculature and improves muscular coordination. By improving muscular coordination and mandibular position, tongue position and respiration are improved and correction of the malocclusion is stable.[52]

Balters developed variations of the bionator that correct most types of skeletal malocclusions, including Class II open and deep bite and Class III malocclusion. Each appliance is designed to reduce muscle activity that may lead to later dentoalveolar instability.[53]

When the bionator was first introduced in the 1950s, many of the ideas proposed by Professor Balters were dismissed by many clinicians as fanciful. Balters thought pa-

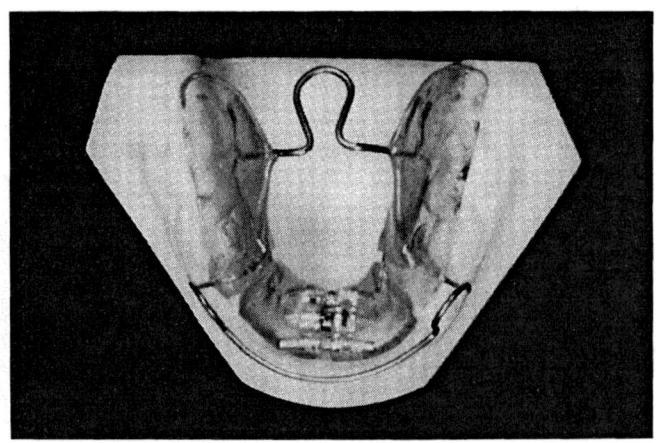

Fig. 1-10 Orthopedic corrector, viewed from above (1982). (Courtesy of Dyna-Flex Orthodontic Laboratories, St. Louis, Mo.)

tients should wear the appliance while following a program of postural exercises and dietary control.

The orthopedic corrector appliance

A later development of the bionator appliance was introduced in 1979 by J. W. Witzig of Minneapolis, Minnesota. The *orthopedic corrector* was designed to alter the functional relationship of the mandible during treatment. Through incorporation into the appliance of expansion screws in the area of the mandibular premolars, the mandible can be repositioned forward as treatment progresses (Fig. 1-10). This variation of the bionator is especially effective for patients with severe overjet, which requires considerable repositioning of the skeletal components, and for older patients who initially may be able to tolerate only slight mandibular repositioning. The orthopedic corrector appliance is also useful for patients with craniomandibular joint disorders. Initially, the mandible can be repositioned forward only slightly in many TMJ patients because of pain and inflammation in the temporomandibular joints. As the patient wears the appliance and muscle and ligament changes take place, the screws can be opened to advance the mandible forward and further reposition the condylar heads.

Although types of appliances have differed, and numerous additional scientists have contributed greatly to the literature, the overall goal has been similar: the development of a systematized approach to early prevention and correction of malocclusion with minimal disruption of healthy tissue.

References

1. Angle, E. H. Treatment of Malocclusion of the Teeth and Fractures of the Maxillae. 6th ed. Philadelphia: S. S. White, 1900, pp. 3–4.
2. Hunter, J. The Natural History of Human Teeth, Explaining Their Structure, Use, Formation, Growth and Disease. London: J. Johnson, 1771.
3. Hunter, J. A Practical Treatise on the Diseases of the Teeth. London: J. Johnson, 1778.
4. Hoffmann-Axthelm, W. History of Dentistry. Chicago: Quintessence Publ. Co., 1981, pp. 362–386.
5. Robin, P. Observation sur un nouvel appareil de redressement. Rev. Stomatol. 9:423–432, 1902.
6. Andresen, V., and Häupl, K. Funktions-Kieferorthopädie. Berlin: Hermann Meusser, 1936.
7. Kingsley, N. W. A Treatise on Oral Deformity with Appropriate Preventive and Remedial Treatment. New York: Appleton & Co., 1880.
8. Angle, E. H. Classification of malocclusion. Dent. Cosmos 41:248–264, 350–357, 1899.
9. Law, W. G. Presidential address. Am. Orthod. 1:130, May 1908.
10. Chapman, H. Early years of the European Orthodontic Society. Trans. Eur. Orthod. Soc. 29–37, 1958.
11. Babcock, J. H. The screw expansion plate. Trans. Br. Soc. Orthod., May-Dec.:3–8, 1911.
12. Nord, C. F. L. Loose appliances in orthodontia. Trans. Eur. Orthod. Soc., 1929.
13. Schwarz, A. M. Gebissregelung mit Platten. Vienna: Urban Schwarzenberg, 1938.
14. Watry, F. M. A contribution to the history of physiotherapeutics in maxillofacial orthopedics. 24th Annual Congress, Trans. Eur. Orthod. Soc. 53–63, 1947.
15. Mershon, J. V. The removable lingual arch as an appliance for the treatment of malocclusion of the teeth. Int. J. Orthod., 1918.
16. Kantorowicz, A. Die Gesichtsanalyse und die orthodontische Physiognomik. Dtsch. Mschr. Zahnheilk. 39:24, 1921.
17. Kantorowicz, A., and Korkhaus, G. Aetiologie der orthodontischen anomalien. Fortschr. Zahnheilk. 1:3, 1925; 2:9, 1926.
18. Schwarz, A. M. Das biologische verhalten orthodontisch beanspruchter zahne. Z. Zahnärztl. Orthop. 4, 1929.
19. Schwarz, A. M. Dologische gesichtspunkte bei der behandlung des distalbisses (Angle-Klasse II). Fortschr. Orthod. 2, 1932.
20. Rogers, A. P. Exercises for the development of the muscles of the face, with a view to increase their functional activity. Dent. Cosmos 60:857–876, 1918.
21. Rogers, A. P. Making facial muscles our allies in treatment and retention. Dent. Cosmos 64:711–730, 1922.
22. Watry, F. M. Die physiotherapeutische Behandlung der kieferdeformitäten. Fortsehr. Orthod. 3:196–200, 318–330, 1933.
23. Andresen, V. Beitrag zur Retention. Z. Zahnärztl. Orthop. 3:121–125, 1910.
24. Andresen, V. The Norwegian System of functional gnatho-orthopedics. Acta Gnathologica 1:5–36, 1936.
25. Andresen, V. Über das sog "Norwegische System" der Funktions-Kieferorthopädie. Dtsch. Zahnärztl. Wschr. 39:235–238, 283–286, 1936.
26. Andresen, V. Det Norske System, Trandlaegebl. Jan., 1937.
27. Andresen, V. The Norwegian System of functional gnatho-orthopedics, antithetical to orthodontia. Acta Gnathologica, Vol. 3, no. 1, 1938.
28. Andresen, V. The Norwegian System of gnathological functional orthopaedics. Acta Gnathologica, Vol. 4, no. 1, 1939.
29. Andresen, V. Ueber das Norwegische System der Funktions-Kieferorthopädie. Schweiz. Mschr. Zahnheilk. 50:3, 1940.
30. Hoffer, O. Indications and contraindications for the "Norwegian" System. 24th Annual Congress, Trans. Eur. Orthod. Soc. 31–33, 1947.
31. Schmuth, G. P. F. Milestones in the development and practical application of functional appliances. Am. J. Orthod. 84:48–53, 1983.
32. Andresen, V. Bio-mekanisk ortodonti et ortodontisk system for privatpraksis og skoletannklinikker. Nor. Tannlaegeforen. Tid. 41:71–93, 442–443, 1931.
33. Andresen, V. Bio-mekanisk ortodonti et ortodontisk system for privatpraksis og skoletannklinikker. Nor. Tannlaegeforen. Tid. 42:131–138, 215–230, 295–312, 1932.
34. Roux, R. Über die Selbstregulation der Lebewesen. Arch. Entw. Mech. Organ. Vol. 13, 1902.
35. Wolff, J. Das Gesetz der Transformation der Knockens. Berlin, 1892.
36. Schwarz, A. M. Wirkungsweise des Aktivators. Fortschr. Kieferorthop. 13:117–138, 1952.
37. Harvold, E. P. The Activator in Interceptive Orthodontics. St. Louis: The C. V. Mosby Co., 1974.
38. Selmer-Olsen, R. En Kritisk betraktning over "Det norske system." Nor. Tannlaegeforen. Tid. 47:85–91, 179–193, 1937.
39. Herren, P. The activator's mode of action. Am. J. Orthod. 45:512–527, 1959.
40. Ahlgren, J. An electromyographic analysis of the response to activator (Andresen-Häupl) therapy. Odontol. Rev. 11:125–151, 1960.
41. Bimler, H.P. Die elastischen Gebissformer. Zahnärztl. Welt. 4: 499–503, 1949.
42. Stockfisch, H. Der Kinetor in der Kieferorthopädie: Die Praxis des Polyvalenten Bimaxillären Apparates und seine rationelle Technik mit Plastik-fertigeilen. Heidelberg: A. Hüthig, 1966.
43. Fränkel, R. The treatment of Class II, Division I malocclusion with functional correctors. Am. J. Orthod. 55:265–275, 1969.
44. Balters, W. Eine Einführung in die Bionator-heilmethod: Ausgewählte Schriften und Vorträge. Heidelberg: C. Herrman, 1973.
45. Bimler, H. P. The Bimler Appliance. pp. 337–500. In T. M. Graber and B. Neumann (eds.) Removable Orthodontic Appliances. Philadelphia: W. B.

Saunders Co., 1977.
46. Häupl, K., Grossman, W. J., and Clarkson, P. Textbook of Functional Jaw Orthopaedics. London: Henry Kimpton, 1952.
47. Stockfisch, H. Class III treatment with the elastic oral adaptor, the function corrector, Kinetor, palatal expansion (splitting the mid palatal suture), light wire and surgical shortening of the tongue. Trans. Eur. Orthod. Soc. 279–294, 1970.
48. Fränkel, R. The theoretical concept underlying treatment with function correctors. Trans. Eur. Orthod. Soc. 233–250, 1966.
49. Fränkel, R. Decrowding during eruption under the screening influence of vestibular shields. Am. J. Orthod. 65:372–406, 1974.
50. Witt, E. Muscular physiological investigations into the effect of bi-maxillary appliances. Trans. Eur. Orthod. Soc. 448–450, 1973.
51. Petrovic, A., Gasson, N., and Oudet, C. Wirkung der ubertriebenen posturalen Vorschubstellung des Unterkiefers auf das Kondylenwachstum der normalen und der mit Washstumshormon behandelten Ratt. Fortschr. Kieferorthop. 36:86–97, 1975.
52. Celestin, L. A. La Méthode Bionator. Paris: Librairie Maloine S. A., 1967.
53. Ascher, F. Praktische Kieferorthopädie. Munich: Urban & Schwarzenerg, 1968.

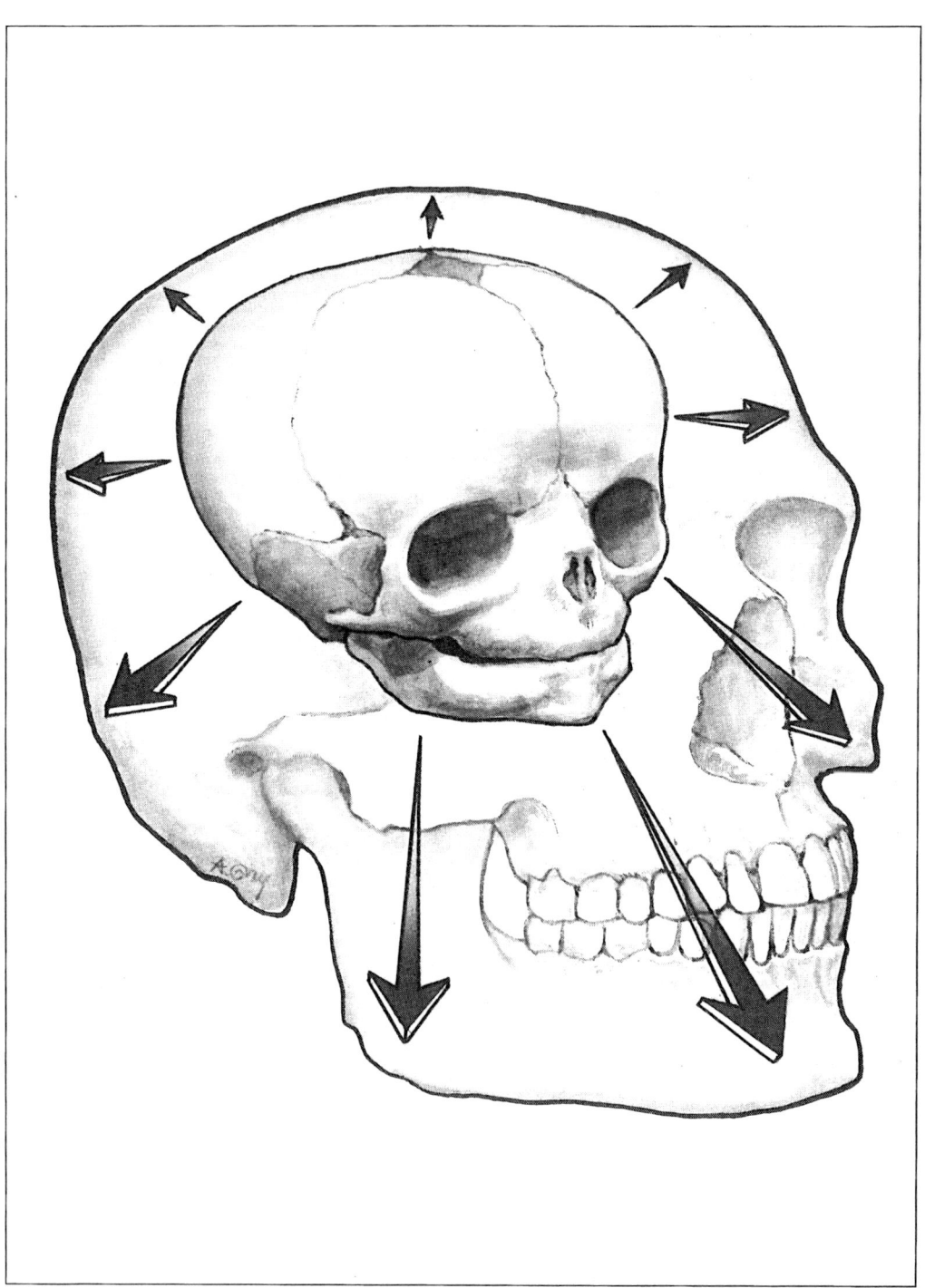

The challenge of maxillofacial orthopedic therapy is to begin with the craniofacial morphology of the neonate and have it evolve into normal adult anatomic characteristics with minimum interference.

Chapter 2

Biological Shaping of the Craniofacial Complex

There is much conjecture and confusion in the study of craniofacial growth and development. Older ideas (e.g., that the length of the mandible is genetically predetermined) are being challenged by clinical experience. The research is incomplete and even contradictory, yet the astute clinician would like to have the best information available. This section correlates the work of some prominent researchers with current clinical techniques (Fig. 2-1).

The continuum of normal biological growth begins in the prenatal period of development and continues throughout the postnatal period. The continuum can be affected by such factors as heredity and environment acting on different sites (e.g., neuromuscular tissue, bone and cartilage, and the dentition). The resulting manifestations occur in the occlusion.

Factors

Prenatal growth—a biological continuum

Facial development is a continuous process spanning the pre- and postnatal periods (Fig. 2-2). From fertilization to progressive onset of cell behavior, the human embryo passes through the series of developmental hurdles.[1-3]

Using cross-sectional growth studies, Burdi[4] has shown that the prebirth profile is relatively stable and that anatomical changes are characterized by progressive enlargement. The continuous developmental process of the midfacial region shows *no significant angular changes with increasing age*. The growth continuum persists from the prenatal *midfacial growth pattern* of increasing size and relative stability of shape,[5,6] to growth and remodeling during early childhood.[7-11]

Since the facial pattern is established prenatally in the second trimester and continues to childhood, the cranial base, from which the face develops, must be in its approximate shape in the first trimester. Indeed, during the first few weeks of life the enlarging forebrain creates the cranial base angle. This angle partially determines the amount of protrusion or retrusion of the mandibular component of the facial profile. The maxilla is suspended from the cranial base and its position in the face is related to the cranial base angle. A large cranial base angle tends to position the maxillary component forward, while a small cranial base angle tends to retrude the maxillary component.

The mandible is suspended from the cranial base at the temporomandibular joint and is generally influenced by the shape of the maxilla. According to Bimler,[12] the location of the temporomandibular joint can determine the type of maxillomandibular rela-

Biological Shaping of the Craniofacial Complex

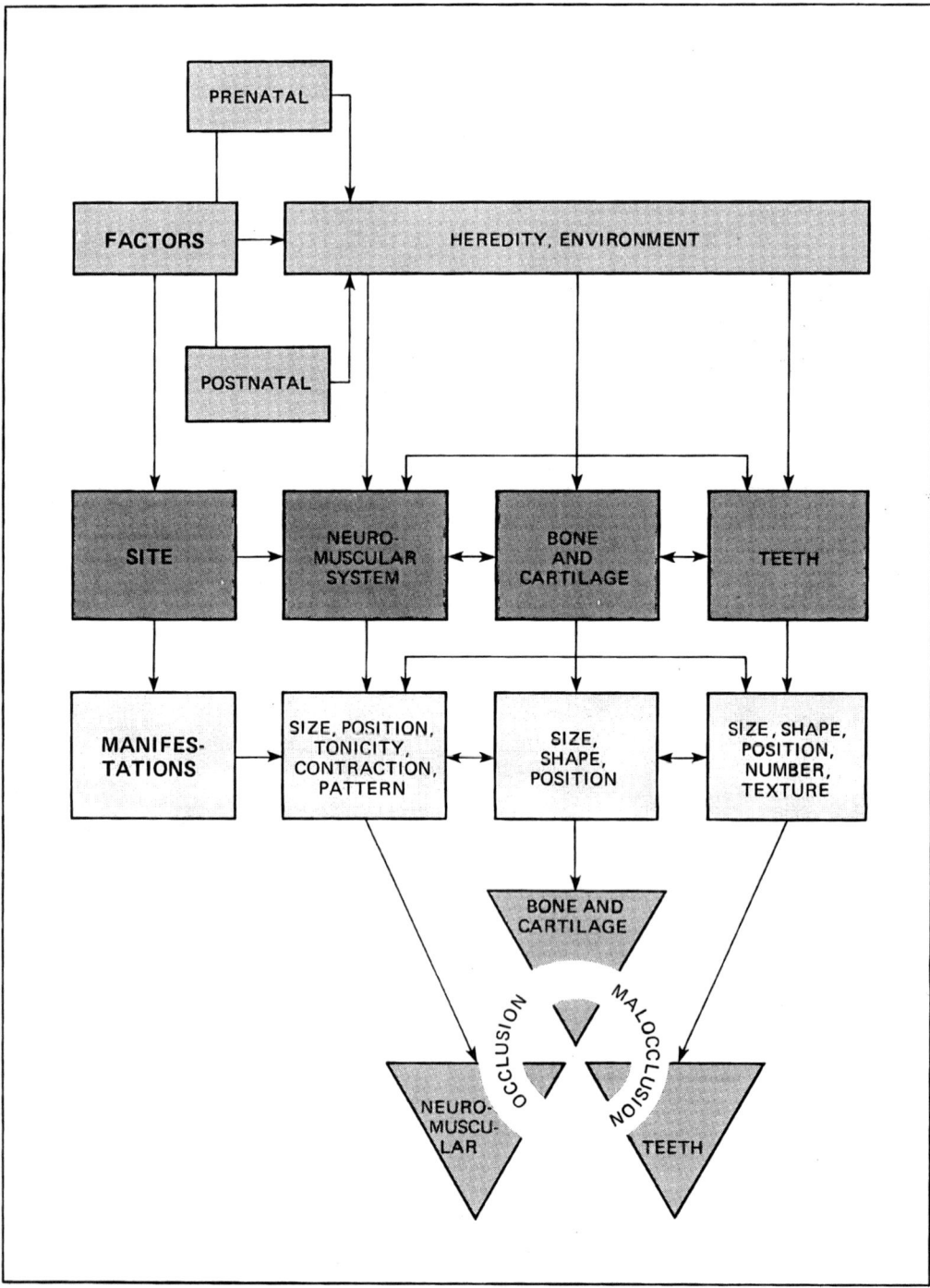

Fig. 2-1 Many factors are involved in growth. Treatment to a normal occlusal result involves intercepting, guiding, and correcting several factors at various sites.

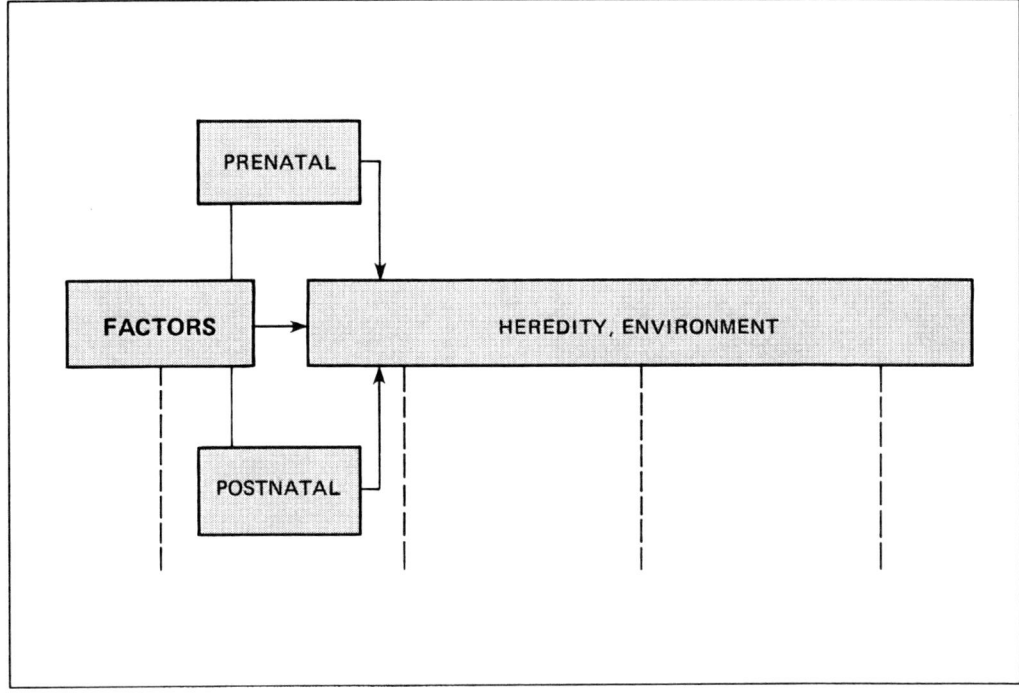

Fig. 2-2 Prenatal and postnatal factors can affect heredity and environment.

tionship: if the temporomandibular joint is positioned too posteriorly, a Class II malocclusion may result; if the temporomandibular joint is positioned too anteriorly, a Class III malocclusion may result (see Fig. 2-3).

Heredity vs. environmental factors

Adaptive growth changes cannot be attributed to either genetic or environmental factors alone: both fluctuate constantly during growth. The interaction of many variables makes it difficult to isolate one organ or structure and define its behavior throughout the craniofacial growth process. Kraus et al.[13] contend that the skull is under rigid genetic control but that environment plays a major role in determining how the bony elements combine to create a harmonious or disharmonious craniofacial skeleton. Genetics and environment are both important factors that determine growth. Defining specific growth theories sheds insight into the thought processes that have motivated researchers in this field.

Sicher[14] suggested that the craniofacial complex is largely controlled by its own genetic information, with remodeling as the only external factor. However, it soon became obvious that many parts of the theory were incorrect (e.g., in microcephaly or hydrocephaly) (Fig. 2-4). Scott later suggested that cartilage and periosteum were purely genetic, while sutures responded to environmental influences from adjacent structures.[15] Moss,[16] basing his work on the original concepts of van der Klaaw,[17] has suggested that there is no *direct* genetic influence on the size, shape, or position of skeletal tissues, except for the initiation of ossification.

Biological Shaping of the Craniofacial Complex

Figs. 2-3a and b The cranial base has a direct effect on the position of the maxillomandibular complex. The flexure of this angle can produce several skeletal patterns.

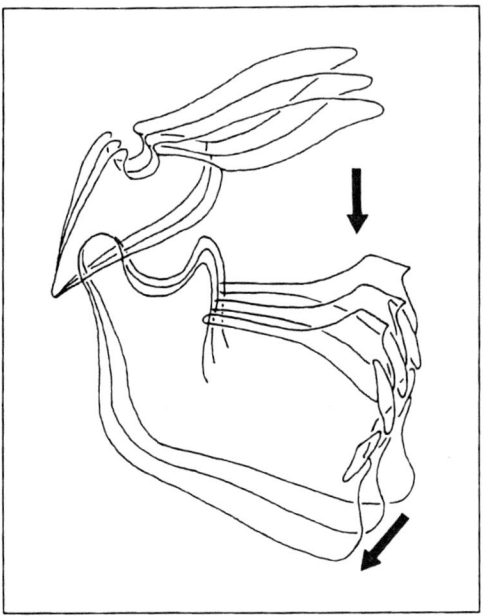
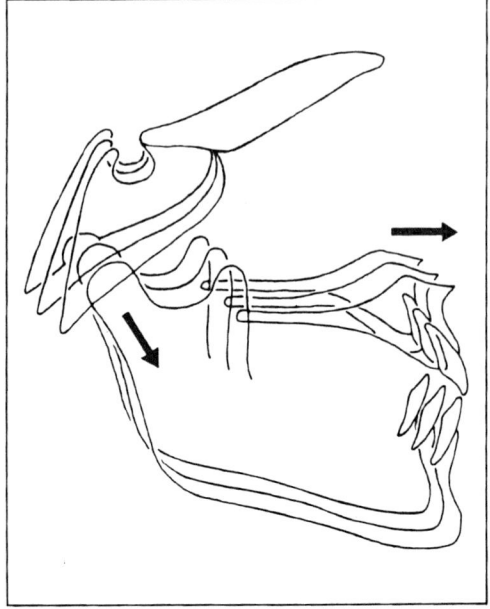

Fig. 2-3a As the nasomaxillary complex is lowered, the entire mandible rotates downward and backward, pivoting on the mandibular condyle. A Class II skeletal pattern may result.

Fig. 2-3b As the middle cranial base angle drops, the mandible is positioned forward, resulting in a tendency toward Class III malocclusion.

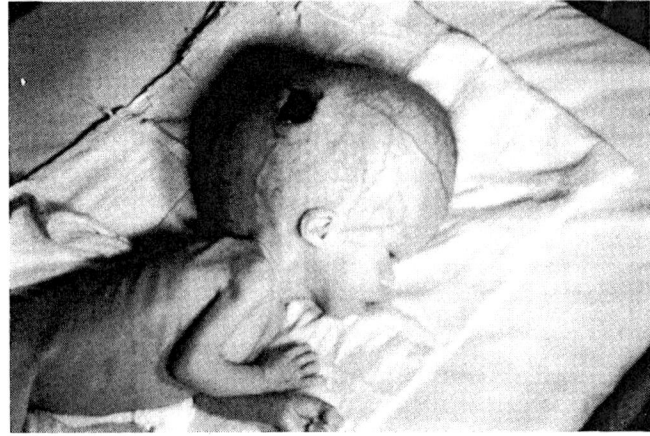

Fig. 2-4 Hydrocephalus. The internal pressure exerted by the cerebrospinal fluid on the developing osseous tissue has enlarged the cranial vault.

Van Limborg[18] has suggested that cartilagenous ossification (cranial base, nasal capsule, etc.) is controlled by genetic factors, while areas of intramembranous growth can be altered by environment.

Although the *general shape* of a bone is determined genetically, a mechanism does exist to adjust its properties to an altered environment. These theories will be applied to maxillofacial appliance treatment of facial skeletal imbalance. On insertion of an appliance to change mandibular position, many changes occur: the muscles gain a new position in space, carrying the mandible with them; tendons, ligaments, vessels, and the airway all acquire new positions; and the condyle is relocated in the fossa. The importance of condylar position is delineated in Chapter 10.

Petrovic et al., in 1981,[19] found that a genetically predetermined *final length* of the mandible did not exist. This was discovered when special orthopedic appliances were used for animals. The mandible was placed in a forward position. Condylar cartilage growth *rate* and *amount* were increased. In the experimental animals, the mandibles lengthened as compared with the mandibles of the control animals. When the appliance was removed on completion of animal growth, no relapse was observed. When the appliance was removed before growth was completed, no significant relapse was detected if good intercuspation had been achieved during the experimental phase. If a good intercuspation had not been achieved, the muscular system imposed an increased or decreased condylar growth rate until a state of intercuspal stability was established. Functional mandibular propulsion involving periodic forward mandibular repositioning appeared to be the best procedure for effecting orthopedic mandibular lengthening.

Balance between form and function is maintained throughout life. Malocclusion represents an attempt to establish a balance between morphogenetic, functional, and environmental forces, and is always in dynamic balance at any particular time. Additional environmental forces that have been shown to influence the growth of the craniofacial complex are nutrition and diet consistency (Chapter 5)[20-26] and mouth breathing (Chapter 13).[27-31]

Site

Neuromuscular system

Neuromuscular function directly affects the growth of the craniofacial skeleton, and certain factors influence craniofacial growth and form (Fig. 2-5):[32]

1. muscular growth
2. muscular migration and attachment
3. variations in neuromuscular function
4. abnormal function, e.g., mouth breathing

Normal muscle function

Wolff's law[33] states that all changes in the function of a bone are attended by definite alterations in both its internal and external structures. Muscular function influences all osseous tissues and is responsible for the proper positioning of the head, neck, and mandible.[34]

Muscles have different types of action and effect on bones. Phasic muscles have high intensity activity for a short period of time, while tonic muscles have low-intensity activity over a longer period of time. In an esthetically balanced face, there is a harmonious relationship between phasic and tonic muscles. The sustained tonic contraction of certain skeletal muscles (e.g., temporalis and orbicularis oris) maintains mandibular and facial position with respect to gravity. Continuous motor adjustments are essential for the maintenance of posture. These adjustments are voluntarily achieved by short-action rapid phasic muscles like

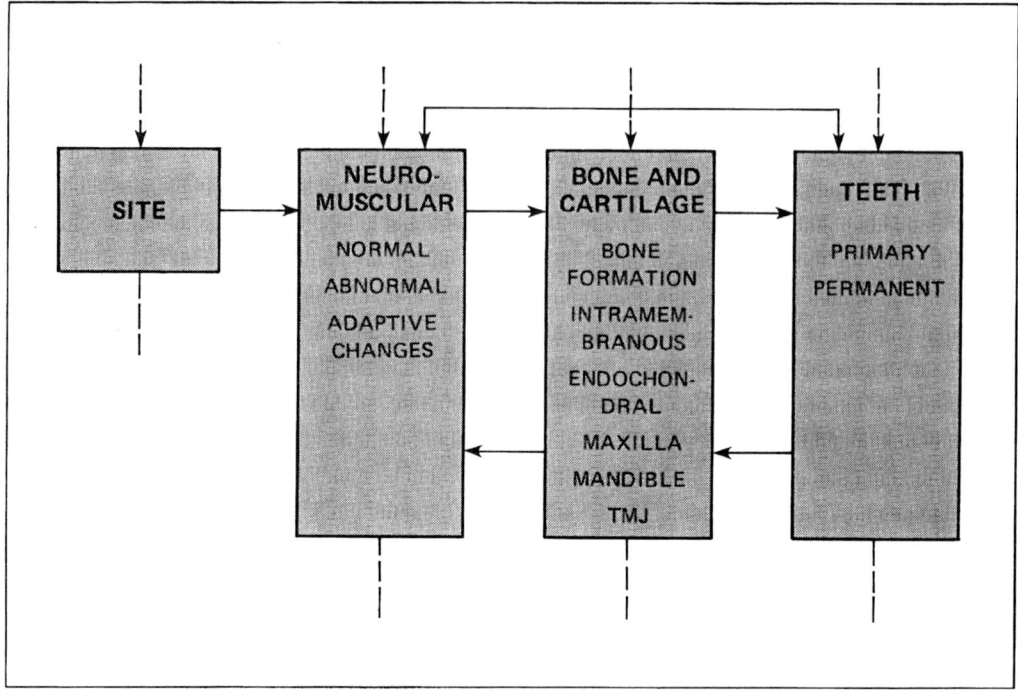

Fig. 2-5 Factors may act on the neuromuscular, osseous, cartilaginous, or dental components.

the lateral pterygoid or masseter muscles.[35]

Mandibular position is related to the position of the tongue and hyoid bone during speech and swallowing (Ingervall et al. 1970).[36] Storey, in 1976,[37] claimed that TMJ receptors strongly influence tongue position. These relationships have been diagrammatically proposed by Simões in 1979[38] as follows:

neck position ⇌ mandibular position
⇅ ⇅
TMJ position ⇌ tongue position

Each time the mandibular position changes, tongue, TMJ, and neck repositioning occurs.

Abnormal muscular function

Some researchers[39,40] have shown that patients with a malocclusion have a pattern of muscular activity different from that found in patients with normal occlusion. Mastication and deglutition were compared in Class I, Class II, and Class III subjects. Synchronized activity between muscles of mastication and facial expression was found in Class I subjects. The upper and lower lips initiated the mastication followed by the suprahyoid muscles (depressors) and the masseter muscles (elevators).

In Class II subjects, the lower lip action appeared first in mastication, followed by the upper lip or depressors, followed by the elevator muscles. No definitive pattern was found among the elevators, depressors, and lips in swallowing.

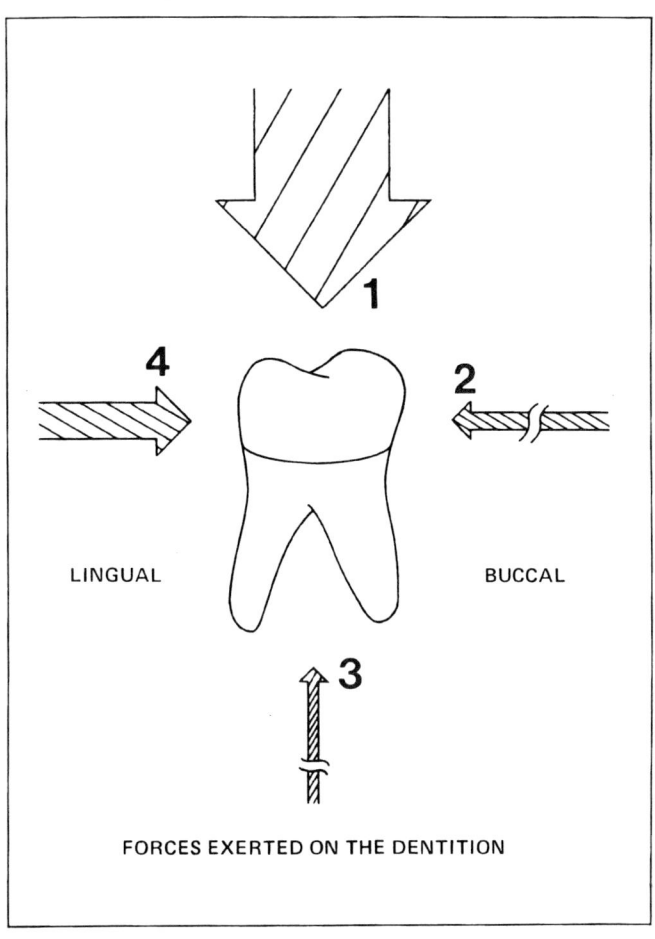

Fig. 2-6 Duration: length of the arrow; frequency: closeness of the line; intensity: width of the arrow (not to scale). (1) Forces of occlusion (2) Buccal musculature (3) Forces of eruption (4) Lingual (tongue) pressure. (Modified from Saadia et al., J. Pedod., Vol. 4, 1980.)

During mastication in Class III subjects, the depressor muscles were activated first. Lip and masseter muscle activation followed. No definitive pattern was found between upper and lower lip activity in swallowing. In addition to the pattern of muscular activity, the duration, intensity, and frequency of the muscle contraction must be quantified.

The teeth are subject to different muscle forces from different directions (Fig. 2-6). The tongue has been found to be two or three times stronger than the perioral musculature, while the forces of occlusion are much stronger than the forces of eruption. The apparent reason that teeth are not intruded and tipped buccally is that the labial and tonic forces counterbalance the dynamic forces exerted by the tongue. Tonic muscles (low intensity and long duration) are more responsible for malocclusion than are phasic muscles because movement occurs as a result of intensity, duration, and frequency, not as a result of intensity alone. Jacobs[41] states that the balance of the labiolingual forces is not determined by the intensity of these forces at a few transient moments, but that muscle performance must be viewed as the result of force over time. Different muscles work together as a unit. It has been found that a weak tonic muscle will have a compensatory hyperactive phasic muscle (e.g., a hypo-orbicularis muscle may result in a hypermentalis muscle, which could with time affect occlusion) (Fig. 2-7).

Any deviation from an optimally balanced muscular state is sufficient to provoke a decrease in the force of occlusion. A decrease in effective contractile activity of the lateral pterygoid muscle may slow growth and cause a condylar imbalance (Fig. 2-8).

Treatment for muscle imbalance is accomplished by breaking the positive feedback mechanism and reestablishing the conditions necessary for functioning of the negative feedback loop (e.g., removing any disturbing factors such as occlusal interferences or abnormal tooth position) (Fig. 2-9).

The homeostatic relationship between soft and hard tissues of the craniofacial complex is found not only in esthetically pleasing faces but also in malocclusion. In spite of the etiological factors that lead to maxillomandibular discrepancy, both the dentofacial and soft tissue component become structurally adapted to each other during the growth and development process and result in a functionally balanced state. This functionally balanced state will last a lifetime unless trauma or therapy intervenes.

When therapy does intervene, what happens to the muscle and osseous components? Protruding the mandible with an orthopedic appliance will stretch some of the masticatory muscles to their physiological limits. These muscles try to regain the rest position but are prevented by the appliance. McNamara[42] has described four physiological adaptations:

1. within the central nervous system
2. within muscle tissue
3. at the muscle bone interface
4. within or between muscle attachments

The earliest and most rapidly occurring adaptive mechanism is altered neuromuscular feedback. Several adaptations within the muscles do occur later. These could be the result of a geometric rearrangement of the fibers, changes in number and length, or changes in muscle physiology.[43] This muscle adaptation will exert a biomechanical force on osseous tissue, which can initiate skeletal change.[44]

Bone formation

Origin of bone cells

Osteogenesis and osteoclasis need three fundamental prerequisites: *(1)* proper cell, *(2)* proper nutrition, and *(3)* proper stimulus. It appears that neither bone formation nor destruction can take place if any of the three is inadequate or absent (Fig. 2-10).[45]

The cells that produce bone are connective tissue cells. The property which most clearly distinguishes bone from other connective tissues is its mineral content. Calcifiable matrix is produced in the enlarging zone of the epiphyseal growth cartilage, and is laid down over the other matrix components. There are three classes of cells: the osteoblasts, the osteocytes, and the osteoclasts. Osteoblasts first lay down collagen and associated polysaccharide, the calcifiable matrix (Fig. 2-15). This calcifies and another strip of collagen is laid down. This phenomenon is repeated to produce the characteristic lamellar structure. Only a small proportion of the osteoblasts covering a bone surface become osteocytes. Many osteoblasts disintegrate after making the required amount of matrix. Osteocytes become imbedded within bony chambers called lacunae (Fig. 2-11). A system of canaliculi links lacunae with each other and with the extracellular and extravascular space of the central canal (Fig. 2-11). These intercellular connections are present at all ages and provide channels for the passage of nutrients necessary for the

Figs. 2-7a to c Patient with hypermentalis activity. Notice the muscle strain while keeping mouth closed. Good posterior occlusion with crowding in the anterior segment.

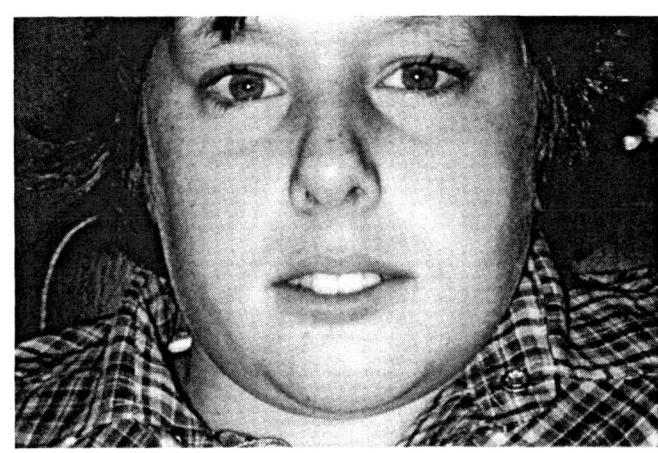

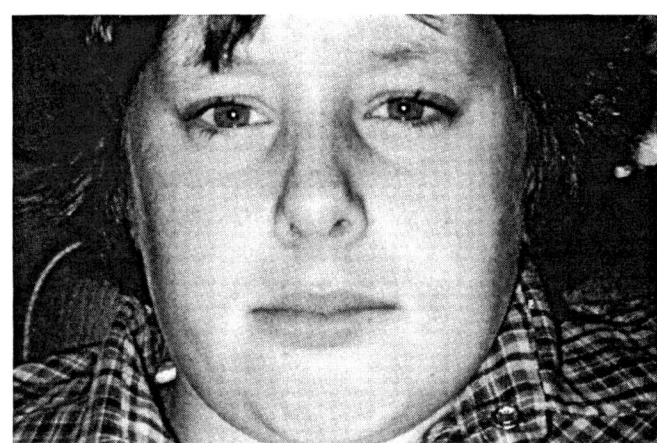

Fig. 2-7b

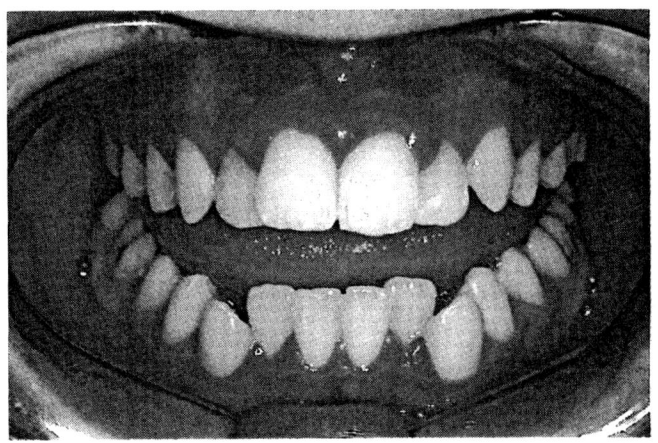

Fig. 2-7c

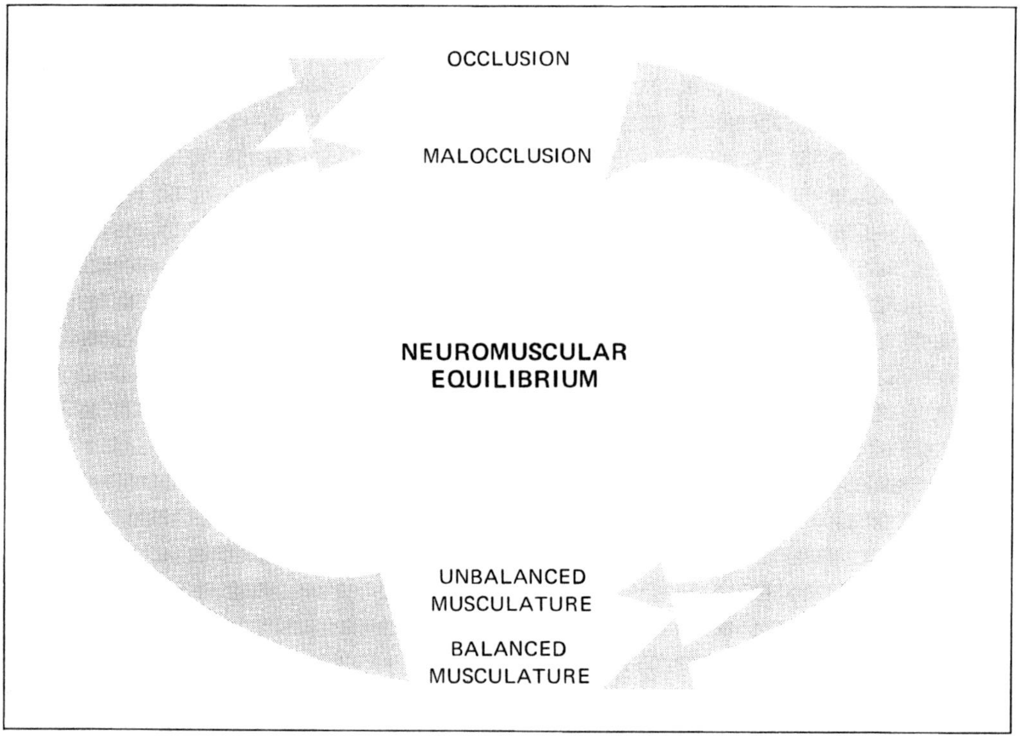

Biological Shaping of the Craniofacial Complex

```
                    OCCLUSION
                   MALOCCLUSION


                 NEUROMUSCULAR
                  EQUILIBRIUM


                   UNBALANCED
                   MUSCULATURE
                    BALANCED
                   MUSCULATURE
```

Fig. 2-8 Muscles are in dynamic balance in occlusion and malocclusion. This balance can be altered physiologically (through growth) and pathologically (as a result of caries-induced migration of teeth or poor restorative dentistry). The change in balance may alter contractile muscular activity, triggering new adaptations of the craniofacial complex and a new state of equilibrium.

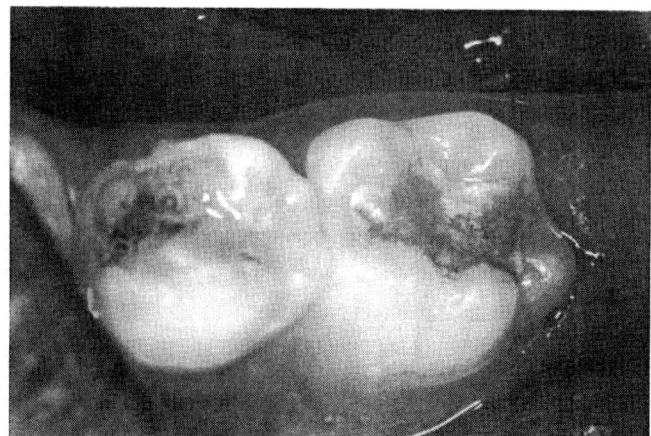

Fig. 2-9 Several problems can alter the propioception of the neuromusculature, e.g., interproximal caries with space loss or iatrogenesis (high contact from amalgam).

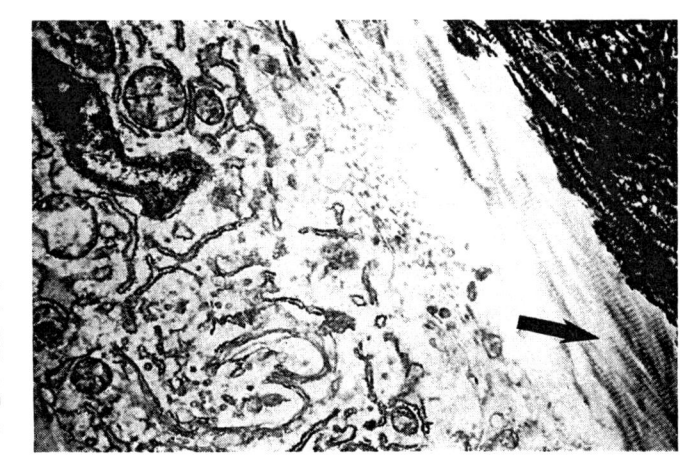

Fig. 2-10 An example of intramembranous ossification. Electron micrograph of a cell which has laid new collagen (striped lines) on the dark bone surface. (Reprinted with permission from Cooper et al., J. Bone Joint Surg., Vol. 48A, 1966.)

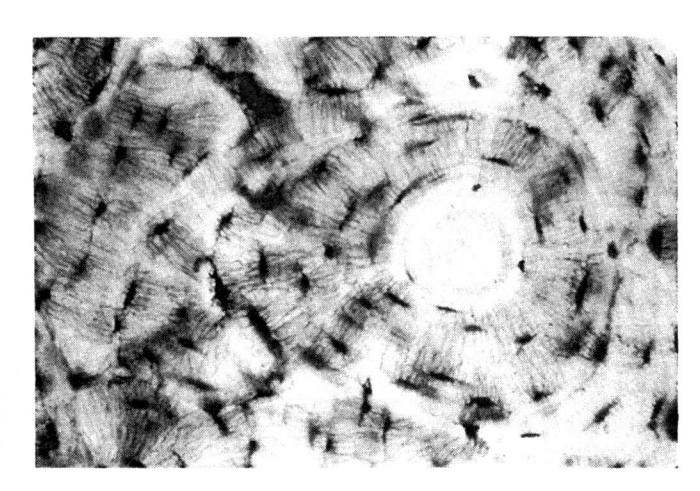

Fig. 2-11a Osteocytes lying in lacunae (dark oval areas). Cells are oriented parallel to the bone lamellae.

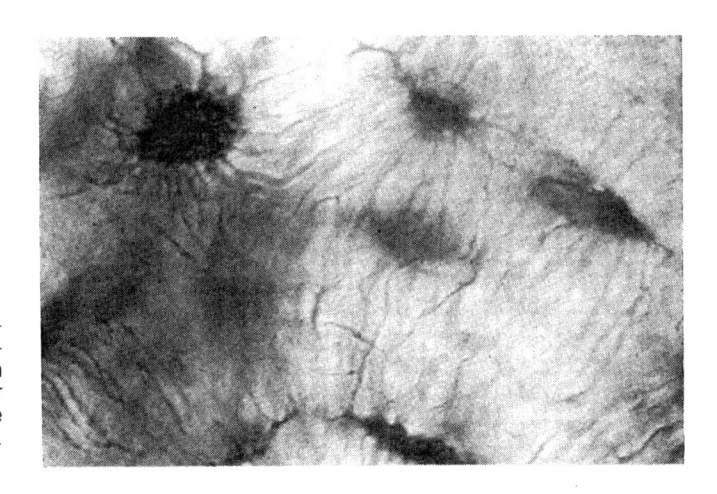

Fig. 2-11b Higher magnification showing the system of canaliculi linking lacunae with each other and with the extracellular and extravascular space of the central canal. (Courtesy of Dr. Reginald R. Cooper.)

Biological Shaping of the Craniofacial Complex

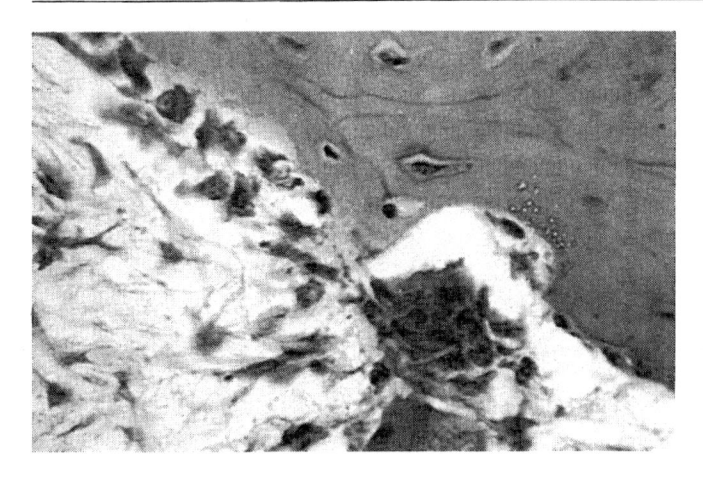

Fig. 2-12a Multinucleated osteoclasts are shown demineralizing the collagenous matrix. The resorptive process creates a Howship lacuna. (Courtesy of Dr. Edmund Cataldo.)

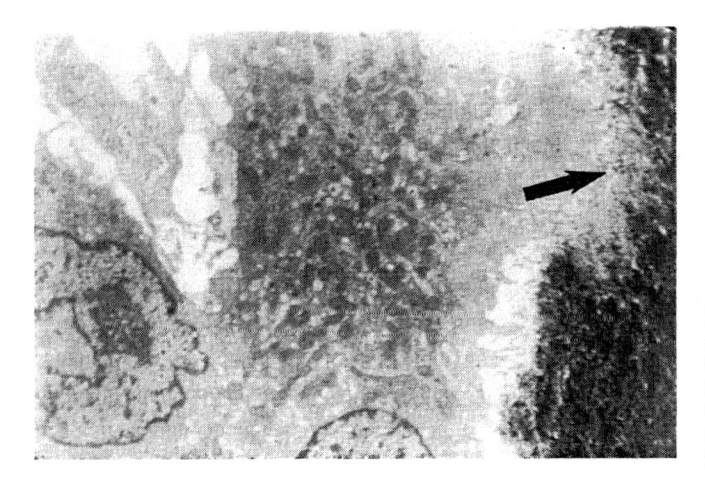

Fig. 2-12b Electron micrograph showing the "brush border" characteristic of these cells. Notice the grey projections of the osteoclast into the darker mineralized bone. (Courtesy of Dr. Reginald R. Cooper.)

maintenance of healthy osteocytes and bone.[46] As the remodeling phenomenon occurs, osteoclasts become responsible for resorption. The resorptive process leads to erosion pits called Howship's lacunae (Figs. 2-12a and b).

As bone starts to remodel, multinucleated osteoclasts demineralize bone and expose the collagenous matrix. The collagen fibrils then undergo phagocytosis from the osteoclasts. Controversy remains about the origin of the main cell types, the osteoblasts and the osteoclasts. It was earlier believed that they shared the same precursors, but now it appears that osteoblasts arise from local mesenchymal cell populations and that osteoclasts are derived from a circulatory monocyte-macrophage cell.[46]

Methods of bone formation

The differentiation of mesenchymal cells to bone can occur by one of two routes. By the first, bone may develop directly from mesenchyme. This process is referred to as intramembranous ossification. The second involves an intervening cartilage model which proceeds to form bone from mesenchymal cells and then itself becomes endochondral bone. Ham and Cormack[47] have

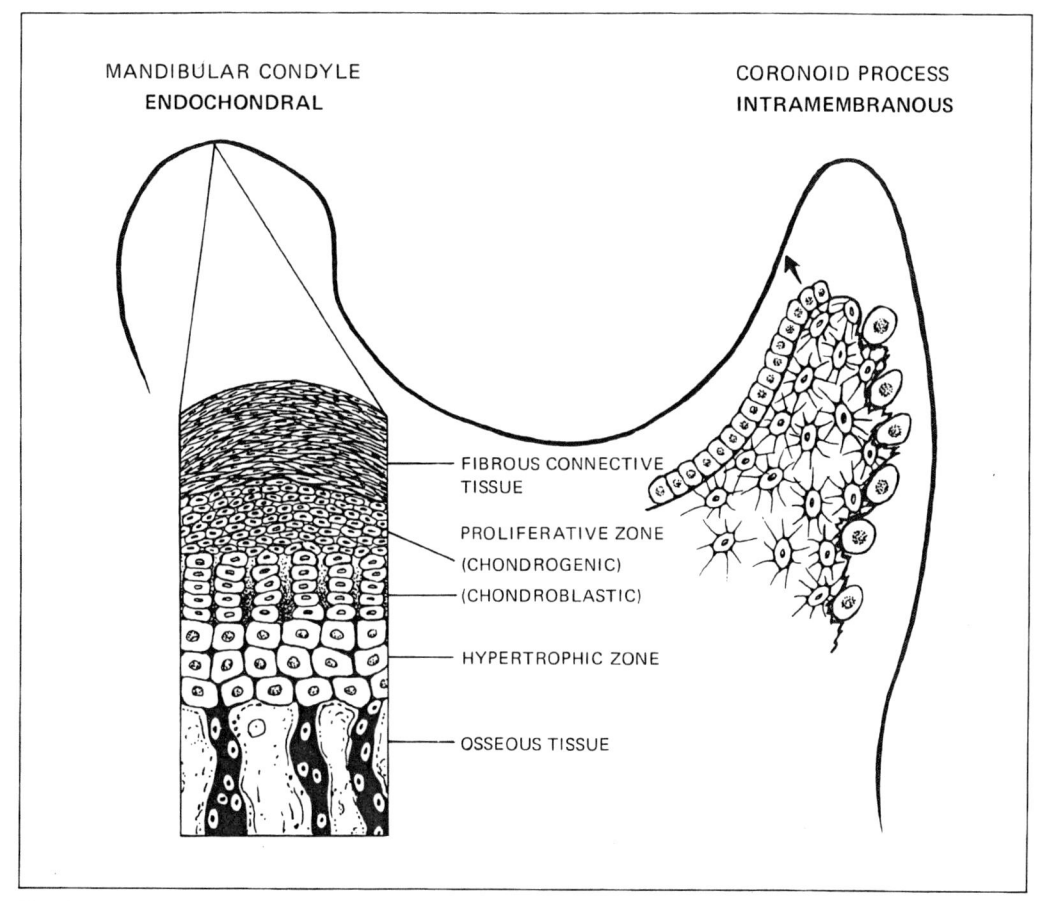

Fig. 2-13 As an organ, bone grows and repairs itself through two basic ossification mechanisms: intramembranous and endochondral. Bone produced by intramembranous ossification is laid down directly by osteoblasts. Endochondral ossification occurs when a preexisting cartilage model is gradually replaced by bone cells and matrix. In the mandible, both phenomena occur side by side.

shown that these two modes of ossification connote only the environment in which bone formation occurs; they do not differ significantly in the kind of bone they form (Figs. 2-13 and 2-14).

Intramembranous growth is produced by the bone-covering membrane (periosteum) on the outer surface, and the lining membrane (endosteum) on the inner surface. It contributes to an increase in diameter in long bones, as well as in most areas of the craniofacial complex. New bone is formed on the periosteal surface. In periosteal bone formation, cartilage is not formed as an intermediate stage in the process. Changes in the shape and distribution of bone tissue occur both before and after remodeling has ceased (Figs. 2-14a and b).[48]

Sutures possess an osteogenic process comparable to periosteal bone growth. As new bone is added to the sutural contact surfaces, the bones are displaced away from each other.[49]

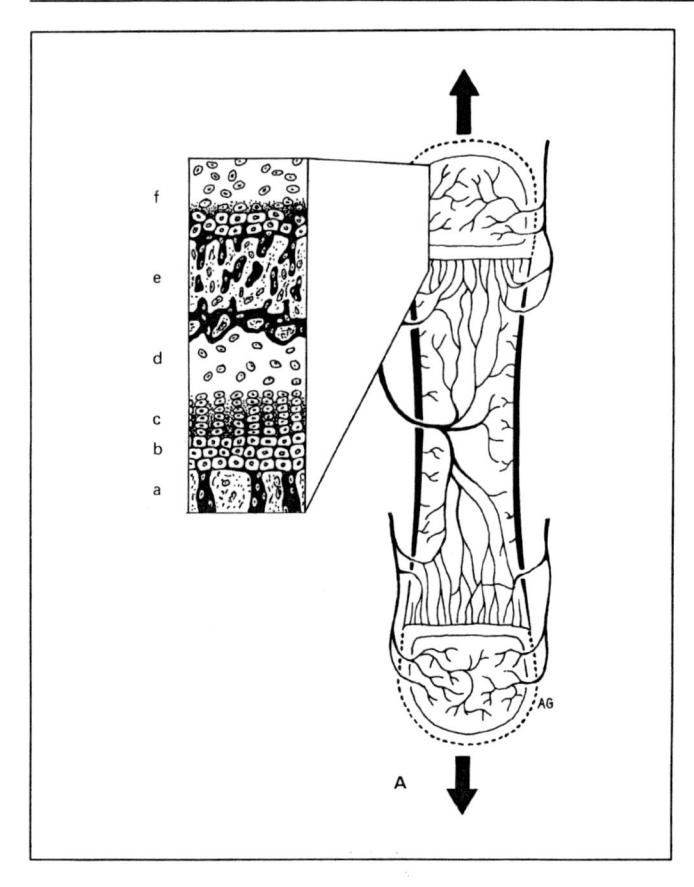

Fig. 2-14a Bone grows *endochondrally* in pressure areas, where the epiphyseal plate cartilage cells proliferate to add length. It is composed of several layers of *(a)* bone, *(b)* chondrogenic zone, *(c)* chondroblastic zone, *(d)* resting zone, *(e)* ossification center in the epiphysis, and *(f)* articular cartilage. The cartilage cells *(d)* closest to the bone undergo hypertrophy and degenerate; the surrounding cartilage matrix calcifies. The vascular components bring with them nutrients, minerals, and primitive mesenchymal cells, which differentiate into osteoblasts and lay down new bone.

Endochondral bone development begins in the human embryo during the seventh or eighth week after conception. Chondroblasts and chondrocytes begin to develop from a central core; they increase in size by a combination of interstitial and appositional growth. This cartilage contains a matrix which is nonvascular and generally noncalcified. The matrix then becomes surrounded by connective tissue called the perichondrium. As the perichondrium thickens, a new vascular system penetrates the central zone, allowing cell differentiation. The differentiated osteoblasts and osteoclasts can then begin converting cartilage to bone. This phenomenon progressively mineralizes the central bony shaft.

Much of this cell division occurs in the ends of the bones (epiphysis). Capillaries later invade the hypertrophic cartilage; bone modeling follows. A section of cartilage remains between the bony compartments, or growth plates. The longitudinal growth comes primarily from the interstitial growth of chondrocytes in the epiphysia growth plate. This growth is accomplished by sequential cell proliferation, maturation, and calcification of the cartilage (Fig. 2-15). Because cartilage does not possess a hard intercellular matrix, it is transformed into bone via a cascade:[46]

Cartilage spicules proliferate and differentiate. ⟶ The cartilaginous matrix calcifies and undergoes vascular invasion. ⟶ Cartilage is resorbed. ⟶ Bone matrix forms

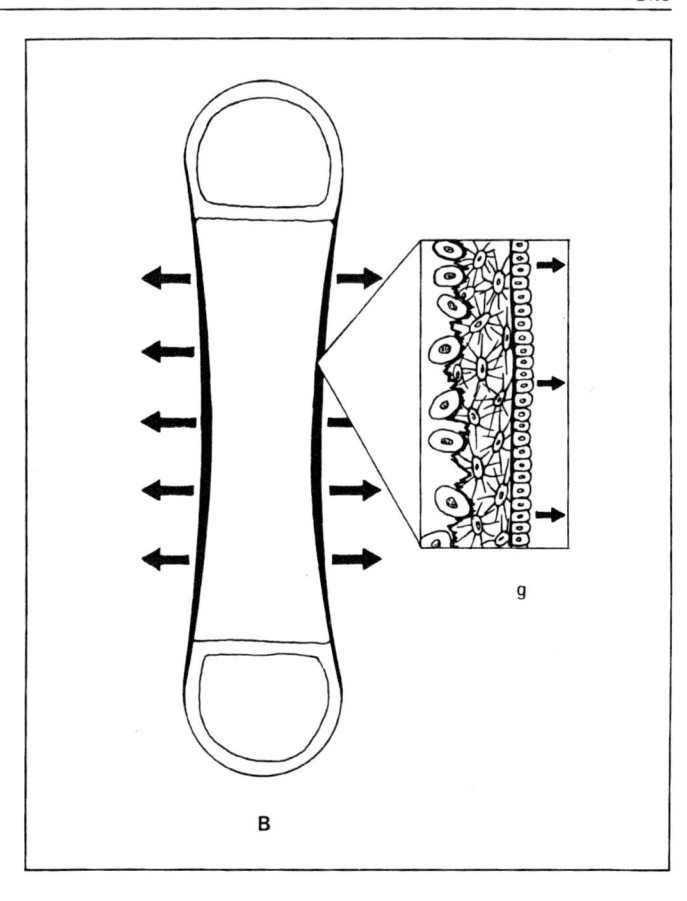

Fig. 2-14b *Intramembranous* growth occurs in tension areas which increase their diameter by apposition of new bone on the subperiosteal surface of bone cortex. This phenomenon is carried out by osteoblasts *(g)*. As active growth ceases, the remodeling phenomenon (apposition and resorption) continues. This remodeling is affected by function.

and mineralizes. ⎯→ Bone undergoes resorption and remodeling. ⎯→ Hematopoiesis occurs.

Bassett[45] has questioned how these cells "know" how, when, and with what orientation to begin or cease their function. Cells in the mesenchymal pool specialize simultaneously as osteoblasts and osteoclasts on adjacent bony surfaces within a few microns of one another.

It is possible that some of the answers were provided in 1892 by Wolff.[33] He suggested that bony trabeculi are oriented to best resist the loads they must support. This theory was complemented in 1920 by Jansen[49] and later by Bassett in 1968:[50]

The form of a bone being given, the bone elements place or displace themselves in the direction of functional forces and increase or decrease their mass to reflect the amount of functional forces.

This implies that the connective tissues could be the mechanism which carry out intrinsic growth changes; bones respond primarily to functional forces.

Connective tissue also acts on the bone and places stress on it. This stress results in electrical energy, which is known to affect bone formation and bone loss. Thus, *mechanical energy is converted into an electrical signal or stimulus, which directs cellular activity.*

Bioelectrical potentials generated by the connective tissues during appliance insertion produce electrical energy through

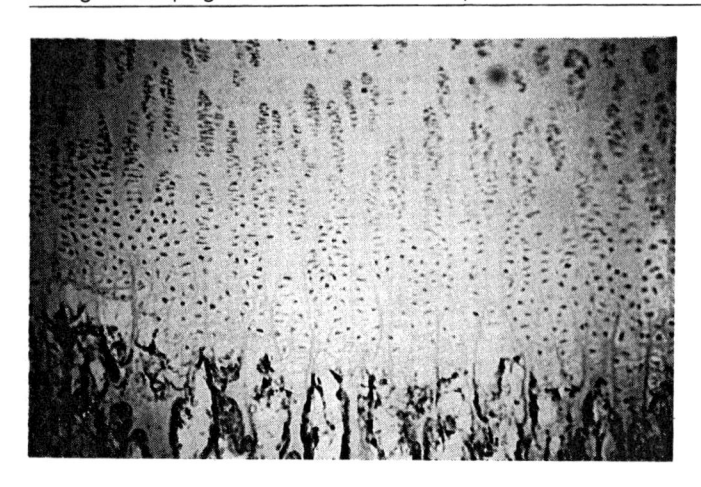

Fig. 2-15 Histologic slide of the epiphyseal growth plate. Proliferating cartilage cells grow farther away from bone (toward the top of the picture). The cartilage cells closest to the bone undergo hypertrophy and degenerate; the surrounding matrix calcifies. (Courtesy of Dr. Reginald R. Cooper.)

physical transduction. It appears that stress potentials in bone show primarily piezoelectric properties. Piezoelectricity is electricity resulting from stress on crystals.

Muscles, vessels, tendons, periosteum, teeth, and cartilage can produce "streaming" potentials that will affect bone behavior directly.[51] The appliances act as transducers converting mechanical energy into electrical responses. Orthopedic appliances that possess little or no acrylic coverage will tend to transmit more energy to these adjacent structures. Acrylic generally absorbs most of the energy produced by the forces which pull the mandible towards the rest position. More energy would be released by minimizing the acrylic coverage in orthopedic appliances. The bioelectrical response would be enhanced and more rapid bone remodeling would occur. Treatment time would be reduced.

Maxillary growth

The total maxillary length increases throughout the growth process (Fig. 2-16).[32,52-54] This increase in maxillary length results from growth at the premaxillary and maxillopalatine sutures as well as from subperiosteal osseous deposition in the alveolus. Björk and Skieller[55] have shown that growth in maxillary length occurs toward the palatine suture and by apposition on the maxillary tuberosities (Fig. 2-17).

The dental arch length (distal of second primary molar to a midpoint between the central incisors) decreases[56,57] as a result of dental migration due to closure of the Leeway spaces, primate spaces, and generalized spacing.

The growth in height of the maxillopalatine complex occurs at the pterygoid processes and in the two lateral squamous sutures between the vertical plates of the palatine bone and maxillae. A combination of sutural and appositional growth of the alveolar process, aided by resorption in the nasal area, permits the maxilla to develop in height.[55]

The vertical growth of the maxilla and mandible separates the arches. The teeth respond by erupting into occlusion thus encouraging alveolar bone growth. The result of this vertical drift[32] is to enlarge the dimension of the nasal chamber by relocating the entire palatal-maxillary complex downward (Fig. 2-18). The maxilla is affected by the structures surrounding it. For example, the cranial base angle affects the positions of the maxilla and mandible and the activity of muscle.[32,58]

Bimler, in 1977,[12] contended that the na-

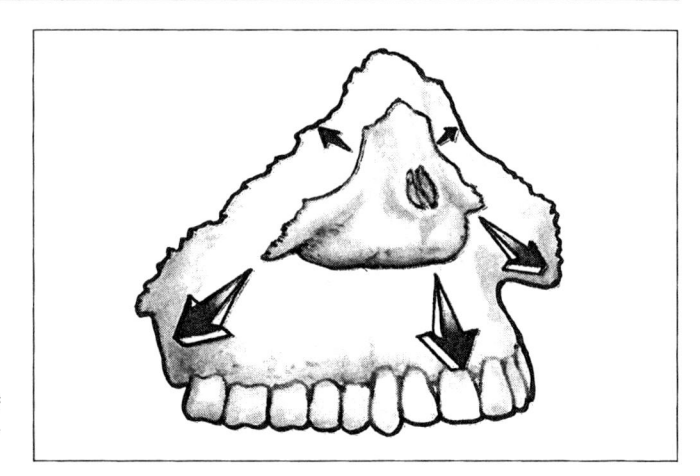

Fig. 2-16 Artist conception of maxillary growth from the neonate to the adult.

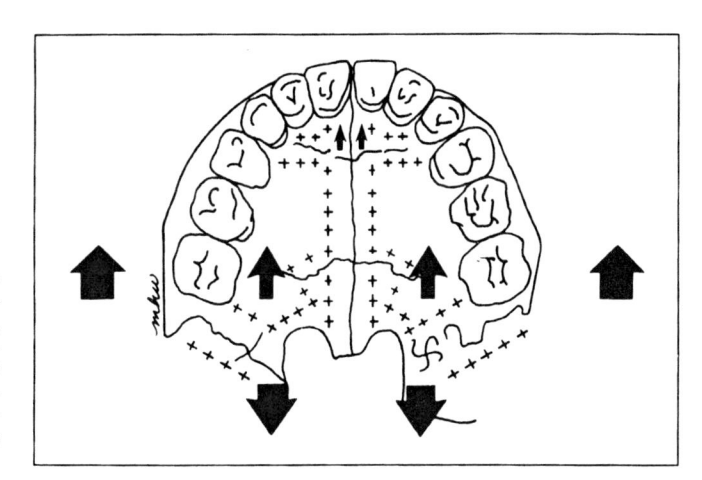

Fig. 2-17 Maxillary length occurs by growth at the premaxillary and maxillopalatine sutures, as well as subperiosteal deposition within the alveolus. As the maxillary arch grows in the posterior direction, the entire complex is displaced in the opposite direction (large arrows).

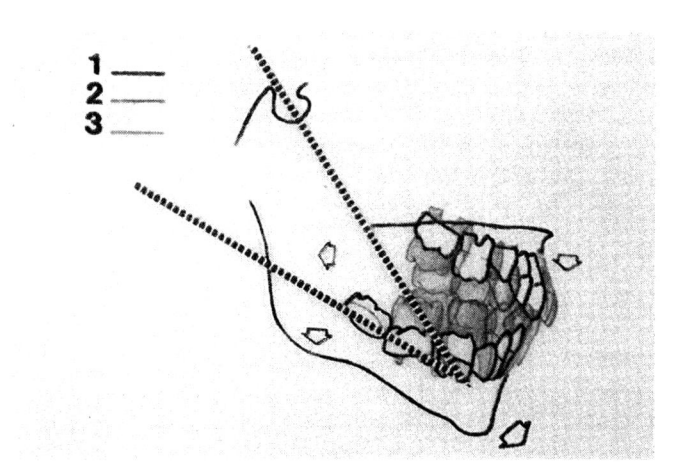

Fig. 2-18 Ages 1, 2, and 3. The teeth will erupt into the vertical separation of the arches.

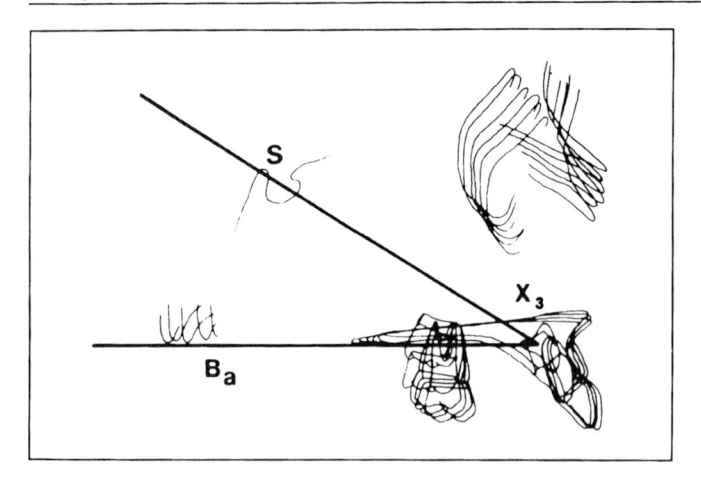

Fig. 2-19 When the growth of the maxilla was monitored from ages 1 to 16, it was found that angle BaX_3S remained stable. Superimposing on BaX_3S, one can notice growth remodeling as well as tooth eruption. (Reprinted with permission from Saadia and White, J. Pedod., Vol. 6, 1982.)

sal floor should be parallel to the Frankfort horizontal plane, but in Class II patients, the palatal plane is frequently inclined forward and downward. This is associated with underdevelopment of the mandible. However, a forward- and upwardly inclined nasal floor is a common sign of underdevelopment of the middle part of the face.

Saadia and White,[52] using symmetric axis geometry from sex-averaged longitudinal data of the Bolton study, compared two cranial points (sella and basion) to two maxillary points (X_3 and X_4). The study period from ages 1 to 16 revealed that angle BaX_3S was stable during the entire growth process (Fig. 2-19). These results suggested that the cranial base and the maxillary arch were interrelated. However, further studies are needed to reconfirm the Enlow analysis of growth equivalence, which suggests that change in one region will produce equivalent changes in corresponding areas elsewhere.[32]

By monitoring the rate of change between the maxilla and mandible, it appears that the mandible grows twice as fast as the maxilla between the ages of 1 and 6 years and one and one-half times as fast as the maxilla between the ages of 7 and 16 years.[59-61] This phenomenon is significant for treatment plans that incorporate maxillofacial orthopedic techniques in young, rapidly growing children.

Biologic continuum of the mandible

The mandible may be thought of as a bent tubular bone. The alveolar process does not form until the teeth begin to develop and erupt (Fig. 2-20). The alveolus is resorbed when the teeth are lost. Areas of muscle attachment at the coronoid processes and the gonial regions become fully differentiated only in response to the development and functioning of the muscles (Fig. 2-21).

Mandibular growth and development are influenced by the maxilla and tongue; the corpus is influenced by the muscles; the ramus by the functioning of the pharynx and tooth eruption. The result is that the *mandibular corpus is the direct structural counterpart of the maxillary corpus*. The mandible is composed of a ramus and corpus; both are independent structures reacting to different stimuli.[32]

As with other bones, the relationship of form to function in the mandible is clear:[62] both the external and internal form of the mandible are directly responsive to the normal pattern of stress. Mandibular form is also closely related to dietary habits,[20-26,63,64] teeth,[20,52,65] and muscle ac-

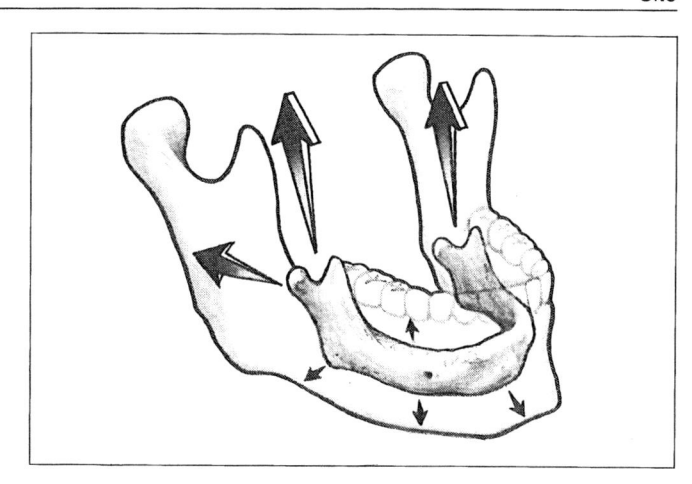

Fig. 2-20 Artist conception of mandibular growth from the neonate to the adult.

tion.[62] Küppers[66] has shown that stress distribution in the mandible during anterior and posterior tooth loading was identical to the distribution of the amount of bone. It was concluded that the volumetric structure of the human mandible was directly related to the distribution of strain. Stress in areas of spongy bone was normally compressive, while the cortical bone was well-adapted to torsion through changes in the cross-sectional shape and thickness distribution.

It is possible to detect significant differences in mandibular function through analysis of osseous structure in past populations. The differences in function are the result of changes in diet and food preparation and of environmental manipulation.

The teeth in the mandible are responsible for the development and preservation of alveolar bone. They also provide "stops" for the tongue to push against. When the teeth contact, intercuspation also exerts forces on the corpus of the mandible and maxilla. These forces affect alveolar bone formation and are transmitted throughout the osseous tissue. Björk[67] has shown a direct relationship between the inclination of the anterior teeth and condylar growth.

It has been shown[52,68] that during the growth process there is first a vertical separation of the bones, followed by tooth eruption. When teeth contact, there is an increase in the vertical opening at the corpus area (mainly in the anterior region). Moss and Picton[69] have suggested that the development of the dentition and the forces of mastication are related to muscle development. If muscles contain the genetic functional determinants of bone growth, a new mandibular position would allow teeth to erupt to a new length and position.

Muscles and the mandible

Any change in the functioning of the musculature has an impact on morphogenesis; the change affects the musculature itself, the skeleton, and the position of the teeth and occlusion. Acceptance of this theory is based on acceptance that:

1. Muscular development depends on use.
2. Interaction occurs between muscular function and bone development as expressed by Wolff's law, which states that the form and structure of a bone represents direct developmental adaptations to the bone's composite of functions.
3. Changes in bone morphology and dental position depend on bone reorganization, i.e., apposition and resorption.

Changes in bone occur when muscular function is altered over a period of time. There must be intensity, frequency, and duration of muscle action for bone formation or resorption to occur.

Biophysical stimuli are transmitted to bone with the following effects:

1. bone modeling and remodeling in the dental alveolus during tooth movement
2. bone apposition during suture expansion in the palate
3. bone apposition in response to elevation of the periosteum

Tension in the periosteal tissue is important to preconditioning of bone for apposition. The architecture of bone is determined by the stress condition established with respect to the attached and adjacent soft tissue in the rest position.

Mandibular ramus

The ramus joins the corpus to the temporomandibular joint. *The structural function of the ramus is to bridge the middle cranial fossa and to connect the corpus to a proper anatomic position.*

The ramus remodels as part of the growth process. Remodeling is aided in part by muscular attachments and pharyngeal function. Enlow[70] has demonstrated four functions of remodeling:

1. The entire ramus is progressively relocated posteriorly by combinations of resorption and deposition on the anterior, posterior, buccal, and lingual surfaces. This relocation provides for posterior growth and elongation of the contiguous corpus. The lengthening of the corpus requires a direct remodeling conversion from ramus into corpus.
2. The ramus progressively increases the horizontal dimensions of the mandible to accommodate the horizontal growth of the middle cranial fossa and pharynx.
3. The ramus lengthens vertically to accommodate the vertical growth of the nasomaxillary complex and dental eruption.
4. The ramus remodels to position the mandibular corpus in proper position with the maxillary corpus.

The ramus has an intrinsic capacity for adaptation as needed. It is influenced by the cranial base, nasomaxillary bones, mandibular corpus, and teeth.

The ramus may undergo two types of remodeling: displacement and rotational. With these changes, the entire mandible alters the functional contacts with the cranial floor and maxilla (Fig. 2-22).

If the cranial base angle is open, the mandible is displaced downward and backward. If the cranial base angle is closed, the mandible is displaced upward and forward (Figs. 2-3a and b). The mandible is displaced downward and backward if the nasomaxillary and dental complexes are vertically elongated. If these complexes are shortened, then the mandible is brought upward and forward. Rotational remodeling of the mandible serves two purposes: first, it allows production of a more upright ramus alignment relative to the corpus; second, it provides ramus-corpus angular adjustments to accommodate the effects of mandibular displacement rotations.

If the mandible is aligned from displacement rotation in an upward and forward direction because of a vertically short midface or a closed cranial base relationship, an upwardly inclined mandibular corpus and occlusal plane will result. Thus, rotational remodeling compensates for the upward inclination by opening the ramus-corpus angular relationship.[70]

The dentition contributes to the closure of the occlusion and occlusal adjustments between the upper and lower bony arches through vertical drift. The result is the curve of Spee.

Site

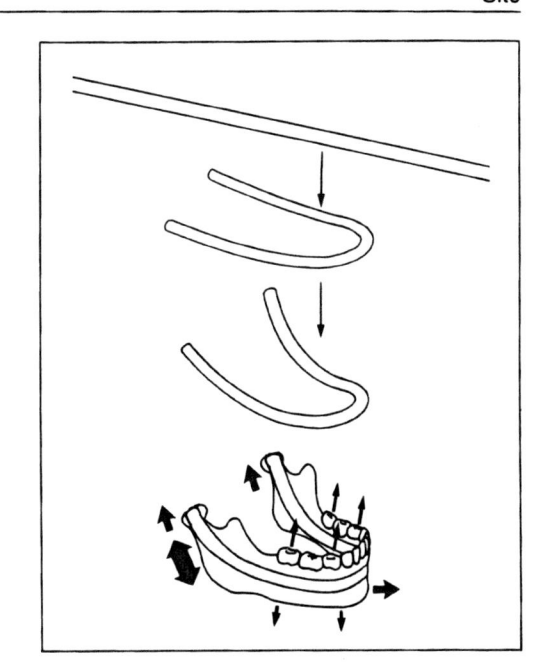

Fig. 2-21 The mandible changes shape constantly during growth; these changes are brought about by function.

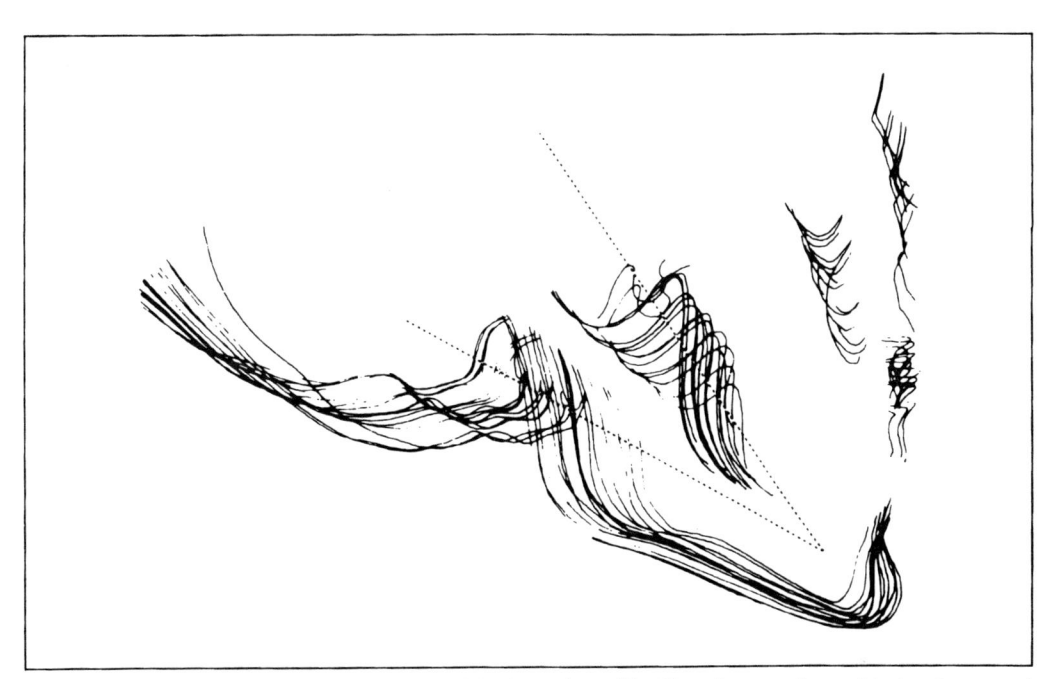

Fig. 2-22 The mandible grows and remodels throughout life. The changes brought about occur at different ages and as a result of different stimuli. In this example, note the growth and remodeling of the mandibular arch (ages 1 to 16). (Reprinted with permission from Saadia and White, J. Pedod., Vol. 6, 1981.)

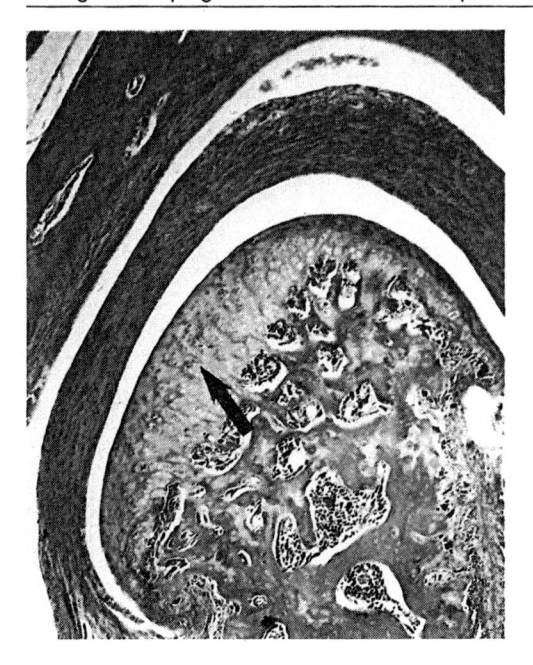

Biological Shaping of the Craniofacial Complex

Fig. 2-23 An example of a low-power section of a young postnatal rat condyle, stained with Mallory's triple. Note the large chondrogenic and hypertrophic zones. Condylar change has been considered the primary center of mandibular growth. Others suggest that the condyle can only grow in response to changes in mandibular position (growth plate).

Mandibular growth

There is much controversy in the literature concerning mandibular and condylar growth. Hunter, in 1771,[71] proposed that the mandible grew by apposition on the posterior border and by resorption on the anterior border. Later, other investigations[72-74] suggested that the condyle was a primary center for mandibular growth. The condylar hypothesis was based on the assumption that this cartilage would serve as an epiphyseal plate.

Does the condyle genetically grow in a superior and posterior direction with the mandible translocated in a downward and forward position? Or is the capsular matrix responsible for mandibular growth? The capsular matrix theory claims that condylar cartilage can grow only in response to changes in mandibular position brought about by the enlargement of the oropharyngeal functioning space.[75-78] These theories are not well-understood (Fig. 2-23). Moss has suggested that it is not known how the tongue or the oral, nasal, and pharyngeal functioning spaces grow, nor is it known where they grow. The process of regulating and controlling epiphyseal growth and development is still unclear.[77]

Functional anatomy of the temporomandibular joint

An understanding of the embryology, histology, and physiology of the temporomandibular joint is helpful for an understanding of the results of maxillofacial orthopedic treatment.

At birth, the joint is characterized by a vascularization of all the components and an anatomic and histologic immaturity. The condyle and the disc are flat, and the articular tubercle is just a small elevation of the zygomatic bone (Fig. 2-24). The mandible is free to move to any direction because there are no interferences. With the eruption of the primary central incisors, the first interferences appear. These teeth prohibit the mandible from sliding forward without

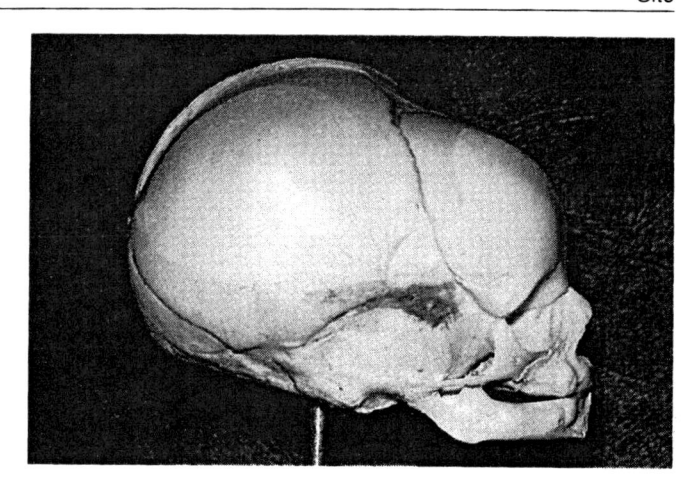

Fig. 2-24 At birth, the condyle and the disc are flat. Notice the craniofacial proportions.

opening. Wright and Moffett[79] have shown that the lateral pterygoid muscle (which attaches to the junction of the condylar head and neck) has a direct effect on the growth of the superior aspect of the condyle. This superior aspect is covered by three tissue layers: a fibrous articular layer, a cellular proliferative layer, and a layer of hyaline growth cartilage. The articular layer covers the superior aspect of the condyle and does not show the presence of chondrocytes. Adjacent is a cellular proliferative layer which undergoes a relatively small amount of mitosis. The innermost layer is hyaline cartilage. This layer can be divided into three distinct zones: the outer zone of cell proliferation, a middle zone characterized by cellular hypertrophy, and the inner layer of calcification and resorption. The mitotic cells are undifferentiated mesenchymal cells. Depending on the environmental stimuli, they can become either osteogenic or chondrogenic (Figs. 2-25a to d).[80]

The lateral pterygoid muscle will act on the innermost layer of hyaline cartilage and on the cellular proliferative layers. These layers give a final characteristic shape to the temporomandibular joint during the first two or three years of life. This joint does not attain its mature anatomical contour until the appearance of the late mixed dentition. While the condyle is growing, the disc will accentuate an S-shaped profile as the articular tubercle develops (Figs. 2-26a and b).

The condylar growth cartilage that was 1.5 mm thick at birth decreases to about 0.5 mm early in the primary dentition. By age 16 the growth cartilage becomes even thinner and a closing plate of bone begins to coalesce below it. Some investigators[79] have found that growth is active until approximately age 21. If further developmental changes occur, they will result from osseous remodeling.

To fully understand TMJ function it should be viewed as a complex joint surrounded by muscles and ligaments that limit and carry the movement. Moss[81] notes that the articular fossa is not a functioning component of the TMJ, nor are the ligaments. The fossa serves as a receptacle for the condyle; the ligaments do not restrict the normal range of motion.

The morphology of the TMJ permits three types of motions, i.e., opening and closing, protrusion and retrusion, and lateral movements. The limit of movement is determined by joint anatomy, and movement is guided by muscles and ligaments. The muscles active during each of these movements are listed in Fig. 2-27.

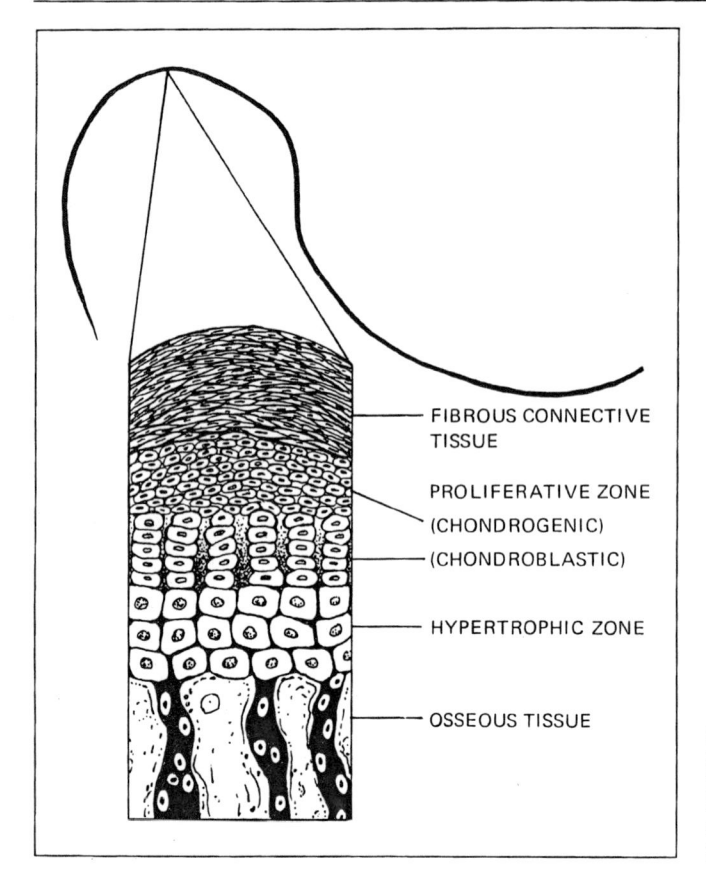

Biological Shaping of the Craniofacial Complex

Fig. 2-25a The superior aspect of the condyle is covered by three tissue layers: a fibrous articular layer, a chondrogenic and chondroblastic zone, and a hypertrophic zone.

Teeth

From birth through the primary dentition

At birth, the width of the primary arch is capable of accommodating the primary incisors only. The greatest increase in mandibular arch width and length occurs before 9 months of age.[8,82,83] This arch length can be adversely affected by oligodontia and other factors (Fig. 2-29).

The primary mandibular central incisor erupts into the oral cavity by the age of 8 months (±2 months) of postnatal life and will exert its influence upon the hard and soft tissues of the oral cavity via functional and static parameters.

The eruption of the primary central mandibular incisors opens the vertical dimension, helping to balance the tonic and phasic muscles. The tongue is forced to readapt to the new space and its movement becomes restricted. The mandible, because of the tooth interference, is hindered from sliding forward without opening. As contact is established with the maxillary teeth, temporomandibular joint remodeling takes place, and occlusion begins. An increase in the vertical dimension affects temporomandibular joint remodeling.

The infantile swallowing pattern ceases with closure of the intermaxillary space. Tooth contact influences the facial musculature to readapt, and regulates forward growth of the mandible. Teeth erupt during

Site

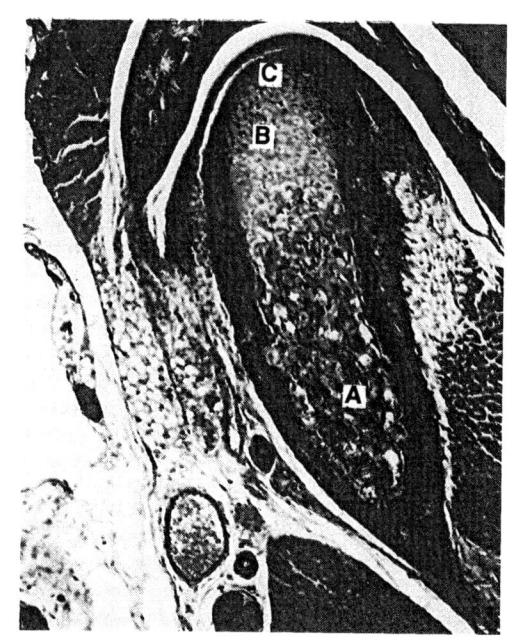

Fig. 2-25b Section through condylar and angular cartilage of a one-week-old rat. Note the well-defined (a) osteogenic zone, (b) hypertrophic zone, and (c) chondrogenic and chondroblastic zone. (Verhoff Stain and eosin × 35.) (Courtesy of Dr. Jack Frommer.)

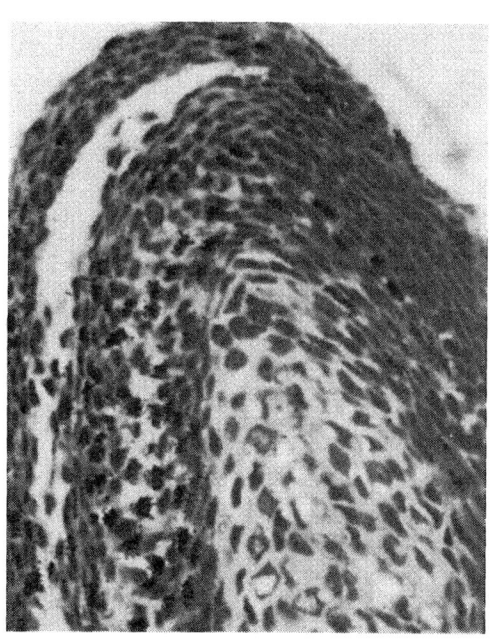

Fig. 2-25c An autoradiograph of the mandibular condyle of a one-day-old mouse, showing a high labeling index (dark cells). ^{3}H+ thymidine picks up those cells which are about to divide. Proliferative activity decreases during early postnatal life.

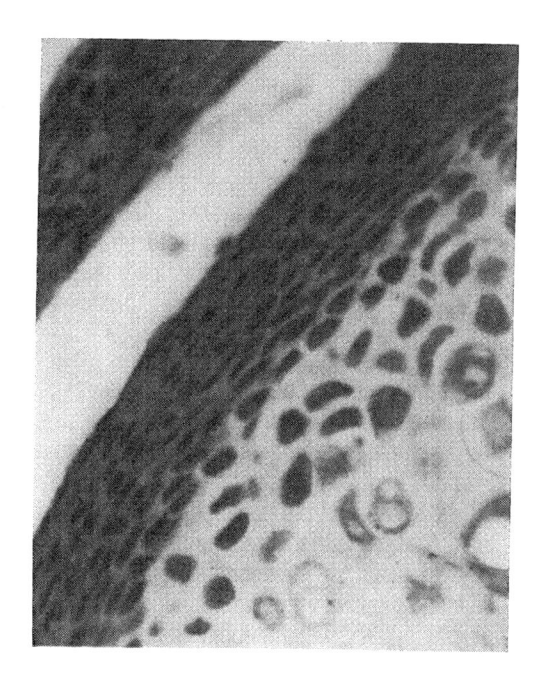

Fig. 2-25d Higher magnification of a 14-day-old mouse condyle (autoradiograph; H & E stain). This example shows no proliferative activity. (Courtesy of Dr. Jack Frommer.)

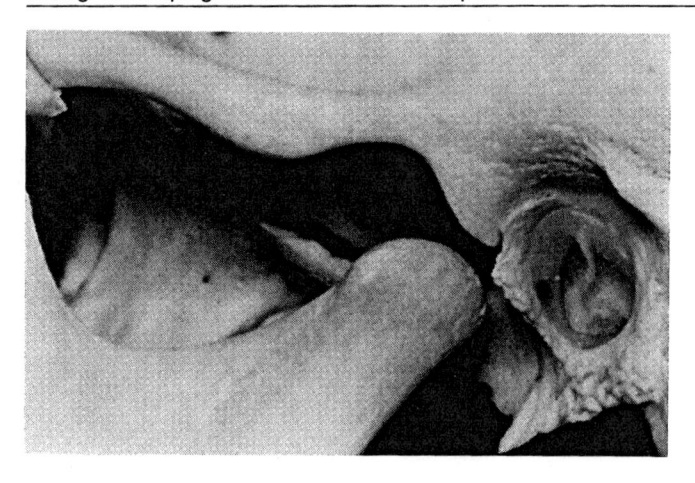

Biological Shaping of the Craniofacial Complex

Figs. 2-26a and b The temporomandibular joint will change its shape constantly during active growth.

Fig. 2-26a Example of a disarticulated temporomandibular joint during the early mixed dentition.

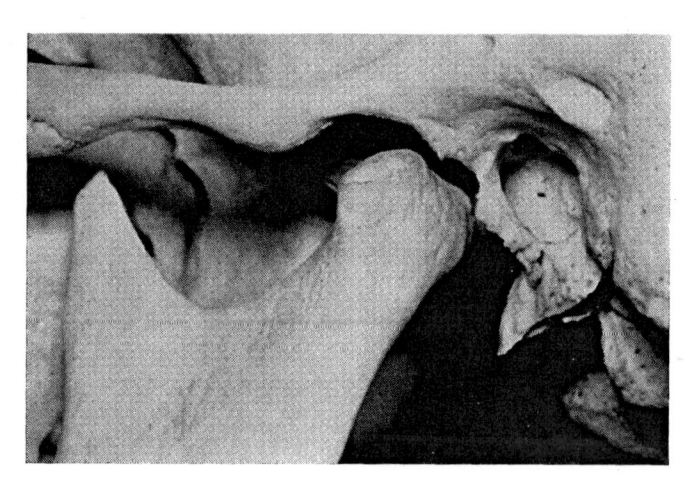

Fig. 2-26b Osseous anatomy of the temporomandibular joint during early adulthood.

a period of very active growth of the facial skeleton. Some investigators contend that they are guided into occlusion from adaptation to the neuromusculature. During the growth process, adaptive changes take place in the craniofacial complex. These changes generally will lead to a normal occlusion as long as there is a normal primary dentition, balanced musculature, and there are no disruptive factors.

There are also dental and skeletal adjustment mechanisms: the muscles of mastication exert an influence through intercuspation, producing growth changes and remodeling in the craniofacial complex.

Transitional stage—mixed to early adolescent dentition

There are two paradoxical dimensional changes in the dental arches during the transition from the mixed dentition to the early adolescent dentition: the circumferences of the maxilla and mandible decrease, while the lengths increase. Fisk[84] and Moorrees[85] reported a mean reduction of about 5 mm in mandibular circumference as the result of the following:

1. late mesial shift of the first permanent molars

FUNCTION OF THE TEMPOROMANDIBULAR JOINT

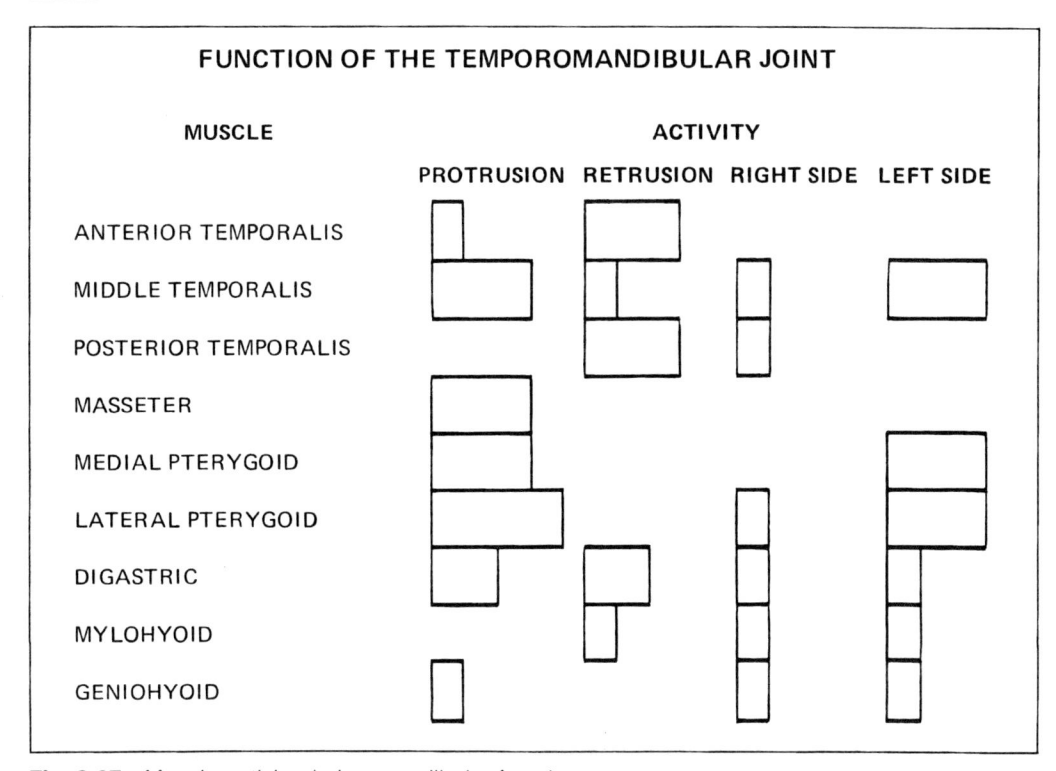

MUSCLE	PROTRUSION	RETRUSION	RIGHT SIDE	LEFT SIDE
ANTERIOR TEMPORALIS				
MIDDLE TEMPORALIS				
POSTERIOR TEMPORALIS				
MASSETER				
MEDIAL PTERYGOID				
LATERAL PTERYGOID				
DIGASTRIC				
MYLOHYOID				
GENIOHYOID				

Fig. 2-27 Muscle activity during mandibular function.

2. mesial drifting of the posterior teeth
3. slight interproximal wear
4. lingual positioning of the permanent incisors (These teeth are wider than the primary incisors yet they occupy a similar position.)

Murray[86] found that four factors contributed to the anteroposterior occlusal adjustment in the transitional dentition:

1. forward growth of the maxilla
2. maxillary leeway space
3. forward growth of the mandible
4. mandibular leeway space (Fig. 2-28)

The skeletal development is more important than the occlusal adjustment in preventing malocclusion. The occlusal relationships are largely the result of skeletal growth. This developmental skeletal morphology is reviewed here.

It has been shown that during the growth process, there is vertical separation of the bones followed by tooth eruption. When anterior teeth erupt, there is an increase in the vertical opening at the corpus.[52,68] The same phenomenon was found by Nanda,[87] who demonstrated that the rate of vertical growth was modified in childhood by the successive shedding of primary teeth and the emergence of permanent teeth.

If the muscle contains the genetic and functional determinants of bone growth, or if muscles are transducers of stimuli, an imbalance in this musculature (depending on the intensity, frequency, and duration of the insult) may lead to an abnormal skeletal configuration. This imbalance can be caused by—or the cause of—an alteration

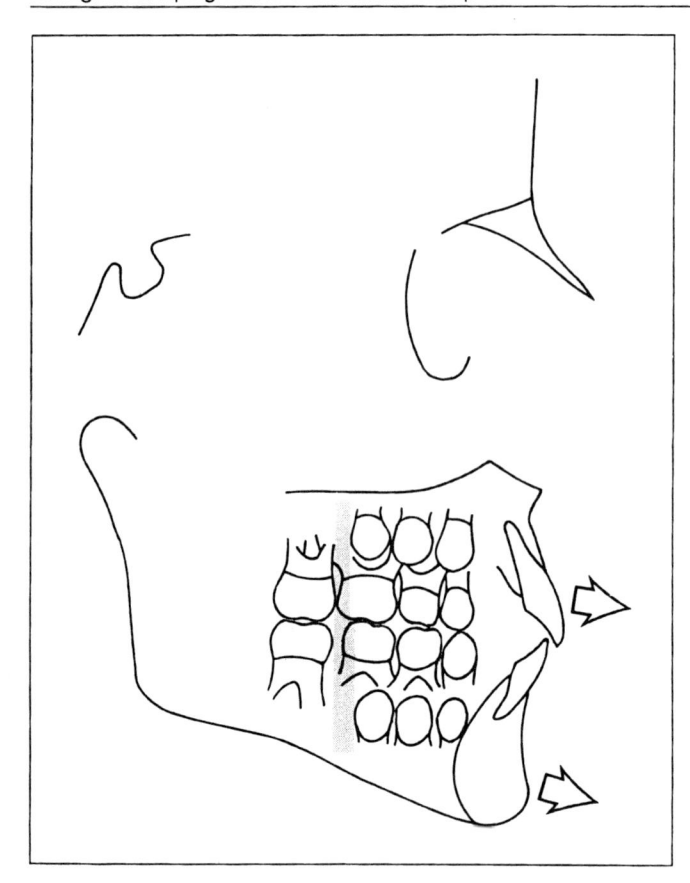

Fig. 2-28 An end-to-end terminal plane relationship in the primary dentition results in a Class I molar relationship in the permanent dentition from the forward growth of the maxilla and mandible and in part from the leeway space. (Modified with permission from Saadia, J. Pedod., Vol. 5, 1981; Oral Health, Vol. 71, 1981.)

in the neuromuscular system. The imbalance could be triggered by injury, disease, occlusion, or environmental factors. Graber[88] suggests that abnormal muscular activity will result in a compensatory response to an abnormal morphogenetic pattern. It is important to realize that malocclusion represents an attempt to establish a balance between morphogenetic, functional, and environmental forces and is always in dynamic balance at any particular time.

It has been shown that the musculature directly affects osseous growth and corroborates Wolff's law: "Function modifies anatomy."[33] The next section will consider some of the effects of imbalance on the development of the craniofacial complex.

Manifestations

Influence of the tongue on the facial osseous components

The tongue has a direct influence on the alteration in shape and position of the maxillary and mandibular arches. Wallace, in 1927,[89] found a direct effect between large and small tongues with correspondingly large and small mandibles: "If the tongue is not the dominant factor in coordinating the growth of the dental arches, at least it helps to coordinate growth."

Harvold[90,91] has shown that induced oral respiration in monkeys can alter muscular balance and result in a skeletal open bite

Manifestations

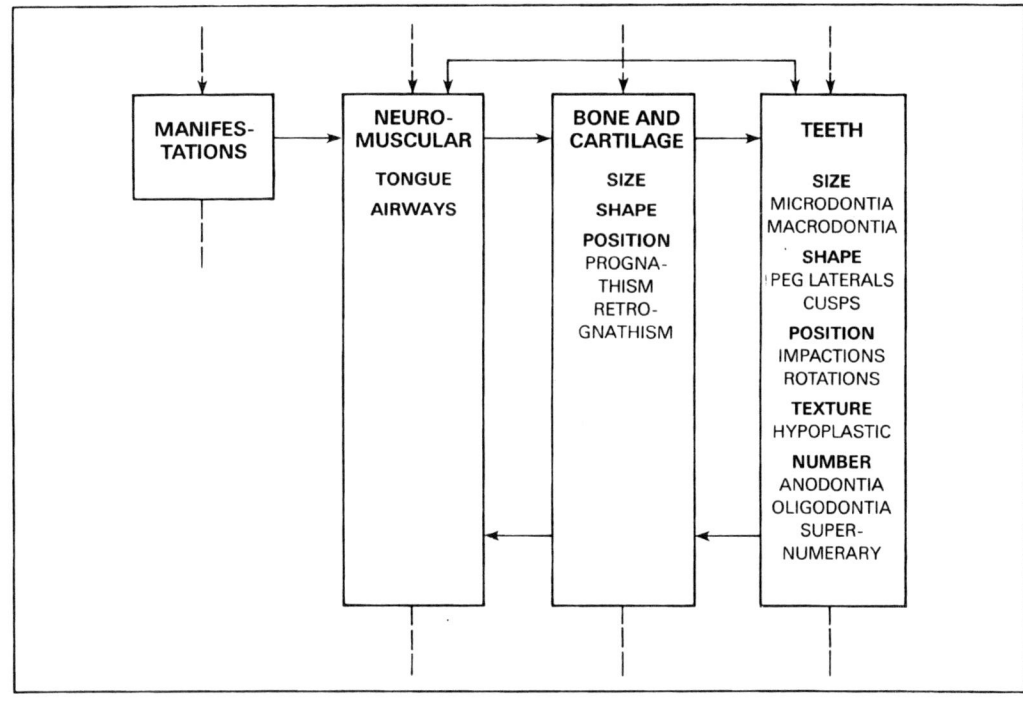

```
                    ↓                  ↓                  ↓                  ↓
┌─────────────────────────────────────────────────────────────────────────────────┐
│  ┌──────────┐     ┌──────────┐    ┌──────────┐    ┌──────────┐                 │
│  │ MANIFES- │ →   │  NEURO-  │ →  │ BONE AND │ →  │  TEETH   │                 │
│  │ TATIONS  │     │ MUSCULAR │    │ CARTILAGE│    │          │                 │
│  └──────────┘     │          │    │          │    │   SIZE   │                 │
│       │           │  TONGUE  │    │   SIZE   │    │MICRODONTIA│                │
│       │           │ AIRWAYS  │    │  SHAPE   │    │MACRODONTIA│                │
│       │           │          │    │ POSITION │    │  SHAPE   │                 │
│       │           │          │    │ PROGNA-  │    │PEG LATERALS│               │
│       │           │          │    │  THISM   │    │  CUSPS   │                 │
│       │           │          │    │ RETRO-   │    │ POSITION │                 │
│       │           │          │    │ GNATHISM │    │IMPACTIONS│                 │
│       │           │          │    │          │    │ROTATIONS │                 │
│       │           │          │    │          │    │ TEXTURE  │                 │
│       │           │          │    │          │    │HYPOPLASTIC│                │
│       │           │          │    │          │    │ NUMBER   │                 │
│       │           │          │    │          │    │ANODONTIA │                 │
│       │           │          │    │          │    │OLIGODONTIA│                │
│       │           │          │    │          │    │ SUPER-   │                 │
│       │           │          │    │          │    │NUMERARY  │                 │
│       │           │          │ ←  │          │ ←  │          │                 │
│       ↓                ↓              ↓                ↓                        │
└─────────────────────────────────────────────────────────────────────────────────┘
```

Fig. 2-29 Examples of the manifestations of factors acting on different sites.

and changes in mandibular morphology. An imbalance between the tongue and the perioral musculature can lead to open bite, narrowed arches, Class II and III malocclusion, or bialveolar retrusion or protrusion.[90-92]

Role of the tongue in regulation of midfacial growth

The tongue has been studied by Stutzmann and Petrovic[93] and Gasson et al.[94] using experimental animals. In partial-glossectomy experiments, the forward growth of the maxilla was considerably less than normal. The growth of the premaxillary suture was significantly and consistently reduced, particularly when tongue resection was extensive. The growth of the maxillopalatine suture also decreased. The authors described the apparent mechanism as a decrease in lingual thrust after partial glossectomy.

In another series of experiments, macroglossia was produced using plastic inserts.[94] Under experimental conditions, the forward growth of the maxilla was stimulated by the thrust of a larger tongue applied *directly* to the maxillary incisors. The effect was not, however, statistically significant. A decrease in the lateral growth rate of the maxilla was observed.

When the tongue was enlarged, it occupied a lower position than normal and did not produce the expected supplementary anterior-posterior growth of the maxilla. The tongue did stimulate the lateral growth of the premaxilla, but not of the maxilla. The pressure from the buccal musculature was

57

Biological Shaping of the Craniofacial Complex

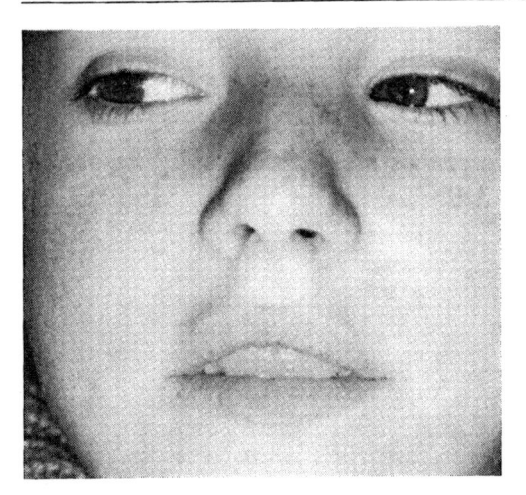

Fig. 2-30 Allergic patient. Notice the underdeveloped upper lip. (Reprinted with permission from Saadia, J. Pedod., Vol. 5, 1981.)

constant, pushing the upper premolars and molars in a palatal direction.

Role of the tongue in mandibular growth

It has been shown that aglossia and hypoglossia can alter mandibular shape, tooth position, and occlusion.[95-97] The tongue influences the rate and extent of mandibular growth. Partial glossectomy in normal young rats resulted in a considerable retardation of condylar, as well as anteroposterior, growth of the mandible. When the same experiment was done with the lateral pterygoid muscle also resected bilaterally, only a negligible retardation of condylar growth was seen.[98]

Stutzmann and Petrovic[98] have shown that an enlarged tongue will result in an increased anteroposterior thrust and a forward protrusion of the mandible. This phenomenon will increase the activity of the lateral pterygoid muscles and stimulate condylar growth.

Respiration and mastication

The nasal cavity is partially formed by the two parts of the maxilla, which also happen to constitute the basal structure for the maxillary dentition and most of the maxilla. The lower limits of the nasal cavity are the upper limits of the oral cavity. Normal breathing is conducive to normal growth of the craniofacial complex and normal development of the occlusion.

Conversely, an altered mode of breathing (e.g., obstructed nasal passages) leads to a lowering of tongue position and occlusal changes in the dentition from the influence of the lip, cheek, and tongue musculature.[99] This change in breathing leads to a change in the balance between tongue and cheek pressure surrounding the maxilla.

The lowered tongue position results in a reduction of buccally directed pressure. If the pressure from the cheek musculature remains unchanged, the maxillary premolars and molars will tend to move in a palatal direction.

Although the nasal airway presents a greater resistance to inspired air than the oral airway, humans generally breathe through the nasal route. However, some individuals breathe through the mouth. Continuous mouth breathing may bring changes in the normal growth of the craniofacial complex.

Johnson[28] has described features common among mouth breathers: facial asymmetry, underdeveloped upper lip and/or nostrils, a thickened and outwardly-rolled lower lip, and lack of tone of the facial musculature (Figs. 2-30 and 2-31).

Linder-Aronson[29] lists the following characteristics of chronic mouth breathers:

1. narrowed maxilla
2. retroclined maxillary-mandibular incisors
3. abnormal palatal vault height
4. tendency for crossbite
5. tendency for overbite

Manifestations

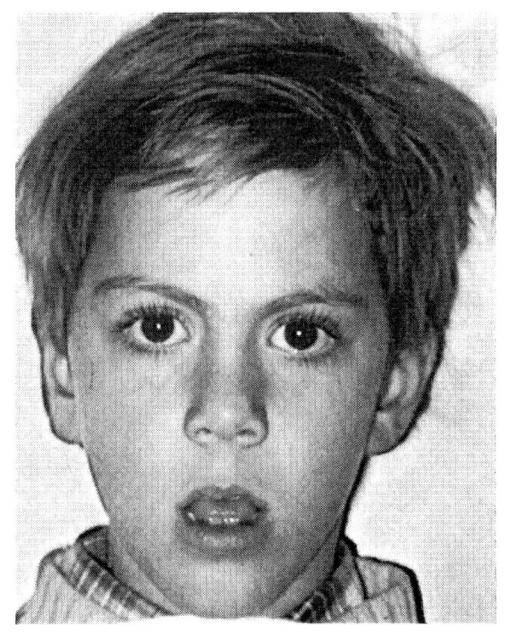

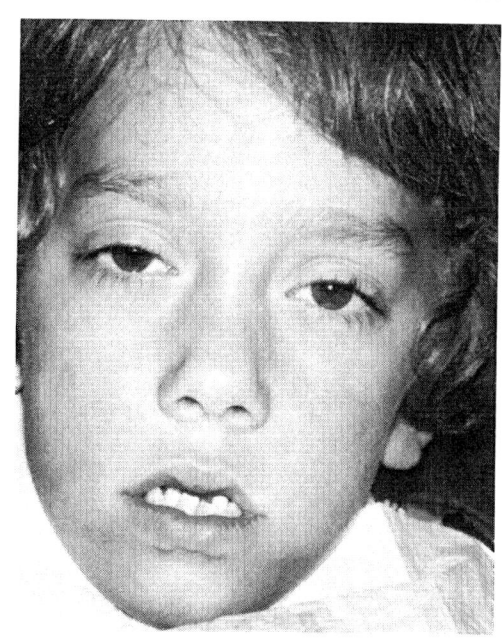

Figs. 2-31a and b Two brothers with characteristic long faces. The allergic adenoids in these patients are causing the blockage of the nasopharyngeal chambers, creating a mouth-breathing pattern.

6. normal anteroposterior relationship between the maxilla and mandible

Etiology

The etiology of nasal airway obstruction may be congenital, acquired, or developed. Congenital problems include large turbinates, choanal atresia, and narrow nasal passages within the maxilla. Small external nares may be inherited. Acquired and developmental problems include:[100]

1. deviated septa
2. extensive nasopharyngeal lymphoid tissue
3. perennial allergic rhinitis
4. neoplasm
5. polyp formation
6. trauma
7. iatrogenic factors

Allergies have long been recognized as an important factor in the creation of malocclusion. Some originate from inhalants found in the normal environment (spores, organic dusts, and microorganisms).[101,102] Certain food allergies (milk, red meat, corn) are also common (Figs. 2-32a and b).

All rapidly growing structures are vulnerable to pathologic changes. Developmental defects can occur during the normal craniofacial growth process. Studies by Todd et al.,[103] Cooke,[104] Marks,[102] Linder-Aronson,[30] and Harvold[90,91] confirm this data. Brash,[105] Huber and Reynolds,[106] Howard,[107] Sillman,[56] and Leech[108] suggest that adenoids and mouth breathing do not interfere directly with facial form and type of malocclusion. Bushey[109] reviews three separate hypotheses proposed by Linder-Aronson:[29]

1. Adenoid enlargement leading to mouth breathing results in a particular type of facial form and dentition.

59

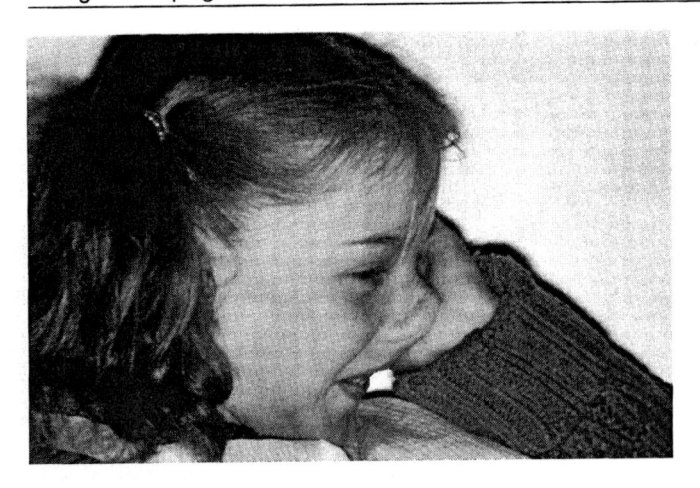

Figs. 2-32a and b Allergic salute of a patient with allergic rhinitis. Notice the short upper lip. (Reprinted with permission from Saadia, J. Pedod., Vol. 5, 1981.)

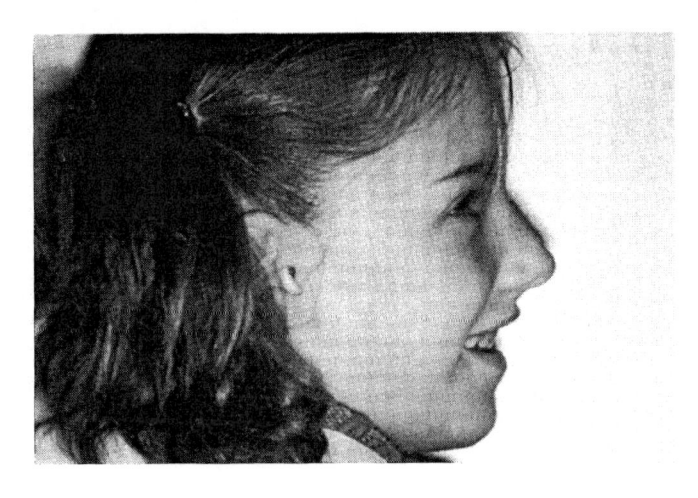

Fig. 2-32b

2. Conversely, enlarged adenoids leading to mouth breathing do not influence facial form and type of dentition.
3. Enlargement of adenoids in certain types of facial structures leads to mouth breathing.

Lymphoid tissue, primarily the tonsils and adenoids, are highly responsive to allergies. At birth the normal lymphoid tissue is small. It increases rapidly in size during childhood and peaks at approximately age 10. The adenoids then begin to atrophy until they shrink to a smaller adult size. The allergic adenoid is swollen and edematous; it can cause blockage of the nasopharyngeal chamber (Figs. 2-33a and b). Children with narrow faces and small nasopharynxes are more inclined to adenoidal obstruction. MacTavish and Matthews[110] recognized that the severity of the malocclusion depends on the degree of obstruction (Table 2-1).

Other important factors are the age of the patient, the frequency, intensity, and duration of the obstruction, and the consequence of any impairment in pulmonary function.[111] Correction of a malocclusion without regard for an obstructed airway will generally result in dental and skeletal relapse.

Manifestations

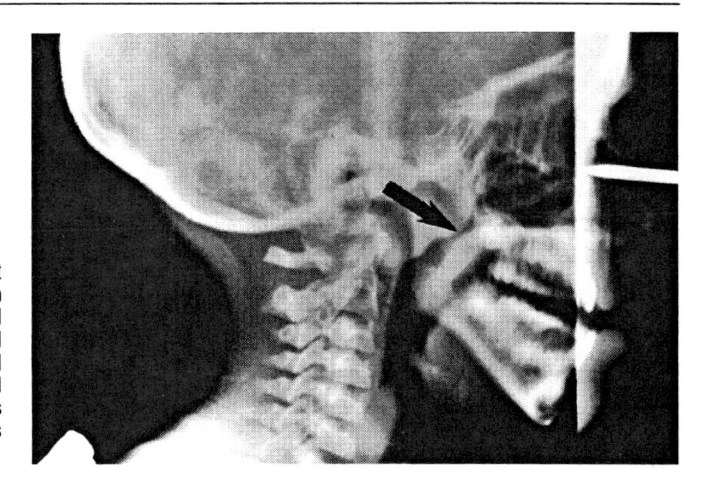

Figs. 2-33a and b Two different growth patterns of patients with blockage of the nasopharyngeal chambers from hypertrophic and edematous pharyngeal lymphoid tissue. Notice the very restricted nasal airway passage. Patients could not keep their mouths closed.

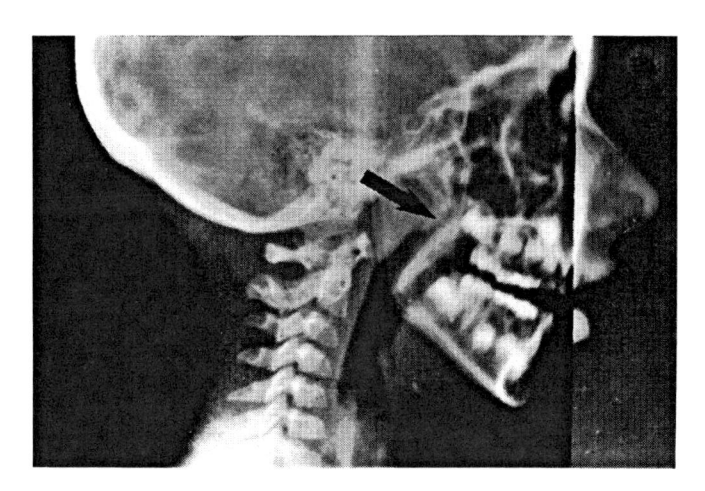

Fig. 2-33b

Table 2-1 Effects of airway obstructions on facial formation

Type of airway	Obstruction	Skeletal change
Broad	None	None
	Partial	None
	Almost complete	Mild
Narrow	None	Mild
	Partial	Moderate
	Almost complete	Severe

There is still controversy as to whether adenoidectomy and/or tonsillectomy can improve oral function by restoring a normal breathing pattern. The paucity of data regarding beneficial growth changes in post-adenoidectomized patients does not permit these procedures to be performed on a routine basis.

Research conducted using better methods of detecting both the oral and nasal airflow will allow better recording of the influence of respiration on the growth of the craniofacial complex.[112]

Bone and cartilage

The relationship of brain form, facial profile,

61

Biological Shaping of the Craniofacial Complex

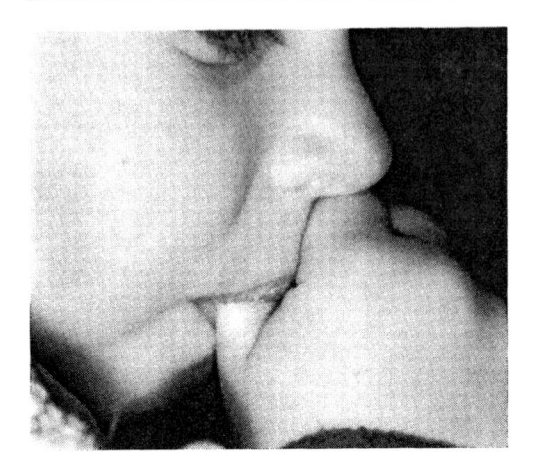

Figs. 2-34a to c Severe Class II in a 3-year-old with a thumb-sucking habit. Notice the large overjet.

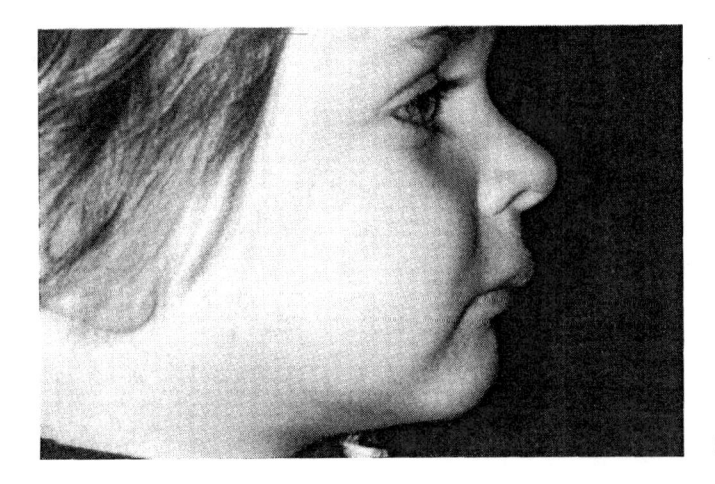

Fig. 2-34b

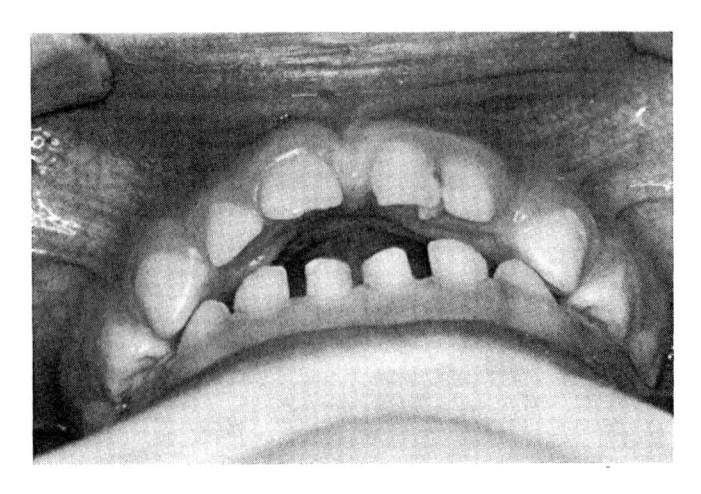

Fig. 2-34c

Manifestations

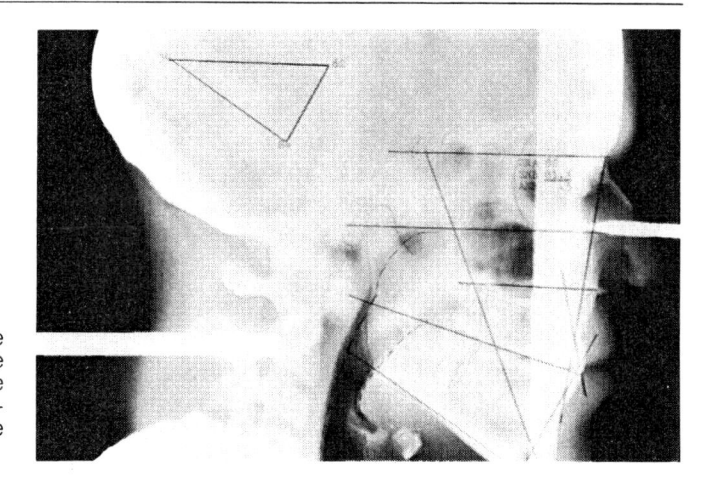

Fig. 2-35 Brachycephalic face on a 16-year-old patient. Notice the more upright position of the cranial base and the more forward relative placement of the mandible.

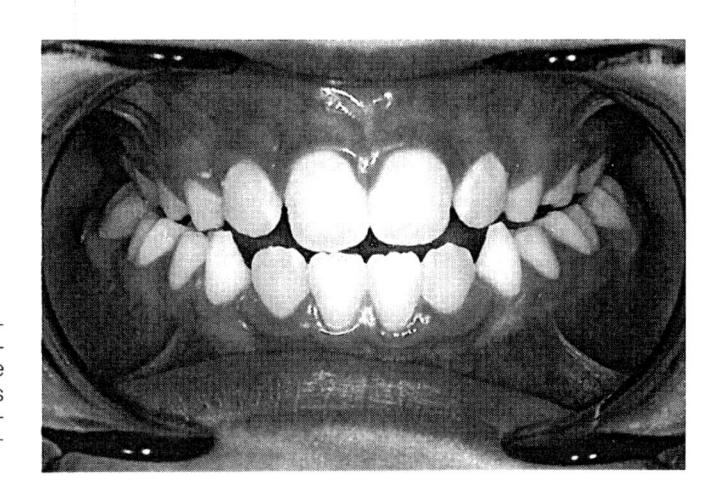

Fig. 2-36a A functional crossbite on a 7-year-old patient. Notice the lack of wear facets on the lower canines. These cusp tips are interfering with normal occlusion and displacing normal closure of the mandible.

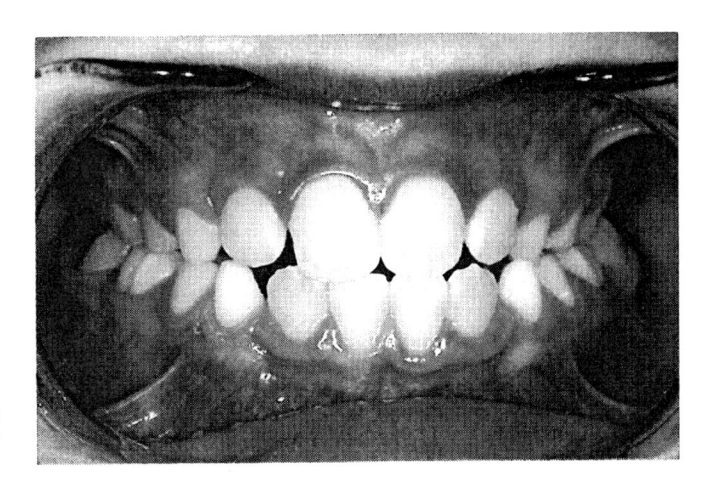

Fig. 2-36b One week after removing the interferences, notice the distal deflection of the mandible.

63

Biological Shaping of the Craniofacial Complex

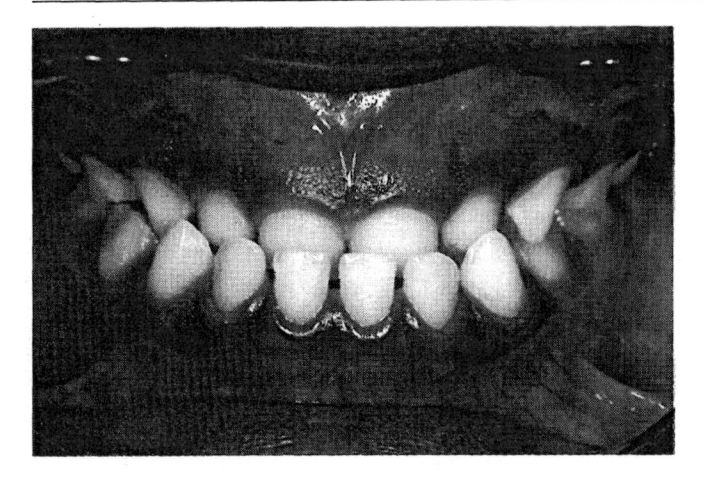

Fig. 2-37a A functional crossbite can mimic the process by which maxillofacial orthopedic appliances trigger mandibular growth. In order to avoid a true Class III malocclusion from developing, every effort should be made to eliminate crossbites as early as possible.

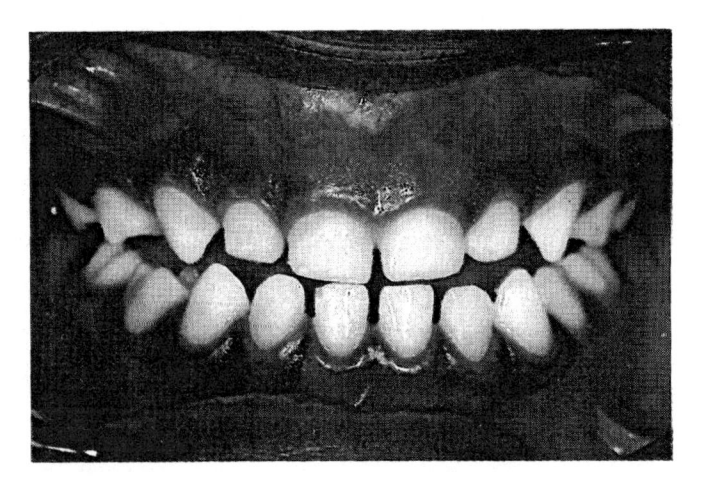

Fig. 2-37b In this patient, mandibular manipulation brought the patient's occlusion to an end-to-end position. The correction could include: *(1)* elimination of the canine interference and *(2)* repositioning the maxillary arch forward to a suitable overjet. The maxillary overbite could then help control mandibular growth.

and occlusal type predisposes the patient to characteristic facial types. For example, dolichocephalics (head form horizontally long and relatively narrow) tend to place the nasomaxillary complex in a protrusive position. This positioning tends to produce a skeletal Class II malocclusion with a retrognathic profile. Habits (digit, pacifier, or blanket sucking) can also contribute to a Class II malocclusion (Figs. 2-34a to c). A Class II, Division 1 malocclusion could be the result or combination of the following:

1. maxillary skeletal protrusion
2. maxillary dentoalveolar protrusion
3. mandibular skeletal retrusion
4. mandibular dentoalveolar retrusion
5. mandibular hyperplasia (long face)
6. mandibular hypoplasia (short face)

The brachycephalic structure (head form rounder with a wider brain) has a more upright cranial base. The result is a relative retrusion of the nasomaxillary complex and a more forward relative placement of the mandible (Fig. 2-35). This developmental form results in a tendency toward Class III malocclusion and a prognathic profile. An anterior interference may produce a functional Class III malocclusion.

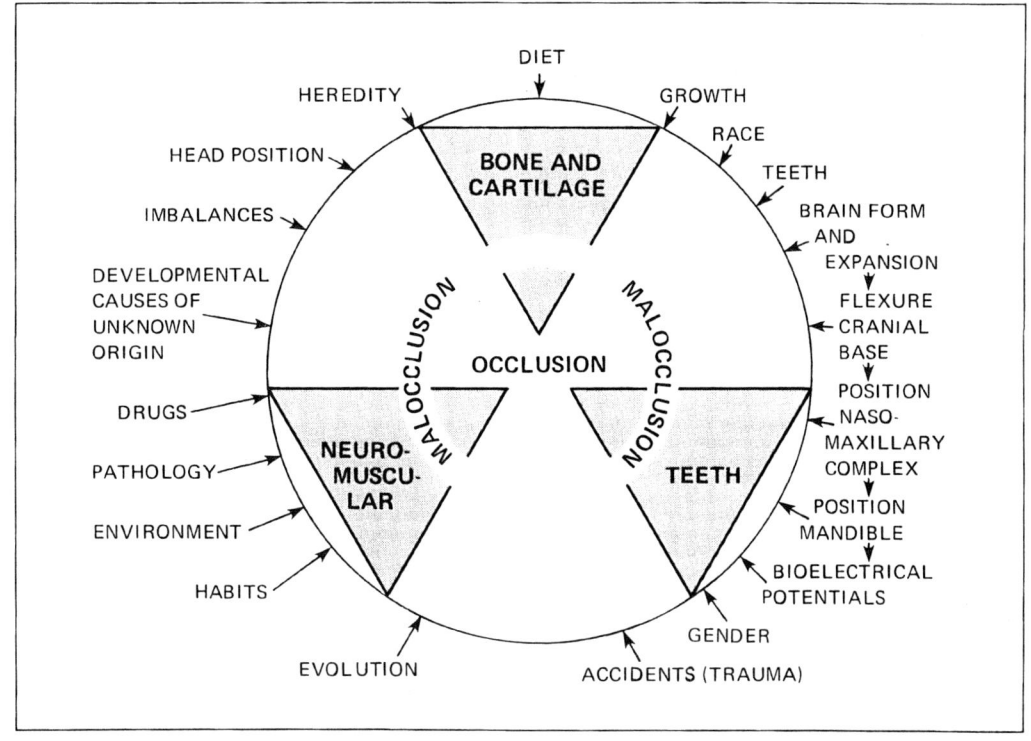

Fig. 2-38 The developing occlusion is affected by a variety of external and internal stimuli.

If untreated, this functional aberration can develop into a true Class III malocclusion. This interference may simulate the action of a mandibular repositioning appliance and trigger condylar growth (Figs. 2-36a and b; 2-37a and b).

Figure 2-38 demonstrates some of the developmental, genetic, and local factors that can alter normal skeletal and occlusal development.

Gross variation in size, shape, position, texture, and number of teeth may cause a malocclusion and indirectly alter osseous growth. A frequent cause of dental crowding is large teeth in normal sized basal arches. Wallace[89] pointed out:

> There are many obvious causes of irregularity of the teeth which may be classed as "accidental." The sequence of events by which they lead to a progressive development of malocclusion must be a matter for expert observation and technical discussion.

Included in this category are supernumerary teeth, unilateral or bilateral absence of individual teeth, ectopic eruption or impaction of individual teeth, and disorders of eruption.

In summary, the dental component has a direct effect on the general form of the arches. *An abnormally positioned tooth should be corrected as soon as possible in order to avoid craniofacial imbalances.*

Some researchers[39,40] have shown that patients with malocclusion have an aberrant pattern of muscular activity compared with patients with normal occlusion. But does the malocclusion produce the abnormal muscular function, or is the abnormal muscular function producing the malocclu-

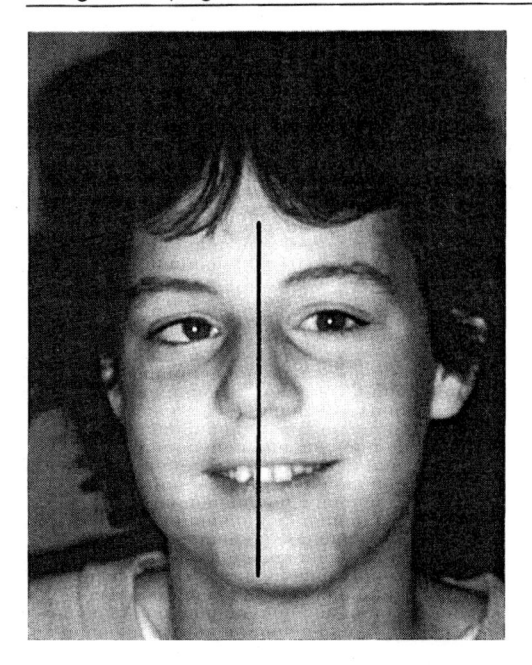

Biological Shaping of the Craniofacial Complex

Fig. 2-39a and b Mild facial imbalance in conjunction with a posterior crossbite in a healthy patient. The muscular imbalance may be creating the crossbite or the crossbite many affect muscular balance. Early correction is indicated.

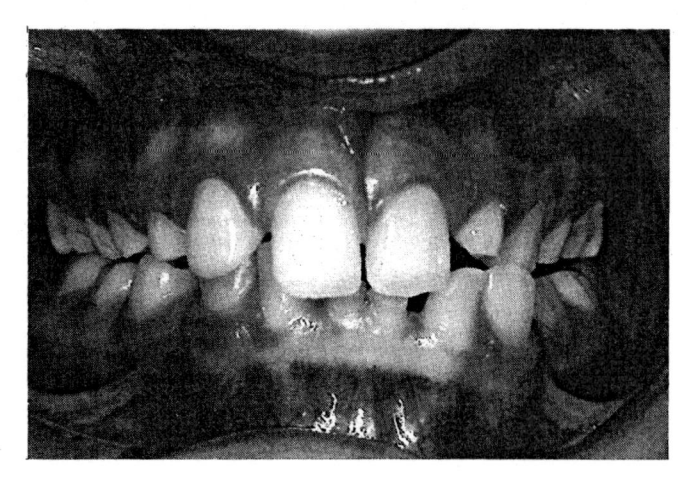

Fig. 2-39b

sion (Fig. 2-39)? Proffit[113] suggests that in the short term, function adapts to changes in form, much more than form adapts to altered function. This phenomenon is brought about by the physiological adaptation and the insensitivity of the teeth to intermittent forces such as chewing, swallowing, and speaking.

Petrovic et al.[65] have shown that unilateral malocclusion (produced by mesialization of the maxillary first molar) or subocclusion (produced by grinding of three maxillary molars) slightly decreased growth of the homolateral condylar and angular cartilages and stimulated growth in the contralateral condyle. The postural and masticatory functioning of the lateral pterygoid muscle is controlled by feedback loops.

Manifestations

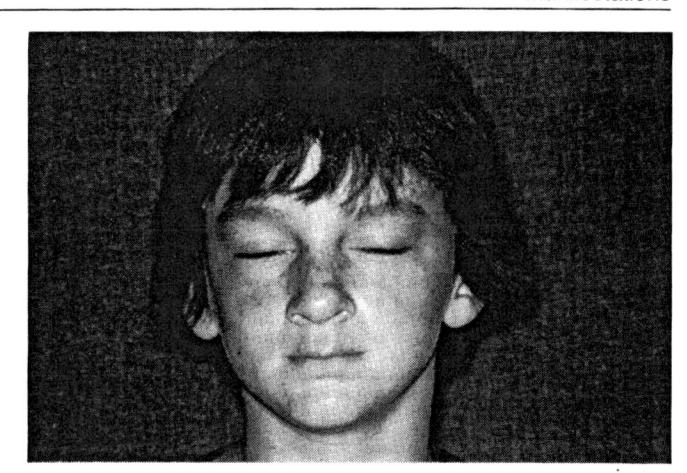

Figs. 2-40a to d Patient with oligodontia and only nine permanent teeth present. Note the pouting, inverted lips, and poor facial esthetics that result from an improper vertical dimension.

A study by Tatum et al.[114] described the dental, occlusal, and cephalometric characteristics of patients with ankylosis of the primary molars. The authors concluded that these patients showed a greater tendency toward crossbites and shorter midfaces than did the normal population.

The shape and structure of the teeth can alter function and facial formation. Several examples can be mentioned; some of them are physiologic, some unfortunately iatrogenic (Chapter 13). A talon cusp on a maxillary incisor may deflect the mandible posteriorly and result in a Class II growth pattern. In dentinogenesis imperfecta and oligodontia, therapeutic intervention is necessary to avoid vertical closure, pouting, inverted lips, poor function, and poor facial esthetics. Treatment may include full tooth coverage and periodic vertical opening to a proper vertical dimension in order to balance the neuromusculature and activate skeletal growth and remodeling (Figs. 2-40a to d).

A direct relationship exists between the musculature and the dentition. In the short term, the musculature reacts to changes in anatomic form, while in the long term the musculature becomes the determinant of facial form.[113]

An occlusal disharmony produced by an

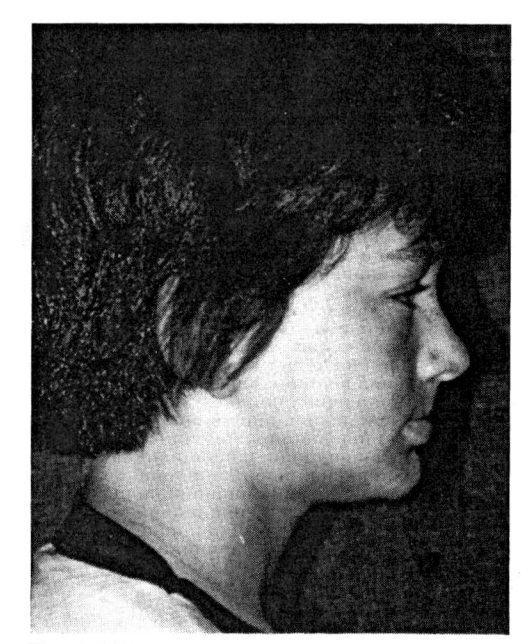

Fig. 2-40b

improper tooth position (e.g., crossbite) or an incorrectly placed dental restoration (high spot on an amalgam) may trigger a deviant muscle feedback mechanism that could lead to an abnormal growth pattern. For proper dentofacial development, treatment may consist of removing occlusal in-

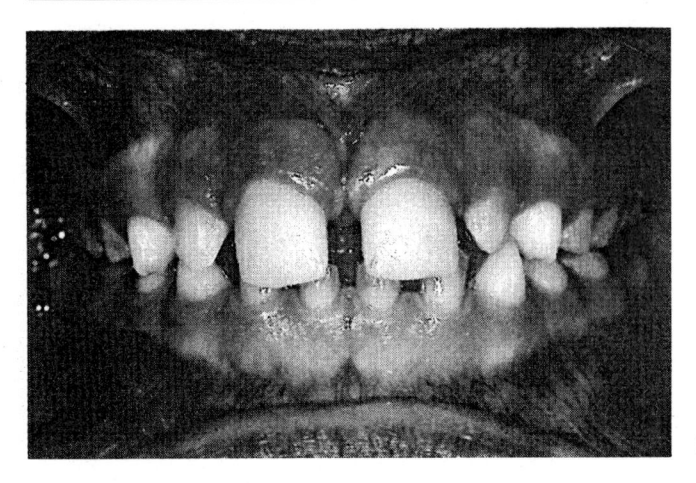

Biological Shaping of the Craniofacial Complex

Fig. 2-40c

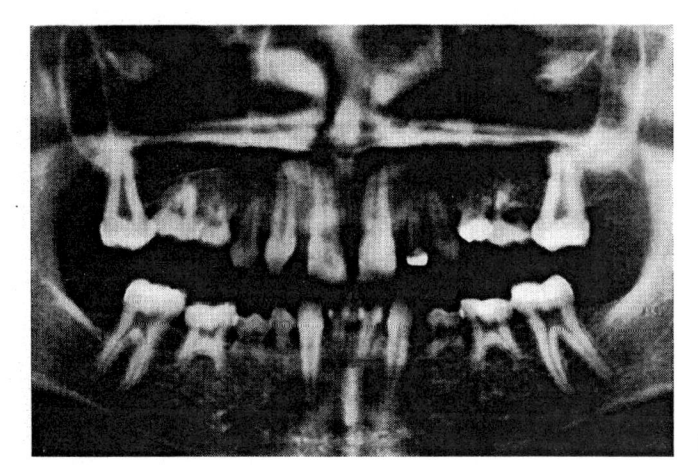

Fig. 2-40d

terferences or adding tooth structure in order to balance the muscle physiologic feedback mechanism and achieve a balanced functional result.

Summary

Influences on the craniofacial structures are so complex that many resulting skeletal types are possible. Because of so many genetic, environmental, and local factors, it is impossible to single out a definitive growth pattern that will apply to each individual. Traditional treatment is generally initiated after most facial growth has been completed. This may prolong treatment of the malocclusion and make definitive treatment more difficult.

This chapter has discussed craniofacial changes from an environmental viewpoint. Dental and skeletal abnormalities should be corrected early. Any deviation from an optimal occlusal state may provoke a change in contractile muscular activity and alter normal growth. Treatment includes breaking any negative occlusal feedback mechanisms and, as early as possible, reestablishing the conditions necessary for normal muscular balance (e.g., correction of crossbite, skeletal retrusion, etc.).

Understanding growth and development may allow future clinicians to diagnose and prevent some forms of malocclusion earlier than was heretofore thought possible.

References

1. Burn, J., Birkbeck, J. A., and Roberts, D. F. Early fetal brain growth. Hum. Biol. 47:511–522, 1975.
2. Holt, A. B., et al. Brain size and the relation of the primate to the nonprimate. In D. B. Cheek (ed.) Fetal and Postnatal Cellular Growth. New York: John Wiley & Sons, 1975.
3. Lemire, R. J., et al. Normal and Abnormal Development of the Human Nervous System. Hagerstown, Md.: Harper and Row Publishers, 1975.
4. Burdi, A. R. Cephalometric growth analyses of the human upper face region during the last two trimesters of gestation. Am. J. Anat. 125:113–122, 1969.
5. Inoue, N. A study of the developmental changes of dentofacial complex during fetal period by means of roentgenographic cephalometrics. Bull. Tokyo Med. Dent. Univ. 8:205–227, 1961.
6. Levihn, W. C. A cephalometric roentgenographic cross-sectional study of the craniofacial complex in fetuses from 12 weeks to birth. Am. J. Orthod. 53:822–848, 1967.
7. Broadbent, B. H. The face of the normal child. Angle Orthod. 7:183–207, 1937.
8. Brodie, A. G. On the growth pattern of the human head from the third month to eighth year of life. Am. J. Anat. 68:209–262, 1941.
9. Oritz, M. H., and Brodie, A. G. On the growth of the human head from birth to the third month of life. Anat. Rec. 103:311–333, 1949.
10. Humphrey, T. The development of oral and facial motor mechanisms in human fetuses and their relation to craniofacial growth. J. Dent. Res. 50:1428–1461, 1971.
11. Mauser, C., et al. A study of the prenatal growth of the human face and cranium. pp. 243–275. In J. A. McNamara (ed.) Determinants of Mandibular Form and Growth. Monogr. no. 4, Craniofacial Growth Series. Ann Arbor: Center for Human Growth and Development, Univ. of Michigan, 1975.
12. Bimler, H. P. The Bimler appliance. In T. M. Graber and B. Neumann (eds.) Removable Orthodontic Appliances. Philadelphia: W. B. Saunders Co., 1977.
13. Kraus, B. S., Wise, W. J., and Frei, R. H. Heredity and the cranio-facial complex. Am. J. Orthod. 45:172–217, 1959.
14. Sicher, H. Oral Anatomy. St. Louis: The C. V. Mosby Co., 1952.
15. Scott, J. H. Dentofacial Development and Growth. Oxford: Pergamon Press, 1967.
16. Moss, M. L. The regulation of skeletal growth. In R. J. Goss (ed.) Regulation of Organ and Tissue Growth. New York: Academic Press, 1972.
17. van der Klaaw, C. J. Size and position of the functional components of the skull. Arch. Neurol. Zool. 91–176, 1948.
18. Van Limborg, J. A new view on the control of the morphogenesis of the skull. Acta Morphol. Neurol. Scand. 8:143–160, 1970.
19. Petrovic, A. G., Stutzmann, J. J., and Gasson, N. The final length of the mandible: is it genetically predetermined? In D. S. Carlson (ed.) Craniofacial Biology. Monogr. no. 10, Craniofacial Growth Series. Ann Arbor: Center for Human Growth and Development, Univ. of Michigan, 1981.
20. Klatsky, M. Studies in the dietaries of contemporary primitive people. J. Am. Dent. Assoc. 36:385, 1948.
21. Watt, D. G., and Williams, C. H. H. The effects of the physical consistency of food on the growth and development of the mandible and the maxilla of the rat. Am. J. Orthod. 37:895–928, 1951.
22. Hiiemae, K. M. Masticatory function in the mammals. J. Dent. Res. 46:883–939, 1967.
23. Barber, C. G., Green, L. J., and Cox, G. J. The effects of the physical consistency of diet on the condylar growth of the rat mandible. J. Dent. Res. 42:848–851, 1963.
24. Henrikson, P. A., Sagnes, S., and Thilander, H. Bone, teeth and muscular function. Calcif. Tissue Res. (suppl.) 22:466–467, 1977.
25. Beecher, R. M., and Corruccini, R. S. Effects of dietary consistency on craniofacial and occlusal development in the rat. Angle Orthod. 51:61–69, 1981.
26. Beecher, R. M., and Corruccini, R. S. Effects of dietary consistency on maxillary arch breadth in macaques. J. Dent. Res. 60:68, 1981.
27. Graber, T. M., and Neumann, B. (eds.) The Fränkel appliance. pp. 526–566. In Removable Orthodontic Appliances. Philadelphia: W. B. Saunders Co., 1977.
28. Johnson, L. R. Habits and their relation to malocclusion. J. Am. Dent. Assoc. 30:848–852, 1943.
29. Linder-Aronson, S. Adenoids: Their effect on mode of breathing and nasal airflow and their relationship to characteristics of the facial skeleton and the dentition. Acta Otolaryngol. (suppl.) 265:3–132, 1970.
30. Linder-Aronson, S. Effects of adenoidectomy on the dentition and facial skeleton over a period of five years. pp. 85–100. In J. Cook (ed.) Transaction of the Third International Orthodontic Confer-

ence. London: Crosby, Lockwood and Staples, 1975.
31. McNamara, J. A., Jr. Influence of respiratory pattern on craniofacial growth. Angle Orthod. 51:269–300, 1981.
32. Enlow, D. H. Handbook of Facial Growth. Philadelphia: W. B. Saunders Co., 1975, pp. 48–185, 284–288.
33. Wolff, J. Das Gasetz der Transformation der Knocher. Berlin: Hirschwald, 1892.
34. Kawamura, Y. Neurogenesis of mastication. In Frontiers of Oral Physiology. Vol. 1. Basel: S. Karger, 1974, pp. 77–120.
35. Jensen, D. The Principles of Physiology. New York: Appleton-Century-Crofts, 1976, pp. 113–121, 156–175.
36. Ingervall, B., Carlsson, G. E., and Helkimo, M. Change in location of hyoid bone with mandibular positions. Acta Odont. Scand. 28:337–361, 1970.
37. Storey, A. Temporomandibular joint receptors. In D. J. Anderson and B. Matthews (eds.) Mastication. Bristol: John Wright & Sons, Ltd. 7:50–58, 1976.
38. Simões, W. A. Some oral neurophysiological resources applied in the use of functional orthopaedic techniques. J. Jap. Orthod. Soc. 38:40–48, 1979.
39. Freeland, T. D. Muscle function during treatment with the functional regulator. Angle Orthod. 49:247–258, 1979.
40. Moss, J. P. An investigation of the muscle activity of patients with Class II, Division I malocclusion and the changes during treatment. Trans. Eur. Orthod. Soc. 51:87–101, 1975.
41. Jacobs, R. M. Muscle equilibrium: Fact or fancy. Angle Orthod. 39:11–21, 1969.
42. McNamara, J. A., Jr. Neuromuscular and Skeletal Adaptations to Altered Orofacial Function. Monogr. no. 1, Craniofacial Growth Series. Ann Arbor: Center for Human Growth and Development, Univ. of Michigan, 1972.
43. McNamara, J. A., Jr., et al. Musculoskeletal adaptation following orthognathic surgery. pp. 91–132. In D. S. Carlson and J. A. McNamara, Jr. (eds.) Muscle Adaptation in the Craniofacial Region. Monogr. no. 8, Craniofacial Growth Series. Ann Arbor: Center for Human Growth and Development, Univ. of Michigan, 1978.
44. Moss, M. L., and Moss-Salentijn, L. The muscle-bone interface: an analysis of a morphological boundary. pp. 38–70. In D. S. Carlson and J. A. McNamara, Jr. (eds.) Muscle Adaptation in the Craniofacial Region. Monogr. no. 8, Craniofacial Growth Series. Ann Arbor: Center for Human Growth and Development, Univ. of Michigan, 1978.
45. Bassett, C. A. L. Biophysical principles affecting bone structure. pp. 1–76. In G. H. Bourne (ed.) The Biochemistry and Physiology of Bone. Vol. III. Development and Growth. New York: Academic Press, 1971.
46. Reddi, A. H. Cell biology and biochemistry of endochondral bone development. Coll. Res. 1:209–226, 1981.
47. Ham, A. W., and Cormack, D. W. Histology. 8th ed. Philadelphia: Lippincott, 1979, pp. 317–390, 430–434.
48. Little, L. Bone Behavior. London: Academic Press, 1973, pp. 2–21, 81–123, 149, 176.
49. Jansen, M. On Bone Formation: Its Relation to Tension and Pressure. New York: Longmans Green, 1920.
50. Bassett, C. A. L. Biologic significance of piezoelectricity. Calcif. Tissue Res. 1:252, 272, 1968.
51. Pidot, A. L., and Diamond, J. M. Streaming potentials in a biological membrane. Nature 201:701–702, 1964.
52. Saadia, A. M., and White, G. E. Analysis of cephalometrics using symmetric axis geometry: maxilla, mandible and craniofacial interrelationships (Part II). J. Pedod. 6:120–147, 1982.
53. O'Reilly, M. A longitudinal growth study: maxillary length at puberty in females. Angle Orthod. 49:234–238, 1979.
54. Savara, B. S., and Singh, I. J. Norms of size and annual increments of seven anatomical measures of maxillae in boys from three to sixteen years of age. Angle Orthod. 38:104–120, 1968.
55. Björk, A., and Skieller, V. Growth of the maxilla in three dimensions as revealed radiographically by the implant method. Br. J. Orthod. 4:52–64, 1977.
56. Sillman, J. H. Dimensional changes of the dental arches: longitudinal study from birth to twenty-five years. Am. J. Orthod. 50:824–842, 1964.
57. Clinch, L. M. An analysis of serial models between three and eight years of age. Dent. Rec. 71:61–72, 1951.
58. Burdi, A. R. Biological forces which shape the human midface before birth. pp. 9–42. In J. A. McNamara, Jr. (ed.) Factors Affecting the Growth of the Midface. Monogr. no. 6, Craniofacial Growth Series. Ann Arbor: Center for Human Growth and Development, Univ. of Michigan, 1976.
59. Carlson, D. S. A serial cephalometric radiographic study of the anteroposterior relation of the maxilla and mandible in individuals with excellent occlusion of the teeth. Am. J. Orthod. 42:787, 1956.
60. Riolo, M. L., et al. An Atlas of Craniofacial Growth. Monogr. no. 2, Craniofacial Growth Series. Ann Arbor: Center for Human Growth and Development, Univ. of Michigan, 1974, pp. 68–186, 355–373.
61. Krogman, W. M. The problem of timing in facial growth with a special reference to the period of the changing dentition. Am. J. Orthod. 37:253–276, 1951.
62. Gans, C. Some limitations and approaches to problems in functional anatomy. Folia. Biotheo. 41–50, 1966.
63. Smith, J. M., and Savage, R. J. G. The mechanics of mammalian jaws. Sch. Sci. Rev. 40:287–201, 1959.

References

64. Hoshi, H. Comparative morphology of the mammalian mandible in relation to food habit. Okajimas Folia. Anat. Jap. 48:333–345, 1971.
65. Petrovic, A. G., Gasson, N., and Schlienger, A. Dissymétrie mandibulaire consécutive a la perturbation occlusale unilatérale provoquée expérimentalement chez le rat. Conception cybernétique des systémes de contrôle de la croissance des cartilages condylien et angulaire. L'Orthod. Fr. 45:409–417, 1974.
66. Küppers, K. Analyse der funktionellen struktur des menschlichen unterkiefers. Ergeb. Anat. Entwick 44:3–91, 1971.
67. Björk, A. Variations in the growth pattern of the human mandible: longitudinal radiographic study by implant method. J. Dent. Res. 42:400–411, 1963.
68. Saadia, A. M., and White, G. E. Analysis of cephalometrics using symmetric axis geometry: method, mandible and superimposition (Part I). J. Pedod. 6:3–25, 1981.
69. Moss, J. P., and Picton, D. C. A. The problems of dental development among children on a Greek island. Dental Practitioner, Dental Record 18:442–448, 1968.
70. Enlow, D. H. Rotations of the mandible during growth. pp. 65–76. In J. A. McNamara, Jr. (ed.) Determinants of Mandibular Form and Growth. Monogr. no. 4, Craniofacial Growth Series. Ann Arbor: Center for Human Growth and Development, Univ. of Michigan, 1975.
71. Hunter, J. The Natural History of the Human Teeth, Explaining Their Structure, Use, Formation, Growth and Disease. London: J. Johnson, 1771.
72. Sarnat, B. G. Facial and neurocranial growth after removal of the condyle in Macaca Rhesus monkey. Am. J. Surg. 94:19–30, 1957.
73. Katz, M., and Kvinnsland, S. Matrix formation in the mandibular condyle of the rat (^{35}S)-Sulfate incorporation studies. Acta Odont. Scand. 37:137–145, 1979.
74. Rushton, M. A. Growth of the mandibular condyle in relation to some deformities. Br. Dent. J. 76:57–68, 1944.
75. Moss, M. L. Functional cranial analysis and the functional matrix. Int. J. Orthod. 17:21–31, 1979.
76. Moss, M. L. Functional cranial analysis of the mandibular angular cartilage in the rat. Angle Orthod. 39:209–214, 1969.
77. Johnston, L. E., Jr. The functional matrix hypothesis: reflections in a jaundiced eye. pp. 131–168. In J. A. McNamara, Jr. (ed.) Factors Affecting the Midface. Monogr. no. 6, Craniofacial Growth Series. Ann Arbor: Center for Human Growth and Development, Univ. of Michigan, 1976.
78. Bernabei, R. L., and Johnston, L. E., Jr. The growth in situ of isolated mandibular segments. Am. J. Orthod. 73:24–35, 1978.
79. Wright, D. M., and Moffett, B. C., Jr. The postnatal development of the human temporomandibular joint. Am. J. Anat. 141:235–250, 1974.
80. Koski, K. The mandibular complex. Trans. Eur. Orthod. Soc. 50:53–67, 1974.
81. Moss, M. L. Functional anatomy of the temporomandibular joint. pp. 73–88. In L. Schwartz (ed.) Disorders of the Temporomandibular Joint. St. Louis: The C. V. Mosby Co., 1959.
82. Richardson, A. S., and Castaldi, C. R. Dental development during the first two years of life. J. Can. Dent. Assoc. 33:418–23, 1967.
83. van der Linden, F. P. G. M. Theoretical and practical aspects of crowding in the human dentition. J. Am. Dent. Assoc. 89:139–153, 1974.
84. Fisk, R. O. Normal mandibular arch changes between ages 9–16. J. Can. Dent. Assoc. 32:652–658, 1966.
85. Moorrees, C. F. A. The Dentition of Growing Child: A Longitudinal Study of Dental Development Between 3 and 18 Years of Age. Cambridge, Mass.: Harvard University Press, 1966.
86. Murray, J. J. Dynamics of occlusal adjustments; a cephalometric analysis. Alumni Bull., School of Dentistry, Univ. of Michigan 61:32–37, 1959.
87. Nanda, R. S. The rates of growth of several facial components measured from serial cephalometric roentgenograms. Am. J. Orthod. 41:658–673, 1955.
88. Graber, T. M. pp. 510–581. In Falkner (ed.) Craniofacial and Dentitional Development in Human Development. Philadelphia: W. B. Saunders Co., 1966.
89. Wallace, J. M. pp. 187–237. In J. C. Brash, et al. (eds.) The Growth and Control of Direction: Physiological and Pathological in the Aetiology of Irregularity and Malocclusion of the Teeth. London: The Dental Board of the United Kingdom, 1956.
90. Harvold, E. P. Experiments on mandibular morphogenesis. pp. 155–178. In J. A. McNamara, Jr. (ed.) Determinants of Mandibular Form and Growth. Monogr. no. 4, Craniofacial Growth Series. Ann Arbor: Center for Human Growth and Development, Univ. of Michigan, 1975.
91. Harvold, E. P. Primate experiments on oral sensation and morphogenesis. Trans. Eur. Orthod. Soc. 49:431–434, 1973.
92. Graber, T. M., and Neumann, B. (eds.) Functional jaw orthopedics: the changes of a concept. pp. 118–132. In Removable Orthodontic Appliances. Philadelphia: W. B. Saunders Co., 1975.
93. Stutzmann, J. J., and Petrovic, A. G. Experimental analysis of general and local extrinsic mechanisms controlling upper jaw growth. pp. 205–238. In J. A. McNamara, Jr. (ed.) Factors Affecting the Growth of the Midface. Monogr. no. 6, Craniofacial Growth Series. Ann Arbor: Center for Human Growth and Development, Univ. of Michigan, 1976.
94. Gasson, N., Stutzmann, J. J., and Petrovic, A. G. Les mécanismes régulateurs de l'ajustement occlusal, interviennent-ils dans le contrôle de la croissance du cartilage condylien? Expériences d'administration d'hormone somatotrope et de résection du cartilage septal chez le jeune rat.

L'Orthod. Fr. 46:77–101, 1975.
95. Salzmann, J. A., and Seide, L. J. Malocclusion with extreme microglossia. Am. J. Orthod. 48:848–857, 1962.
96. Roth, J. B., Sommer, A., and Strafford, D. Microglossia, micrognatia. Clin. Pediatr. 11:357–359, 1972.
97. Kuroda, T., and Ohyama, K. Hypoglossia: case report and discussion. Am. J. Orthod. 79:86–94, 1981.
98. Stutzmann, J., and Petrovic, A. G. Le muscle ptérygoidien éxterne, un relais de l'action de la langue sur la croissance du condyle mandibulaire. Données éxperimentales. L'Orthod. Fr. 45:385–399, 1974.
99. Yip, A. S., and Cleall, J. F. Cinefluorographic study of velopharyngeal function before and after removal of tonsils and adenoids. Angle Orthod. 41:251–263, 1971.
100. Rubin, R. M. Facial deformity: a preventable disease? Angle Orthod. 49:98–103, 1979.
101. Ward, G. W., Jr. Hypersensitivity lung diseases (extrinsic alveolitis). pp. 86–93. In Mitchell (ed.) Synopsis of Clinical Pulmonary Disease. The C. V. Mosby Co., 1974.
102. Marks, M. B. Allergy in relation to orofacial dental deformities in children. J. Allergy 36:293–302, 1965.
103. Todd, T. W., Cohen, M. D., and Broadbent, B. H. The role of allergy in the etiology of orthodontic deformity. J. Allergy 10:216, 1939.
104. Cooke, R. A. The role of allergy in medico-dental problems. pp. 134–140. In Anderson (ed.) Allergy. Baltimore: Waverly Press, 1940.
105. Brash, J. C. The Aetiology or Irregularity and Malocclusion of the Teeth. London: The Dental Board of the United Kingdom, 1929, pp. 212–222.
106. Huber, R. E., and Reynolds, J. W. A dentofacial study of male students at the University of Michigan in the physical hardening program. Am. J. Orthod. Oral Surg. 32:1–21, 1946.
107. Howard, C. C. Inherent growth and its influence on malocclusion. J. Am. Dent. Assoc. 19:642–650, 1932.
108. Leech, H. L. A clinical analysis of orofacial morphology and behavior of five hundred patients attending an upper respiratory research clinic. Dent. Pract. 9:57–68, 1968.
109. Bushey, R. S. Adenoid obstruction of the nasopharynx. pp. 199–232. In J. A. McNamara, Jr. (ed.) Naso-respiratory Function and Craniofacial Growth. Monogr. no. 9, Craniofacial Growth Series. Ann Arbor: Center for Human Growth and Development, Univ. of Michigan, 1979.
110. MacTavish, W. K., and Matthews, R. L. Airways: the key to early facial growth and malocclusions. 33rd Annual Mtg. American Academy of Pedodontics, San Francisco, 1980. Personal communication.
111. Saadia, A. M. Airway obstruction and facial form: a review. J. Pedod. 5:222–239, 1981.
112. Gurley, W. H., Vig., P. S., and Sheets, M. A technique for the simultaneous measurement of nasal and oral respiration. Am. J. Orthod. 82:33–41, 1982.
113. Proffit, W. R. The facial musculature in its relation to the dental occlusion. pp. 73–89. In D. S. Carlson and J. A. McNamara, Jr. (eds.) Muscle Adaptation in the Craniofacial Region. Monogr. no. 8, Craniofacial Growth Series. Ann Arbor: Center for Human Growth and Development, Univ. of Michigan, 1978.
114. Tatum, B., et al. An occlusal and cephalometric analysis of pediatric patients with ankylosis. J. Dent. Res. 61:341, 1982.

Chapter 3

Craniofacial Response to Maxillofacial Orthopedic Therapy

The reduction of overbite and overjet in Class II malocclusion can occur rapidly. However, how bone growth is stimulated and directed is still controversial. The correction of the malocclusion may be the result of the activation of condylar growth, a retraction of the maxillary arch, tipping or migration of the dentoalveolar process, or any combination of the above.

Maxillofacial orthopedic technique is directed at the cause of the malocclusion. The skeletal malformation is not camouflaged by moving teeth into a position that may be more esthetic but that is improperly functioning. This chapter reviews the response of maxillofacial orthopedic therapy on the craniofacial complex in experimental animals and clinical patients (Fig. 3-1).

Dentoalveolar changes

Some researchers deny that orthopedic appliances have an effect on growth stimulation and instead contend that any resulting changes are of dentoalveolar origin. Harvold and Vargervik,[1] and Bimler[2] showed that no significant growth of the mandible occurred during activator or Bimler appliance therapy. The primary factor in the correction of Class II malocclusion was a reduction of the forward growth of the maxilla. Stöckli and Dietrich[3] stressed that activator treatment lacks the potential to induce tissue response from the condylar cartilage. The primary change noted was a decrease in the Sella-Nasion-Point A measurement. Sella-Nasion-Point B measurement did not increase beyond normal limits. Woodside,[4] using an extremely open construction bite registration, found that vertical opening of the activator restricts the forward development of the midfacial area at subnasale. These results suggest that the activator may act as a form of headgear. The strong retracting force should direct the developing maxilla distally.[1,3-7]

Sergl,[8] and Reey and Eastwood[9] found an increase of the Sella-Nasion-Point B angle in the correction of patients with Class II, Division 1 malocclusion. This was attributed to the combined effect of mandibular relocation and dental compensation (i.e., retraction of the maxillary incisors).

An animal study, using vestibular shields, showed no histological evidence of regional, alveolar, or palatal growth changes between the experimental and control groups. The author suggests that normal skeletal relationships cannot be altered beyond prescribed growth boundaries by means of vestibular shields.[10]

A recent study[11] reported on changes in width resulting from the use of the Fränkel appliance. Sixty treated Class II, Division 1 malocclusions were compared with those in 47 untreated patients. The authors showed

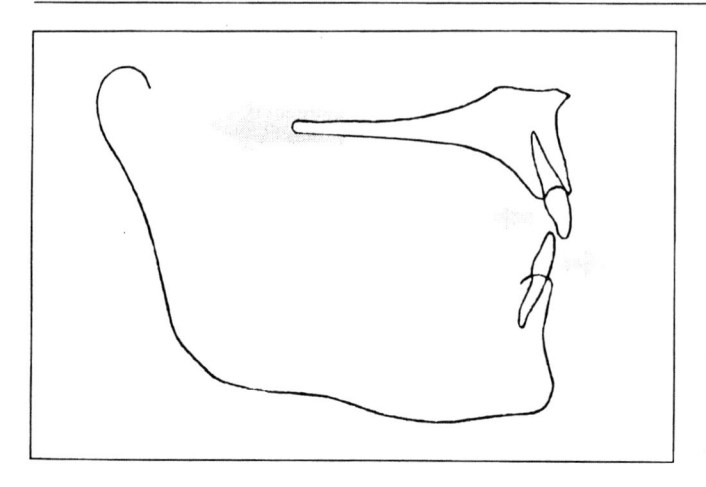

Fig. 3-1 Orthopedic appliance therapy in the correction of Class II malocclusion has been associated with maxillary retraction (large arrow) and/or tipping of the anterior teeth.

that expansion of the maxillary and mandibular arches occurred routinely in patients wearing the appliance. The principle dental improvement was generally noticed in the molar and premolar region.

Janson[12] found that the effects of the bionator on osseous tissue were insignificant. The primary changes were retrusion of the upper incisors and protrusion of the lower incisors. Wieslander and Lagerström[13] reported that the activator was effective on dentoalveolar tissue, with a major favorable change in the position of the upper incisors. The lower incisors were slightly intruded, but there was no significant incisor protrusion. Meikle[14] states that the condyle does not control the growth of the entire mandible, but is an essential element for normal mandibular development (Fig. 3-2).

Condylar changes

Animal studies have shown that mechanical environmental stimuli will produce proliferative activity in condylar cell growth. Elgoyhen et al.[15] and McNamara et al.[16-18] produced mandibular protrusion with cast gold or ticonium inlays cemented on the maxillary and mandibular dentitions. Appliances were made to displace the mandible approximately 4 mm anteriorly and 3 mm inferiorly. Other studies by Charlier et al.[19-21] and Petrovic et al.[22-25] used Sprague-Dawley rats. Removable appliances that rested on the entire maxilla were inserted. These appliances acted as inclined planes. The animal had to propulse the mandible forward in order to accomplish mouth closure. Another method used to produce mandibular hyperpropulsion was to move the mandibular incisors forward of the maxillary incisors by extraoral elastic traction. The appliance produced a distortion in the normal functional pattern. At the end of the experimental period, the investigators found that mechanical stimuli produced proliferative cell activity and condylar growth.

The growth of this mandibular cartilage was more directed than regulated.[26] It has been shown by Charlier et al.[20] that growth hormone stimulates cellular proliferation in both prechondroblastic and chondroblastic layers. The essential mediator in the controlling process of condylar bone is the lateral pterygoid muscle.[16,19-20,22-25,27-29] Petrovic and Stutzmann,[22] and Charlier et al.[20] found that the resection of the lateral pterygoid muscle produced a significant de-

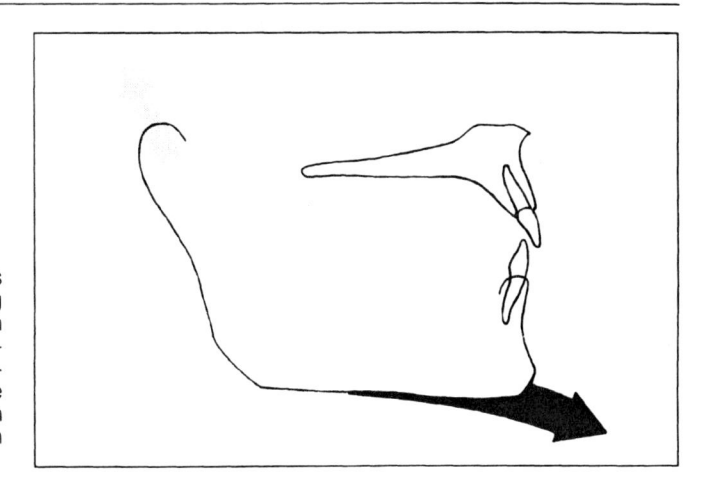

Fig. 3-2 Condylar response as the main factor of correcting mandibular retrusion has been associated with maxillofacial orthopedic therapy. As the mandible is displaced forward by the appliance (black arrow), growth occurs in the opposite direction (shaded arrow).

crease in the multiplication of prechondroblasts in the homolateral chain process that controls the growth of the condylar cartilage in the mandible. The lateral pterygoid muscle is a definite link in the action that regulates the growth of condylar cartilage. During forward positioning of the mandible,[20,30] an increase was noted in the mitotic activity of the prechondroblasts. Petrovic et al.[23] have stated with the findings from rat studies that a postural hyperpropulsion can provoke a decrease in the number of serially arranged sarcomers and an increase in proliferative condylar activity. The opposite changes occurred when the mandible was drawn posteriorly with a chin cup. The addition or removal of the serially arranged sarcomers is the result of physiological fiber changes in a new anatomical length. The adaptive response of the prechondroblastic-chondroblastic layer could be related to the new functional activity of the muscles of mastication. Several investigators[17,21-22] using young rats have stated that the functional protrusion of the mandible led to an extreme thickening of the prechondroblastic-chondroblastic layer and to an increase in bone deposition along the posterior border of the ramus below the condylar cartilage. These adaptive changes are primarily localized in the posterior and superior condylar area and are time-dependent. Adaptive responses were observed at two weeks. Extreme hyperplasia of the growth cartilage layer and hypertrophy of individual chondrocytes were noted during the first six weeks in the posterior region of the mandibular condyle. After this time, a gradual diminution of the response of the normal cartilage was noted until 24 weeks, when the thickness of the prechondroblastic-chondroblastic layer returned.

Stöckli and Willert[31] noted a reaction toward compensation with respect to the altered topographic relationship in the temporal portion of the temporomandibular joint. Koski,[27] in a roentgenographic and histological analysis of the temporomandibular joint after functional therapy, found an increase in the activity of condylar tissue, but transformation of the structural components of the joint in the temporal bone were minimal.

Timing of treatment

McNamara has stressed the importance of the relationship between age and tissue response.[18] He found that marked skeletal

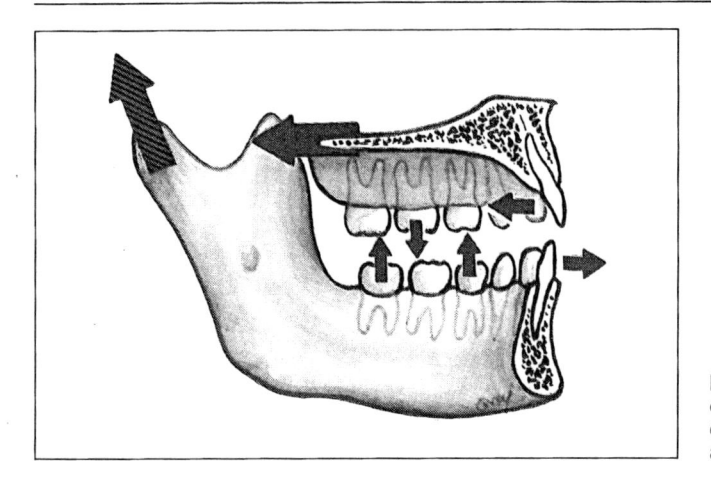

Fig. 3-3 Some responses associated with maxillofacial orthopedic therapy in the correction of anteroposterior discrepancies.

adaptations occurred in young animals, while dentoalveolar adaptation prevailed in adult animals. Carlson et al.[32] found that the prechondroblastic-chondroblastic condylar cartilage increases sharply in size in the neonatal and juvenile age groups and decreases in older age groups. This suggests that in infants or young patients, greater vertical osseous growth should occur. In older patients, the direction of mandibular growth is more horizontal.

Baume[33,34] has shown that the younger the patient, the greater and faster the growth response of the condyles. He also reported that condylar cartilage never loses its growth potential.

Reey and Eastwood,[9] Hausser,[35] Janson,[12] and Stockfisch[36] suggest beginning activator and kinetor treatment during the mixed dentition period, i.e., during premolar exchange. Deffez and Fellus[37] insist that malocclusion should be treated as soon as the primary teeth are present in the arch. Reey and Eastwood[9] suggest that, in order to take advantage of cooperation, fast osseous remodeling, and tissue response, treatment should begin when the patient can tolerate the appliance. Baume et al.[33] reported a case of an infant with Pierre Robin syndrome who was treated successfully with an orthopedic appliance. The treatment result included a growth spurt of the condyle and forward displacement of the fossa. Functional appliances are generally used to correct deficiencies and not excesses (Figs. 3-3 and 3-4) (Chapter 4).

The developing facial structures do not follow an inevitable growth pattern. Growth direction can be changed permanently by the application of forces which induce translation and/or change hard tissue and muscular relationships.[38,39]

Neuromuscular response

Simões[40] has argued that stomatognathic equilibrium should be obtained by "correct neural excitation of the temporomandibular joints, muscles, periodontium, and mucosa." This excitation is "provoked by stimuli given through orthopedic appliances applied within patterns of time, intensity, and quality, using the quickest conduction velocity in each case." Neural excitation is common to maxillofacial orthopedic techniques, and the techniques used to correct skeletal deficiencies are similar except in the quality and intensity of the exteroception and proprioception (Fig. 3-5).

The bionator appliance (a modified Balters appliance) stimulates the periodontium, the tongue, and the frontal palatal

Muscular Changes During Maxillofacial Orthopedic Therapy

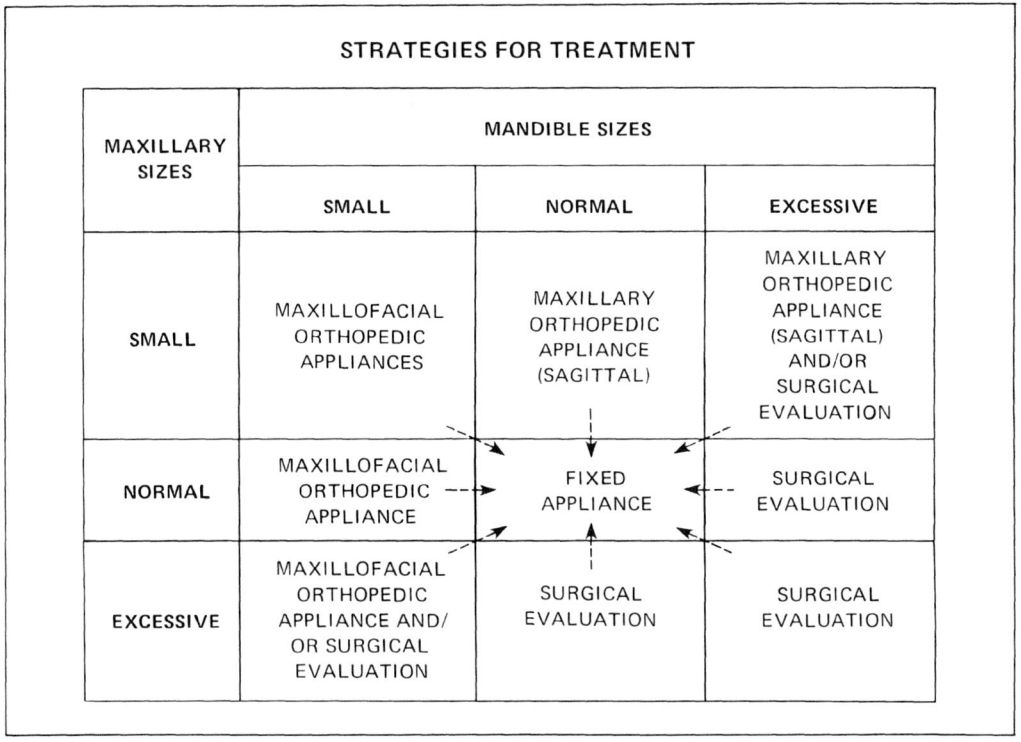

STRATEGIES FOR TREATMENT

MAXILLARY SIZES	MANDIBLE SIZES		
	SMALL	NORMAL	EXCESSIVE
SMALL	MAXILLOFACIAL ORTHOPEDIC APPLIANCES	MAXILLARY ORTHOPEDIC APPLIANCE (SAGITTAL)	MAXILLARY ORTHOPEDIC APPLIANCE (SAGITTAL) AND/OR SURGICAL EVALUATION
NORMAL	MAXILLOFACIAL ORTHOPEDIC APPLIANCE	FIXED APPLIANCE	SURGICAL EVALUATION
EXCESSIVE	MAXILLOFACIAL ORTHOPEDIC APPLIANCE AND/OR SURGICAL EVALUATION	SURGICAL EVALUATION	SURGICAL EVALUATION

Fig. 3-4 Maxillofacial orthopedic appliances are generally used to correct deficiencies; a thorough evaluation is required in order to gain full advantage of therapy. Teeth may have to be leveled, aligned, or rotated with a fixed technique prior to, during, or after treatment.

mucosa, while acting simultaneously on other structures. The Fränkel appliance acts primarily on the tongue, the oral vestibular muscles, and the mucosa, and secondly on the sensorial mechanism of the temporomandibular joint and periodontium. The Bimler appliance affects the temporomandibular joint, periodontium, incisive proprioception, and, to a lesser degree, the muscles of propulsion and the frontal palatal mucosa.

Muscular changes during maxillofacial orthopedic therapy

The bionator is somewhat directed, and the Fränkel regulator almost completely directed toward the nonskeletal tissues. Treatment consists of interrupting the abnormal muscle function and promoting harmonious functional patterns to effect a balance between the phasic and tonic muscles. This is done by means of an activating bite through which the mandible will adapt to a new three-dimensional relationship to the maxilla: horizontal, vertical, and sagittal.

The extent of the translocation depends on the appliance utilized and the severity of

PROPRIOCEPTION		
BIMLER	FRANKEL	BALTERS
TMJ	TMJ	TMJ
PERIODONTIUM	PERIODONTIUM	PERIODONTIUM
TONGUE	TONGUE	TONGUE
INCISIVE	INCISIVE	INCISIVE
MUSCLES LATERAL AND PROTRUSIVE	MUSCLES LATERAL AND PROTRUSIVE	MUSCLES LATERAL AND PROTRUSIVE
MUSCLES ORAL VESTIBULE	MUSCLES ORAL VESTIBULE	MUSCLES ORAL VESTIBULE
EXTEROCEPTION		
MUCOSA ORAL VESTIBULE	MUCOSA ORAL VESTIBULE	MUCOSA ORAL VESTIBULE
MUCOSA FRONTAL PALATE	MUCOSA FRONTAL PALATE	MUCOSA FRONTAL PALATE

Fig. 3-5 Proprioceptive and exteroceptive effects produced by different maxillofacial orthopedic appliances. (Adapted from Simões, W. A. J. Japan Orthod. Soc. 38, 40–48, 1979.)

the problem.[15,41] Herren concluded that the mode of action of the appliance is the same regardless of the degree of vertical mandibular displacement, but it is known that more pronounced displacement will generate forces more constant in direction and of greater intensity.[41] Woodside[4] found that these forces would restrict the forward development of the midfacial area. The more the vertical dimension was opened, the more downward displacement was obtained in the midface and subnasale.

On insertion of the appliance, the mandible is deviated by isotonic muscle contraction as an intermaxillary force begins to build. Isometric tonic contraction succeeds when the mandible is prevented from reaching the rest position. This stretch or myostatic reflex is triggered as a defense mechanism so that the muscles resist any further stretch.[9,41] Findings by McNamara,[16-18] Petrovic and co-workers,[19,20,22-26,30] and others[15,31,42] demonstrate that a new closing pattern will induce musculoskeletal adaptations. The appliance will transform mechanical energy into neural excitation. The impulses generated by the appliance through the muscles, the periodontal membrane, and the temporomandibular joint will be received by the central nervous system and a new response will be transmitted to the receptors, activating skeletal remodeling.

Thus, excitation and information are the basis of growth and development.[9,41,43] The new position of the mandible and the muscular changes adapt the masticatory apparatus to a new maxillomandibular relationship. The teeth are moved by forces generated by the musculature and transmitted via the appliance.

The anatomical change produced by muscular function and structure ensures permanent retention of the improvement achieved in occlusion and craniofacial growth.[44] There is general agreement that posttreatment relapse is minimal,[13,31,45,46] although some researchers have found relapse.[47,48]

There is some debate on the length of retention. Some clinicians will recommend no retention, while others recommend use of the appliance at night as a retainer until the eruption of the second molars. During treatment, however, the patient usually wears the appliance 24 hours a day.[44] Witt[29] found that, during use of the bionator appliance, muscle forces measured during speech were much less than those measured during sleep. Myotonic twitches of the atonic musculature were transmitted to the dentition via the appliance. Forces exerted on the teeth varied with the sleeping posture and the level of sleep.

Those forces that pull the mandible toward the rest position were absorbed by the appliance and transmitted to the teeth and the alveolar processes. In addition, the appliance prevented the mandible from being transferred to an eccentric position.[29,41]

Muscular changes will have a direct influence on the condyle by altering mandibular growth.[13,15,18-20,23,30,31,42] This has also been shown by Freeland,[49] using the functional regulator of Fränkel.

Moss[47] found that Class II, Division 1 patients had a pattern of muscle activity different from that of patients with normal occlusion. Patients with normal occlusion showed a high degree of correlation among the activities of all muscles. The activity of the anterior temporalis muscle and that of the anterior masseter muscle were equal and greatest. The posterior temporalis activity was next largest and the posterior masseter was least. In Class II, Division 1 patients, Moss found that anterior temporalis and masseter activity were slightly greater than in patients with normal occlusion. After the malocclusion had been corrected using orthopedic appliances, these muscle activities were decreased. There was an improvement in the correlation of muscle activity but anterior temporal activity was still not correlated with anterior masseter activity. When the patients were out of retention masseter activity decreased and posterior temporal activity increased slightly. Witt[29] found that the reorganization of the musculature occurred faster and to a much greater extent with the bionator than with the classical activator.

In six- and 12-month studies of Class II patients using the Fränkel appliance, Freeland[49] found a decrease in muscle activity, while Class III patients showed an increase in muscle activity, principally in the lower lip and suprahyoid muscle group. Freeland also found that Class II patients who exhibited the greatest changes in muscular behavior also had the greatest changes in skeletal and dental relationships. But the opposite happened in Class III patients: the greatest dental and skeletal changes brought about the least amount of muscular activity.

Summary

Malocclusion should be corrected early. Even the slightest deviation from an optimal occlusal state is sufficient to provoke a decrease in contractile muscle activity and retard normal growth. Treatment includes breaking the positive occlusal feedback mechanism and reestablishing conditions necessary for normal behavior (e.g., correct occlusal interferences, abnormal tooth position, or skeletal discrepancies). The longer the occlusal discrepancy exists, the longer the negative neuromuscular influence will prevail. This may produce negative craniofacial growth patterns, making later correction more difficult.

The facial skeleton responds dynamically to the application of maxillofacial orthopedic techniques. Appliances act as transducers changing mechanical energy into neural excitation. This neural energy affects the temporomandibular joint, muscles, periodontium, mucosa, and teeth.

General agreement exists regarding the orthopedic result of treatment for skeletal discrepancies to achieve normal occlusion. The orthopedic correction could be from any of the following: condylar growth, maxillary retraction, mesial migration of anterior mandibular teeth, distal migration of the maxillary teeth, tipping of the occlusal plane, or some combination of the above. The appliances discussed in this chapter are generally used to correct deficiencies and not excesses (Chapter 4). Treatment should begin as soon as the patient can tolerate the appliance in order to reestablish conditions necessary for normal tissue remodeling and osseous growth.

Maxillofacial orthopedic treatment success depends on four primary factors: patient cooperation, appliance selection, type of malocclusion, and genetic predisposition for growth.

References

1. Harvold, E. P., and Vargervik, K. Morphogenetic response to activator treatment. Am. J. Orthod. 60:478–490, 1971.
2. Bimler, H. P. Dynamic functional therapy. Trans. Eur. Orthod. Soc. 49:451–456, 1973.
3. Stöckli, R. W., and Dietrich, U. Sensation and morphogenesis, experimental and clinical findings following functional forward displacement of the mandible. Trans. Eur. Orthod. Soc. 49:435–447, 1973.
4. Woodside, D. G. Some effects of activator treatment on the mandible and midface. Trans. Eur. Orthod. Soc. 49:443–447, 1973.
5. Tulley, W. J. Introduction of myofunctional seminar. Trans. Eur. Orthod. Soc. 49:425–426, 1973.
6. Luder, H. U. Effects of activator treatment: evidence for the occurrence of two different types of reaction. Eur. J. Orthod. 3:205–222, 1981.
7. Forsberg, C. M., and Odenric, L. Skeletal and soft tissue response to activator treatment. Eur. J. Orthod. 3:247–253, 1981.
8. Sergl, H. G. The treatment of Class II, Division 1 cases with functional orthopedic appliances. Trans. Eur. Orthod. Soc. 52:119–125, 1976.
9. Reey, R. W., and Eastwood, A. The passive activator: case selection treatment response and corrective mechanics. Am. J. Orthod. 73:378–409, 1978.
10. Popovic, L. Transverse growth changes in rabbit maxilla utilizing vestibular shields. Am. J. Orthod. 80:447, 1981.
11. McDougall, P. D., McNamara, J. A., Jr., and Dierkes, J. M. Arch width development in Class II patients treated with Fränkel appliance. Am. J. Orthod. 82:10–22, 1982.
12. Janson, I. A cephalometric study of the efficiency of the bionator. Trans. Eur. Orthod. Soc. 53:283–295, 1977.
13. Wieslander, L., and Lagerström, L. The effect of activator treatment on Class II malocclusions. Am. J. Orthod. 75:20–26, 1979.
14. Meikle, M. C. The role of the condyle in the postnatal growth of the mandible. Am. J. Orthod. 64:50–62, 1973.
15. Elgoyhen, J. C., Moyers, R. E., McNamara, J. A., Jr., and Riolo, M. L. Craniofacial adaptations to protrusive function in young rhesus monkeys. Am. J. Orthod. 62:469–480, 1972.
16. McNamara, J. A., Jr., and Carlson, D. S. Quantitative analysis of temporomandibular joint adaptations to protrusive function. Am. J. Orthod. 76:593–611, 1979.
17. McNamara, J. A., Jr., Connely, T. G., and McBride, H. C. Histological studies of temporomandibular adaptations. pp. 209–227. In J. A. McNamara, Jr. (ed.) Determinants of Mandibular Form and Growth. Monogr. no. 4, Craniofacial Growth Series. Ann Arbor: Center for Human Growth and Development, Univ. of Michigan, 1975.
18. McNamara, J. A., Jr. Neuromuscular and skeletal adaptations to altered function in the orofacial region. Am. J. Orthod. 64:578–606, 1973.

References

19. Charlier, J. P. Les facteurs mécaniques dans la croissance de l'arc basal mandibulaire a la lumière de l'analyse des caractères structuraux et des propriétés biologiques du cartilage condylien. L'Orthod. Fr. 38:177–186, 1967.
20. Charlier, J. P., Petrovic, A. G., and Herrmann, J. Déterminisme de la croissance mandibulaire: effets de l'hyperpropulsion et de l'hormone somatotrope sur la croissance condylienne de jeunes rats. L'Orthod. Fr. 39:567–579, 1968.
21. Charlier, J. P., Petrovic, A. G., and Stutzmann, J. Effect of mandibular hyperpropulsion on the prechondroblastic zone of young rat condyle. Am. J. Orthod. 55:71–74, 1969.
22. Petrovic, A. G., and Stutzmann, J. Le muscle ptérigoïdien externe et al croissance du condyle mandibulaire. Recherches expérimentales chez le jeune rat. L'Orthod. Fr. 43:271–276, 1972.
23. Petrovic, A. G., Oudet, C., and Gasson, N. Effets des appareils de propulsion et de rétropulsion mandibulaire sur le nombre de sarcomères en série du muscle ptérigoïdien externe et sur la croissance du cartilage condylien du jeune rat. L'Orthod. Fr. 44:191–212, 1973.
24. Petrovic, A. G., Gasson, N., and Schlienger, A. Dissymétrie mandibulaire consécutive á la pérturbation occlusale unilatérale provoquée expérimentalement chez le rat. Conception cybernétique des systémes de contrôle de la croissance des cartilages condylien et angulaire. L'Orthod. Fr. 45:409–417, 1974.
25. Petrovic, A. G., Stutzmann, J., and Oudet, C. Control processes in the postnatal growth of the condylar cartilage of the mandible. pp. 101–153. In J. A. McNamara, Jr. (ed.) Determinants of Mandibular Form and Growth, Monogr. no. 4, Craniofacial Growth Series. Ann Arbor: Center for Human Growth and Development, Univ. of Michigan, 1975.
26. Petrovic, A.G. Control of postnatal growth of secondary cartilages of the mandible by mechanisms regulating occlusion. Cybernetic model. Trans. Eur. Orthod. Soc. 44:69–75, 1974.
27. Koski, K. The mandibular complex. Trans. Eur. Orthod. Soc. 50:53–67, 1974.
28. Wright, D. M., and Moffett, B. C., Jr. The postnatal development of the human temporomandibular joint. Am. J. Anat. 141:235–250, 1974.
29. Witt, E. Muscular physiological investigations into the effects of bi-maxillary appliances. Trans. Eur. Orthod. Soc. 49:448–450, 1973.
30. Charlier, J. P., Petrovic, A. G., and Linck, G. La frondre mentonnière et son action sur la croissance mandibulaire. Recherches expérimentales chez le rat. L'Orthod. Fr. 40:99–113, 1969.
31. Stöckli, P. W., and Willert, H. G. Tissue response in the temporomandibular joint resulting from an anterior displacement of the mandible. Am. J. Orthod. 60:142–155, 1971.
32. Carlson, D. S., McNamara, J. A., Jr., and Jaul, D. H. The histological analysis of the growth of the mandibular condyle in the rhesus monkeys. Am. J. Anat. 151:103–118, 1978.
33. Baume, L. J., Häupl, K., and Stellmach, R. Growth and transformation of the temporomandibular joint in an orthopedically treated case of Pierre Robin Syndrome. Am. J. Orthod. 45:901–916, 1959.
34. Baume, L. J. Principles of cephalofacial development revealed by experimental biology. Am. J. Orthod. 47:881–900, 1961.
35. Hausser, E. Functional orthodontic treatment with the activator. Trans. Eur. Orthod. Soc. 49:427–430, 1973.
36. Stockfisch, H. The kinetor. Trans. Eur. Orthod. Soc. 49:457–460, 1973.
37. Deffez, J. P., and Fellus, P. Modification précoce de la posture mandibulaire, son retentissement sur la croissance, son utilization thérapeutique. Am. J. Orthod. 75:218, 1979.
38. Storey, E. Tissue response to the movement of bones. Am. J. Orthod. 64:71–74, 1973.
39. Harris, J. E. A cephalometric analysis of mandibular growth rate. Am. J. Orthod. 48:161–174, 1962.
40. Simões, W. A. Some oral neurophysiological resources applied in the use of functional orthopaedic techniques. J. Japan Orthod. Soc. 38:40–48, 1979.
41. Graber, T. M., and Neumann, B. (eds.) Functional jaw orthopedics: the changes of a concept. pp. 118–132. In Removable Orthodontic Appliances. Philadelphia: W. B. Saunders Co., 1975.
42. Graber, T. M. The alterability of mandibular growth. pp. 229–241. In J. A. McNamara, Jr. (ed.) Determinants of Mandibular Form and Growth. Monogr. no. 4, Craniofacial Growth Series. Ann Arbor: Center for Human Growth and Development, Univ. of Michigan, 1975.
43. Simões, W. A. Reports on functional orthopedic techniques. J. Pedod. 4:32–62, 1979.
44. Ahlgren, J. Early and late electromyographic response to treatment with activators. Am. J. Orthod. 74:88–93, 1978.
45. Ahlgren, J. A longitudinal clinical and cephalometric study of 50 malocclusion cases treated with activator appliances. Trans. Eur. Orthod. Soc. 48:285–293, 1972.
46. Dougherty, H. Failures in orthodontics. Trans. Eur. Orthod. Soc. 49:231–240, 1973.
47. Moss, J. P. An investigation of the muscle activity of patients with Class II, Division 1 malocclusion and the changes during treatment. Trans. Eur. Orthod. Soc. 51:87–101, 1975.
48. Pancherz, H. Relapse after activator treatment. A biometric, cephalometric and electromyographic study of subjects with and without relapse of overjet. Am. J. Orthod. 72:499–512, 1977.
49. Freeland, T. D. Muscle function during treatment with functional regulator. Angle Orthod. 49:247–258, 1979.

Part 2

Evaluation

Chapter 4

Examination and Diagnosis for Malocclusion

Initial personal contact

As the patient enters the examination room, the gait and standing posture are observed. Is the posture erect, or is the head tilted slightly to one side? Does the body frontal or posterior view demonstrate any scoliosis? Does the body profile view demonstrate any increased spinal curvature (kyphosis)? The size and height of the eyes, eyebrows, shoulders, and hips are evaluated. A tilt to one side could indicate a leg length discrepancy, abnormal spinal curvature, temporomandibular joint disorder, or a combination of these signs. Is there any limp or sense of hesitation? Tactile sensation can divulge further information: shake hands with new patients. This initial inspection may take only 30 seconds to a minute. However, it is time well spent if some important conclusions can be made concerning the patient's overall attitude to treatment. Treatment with removable orthopedic appliances requires good patient cooperation and dedication to participate in the treatment program.

Patient feedback

Patients should be encouraged to tell something about themselves. Part of being an effective clinician is being an effective listener. The patient's sense of self-worth can be determined while listening to the chief complaint. Consider the following questions:

1. How does the patient feel about the malocclusion?
2. Is the voice quiet, flat, or monotone; or is there a feeling of animation or nervousness?
3. Does the patient show a real self-interest in correcting the malocclusion, or is the parent the one primarily interested in treatment?
4. Is there any peer pressure?
5. Have friends had experience with orthopedic appliances?

Perception and evaluation of patient confidence are essential. Some appliances can bring ridicule from less-than-well-intentioned classmates.

If a child enters the examination room with reluctance, speaks only when spoken to, and stares at the floor, then one should proceed with caution and perhaps postpone treatment until the individual matures.

When there are doubts about the probable success of treatment, it is wise to assess the motivation of the patient. Highly goal-oriented patients are more likely to cooperate with treatment than patients with limited expectations.[1] Motivation and cooperation may be difficult to assess unless the patient has been treated over a period of time. Clinical judgment based on experience will help assess the desire for treatment for new patients. It is impossible to eliminate all high-risk patients from clinical practice, but a negative attitude about treatment would suggest considering an alternate treatment plan. In a postretention analysis of treatment problems and failures, Berg found that patient cooperation was the primary obstacle to successful treatment.[2]

History

Before a detailed oral examination, previous parental experience with malocclusion should be determined.

The following questions should be asked:

1. Have any siblings had treatment for malocclusion?
2. Has this child had any other consultations for treatment of malocclusion?
3. Have you had any experience with malocclusion treatment for yourself?

The answers to the above can give a starting point and perspective for beginning a discussion of maxillofacial orthopedic treatment.

If the parent or any siblings have been treated for malocclusion, ask the following questions:

1. Was any part of the treatment difficult or unpleasant?
2. Was there any pain during treatment?
3. Were there headaches, jaw clicking, or other temporomandibular joint symptoms?
4. Were there any problems with gingival disease, caries, or decalcification?
5. Was there any relapse?

If the parent or sibling has had a generally positive treatment experience, introducing orthopedic techniques will be easier.

The historical survey includes a discussion of past and present oral habits. A thumb- or finger-sucking habit can change the facial skeleton. Melsen et al.,[3] Larsson,[4-6] and Subtelny and Subtelny[7] have found sucking habits to have significant influence in the etiology of malocclusion. Even sucking habits of short duration or pacifier use were found to advance the development of malocclusion symptoms. The intensity and length of time of the habit will determine the severity of posterior crossbite, deep palatal vault, retruded and crowded lower incisors, or flaired maxillary anterior teeth. Compulsive blanket sucking and pencil chewing can also adversely affect the facial skeleton (Figs. 4-1 to 4-3).

Continuous playing of certain musical wind instruments will interfere with normal growth of facial hard tissue structure and may cause significant anterior tooth movement.[8-11] Some wind instruments may aid in the correction of malocclusion (e.g., trumpets and horns help to reduce overjet).[12]

Functional orthopedic appliances automatically discourage most digit habits and help correct abnormal osseous growth (overjet) resulting from playing single-reed musical instruments such as the clarinet or saxophone.

A review of the medical history from the parental consent form may reveal systemic disease that might compromise treatment. For example, oral tissues do not tolerate appliance intrusion well if the patient has uncontrolled diabetes.

Soft tissue and temporomandibular joint evaluation

An evaluation of the soft tissue musculature

Soft Tissue and Temporomandibular Joint Evaluation

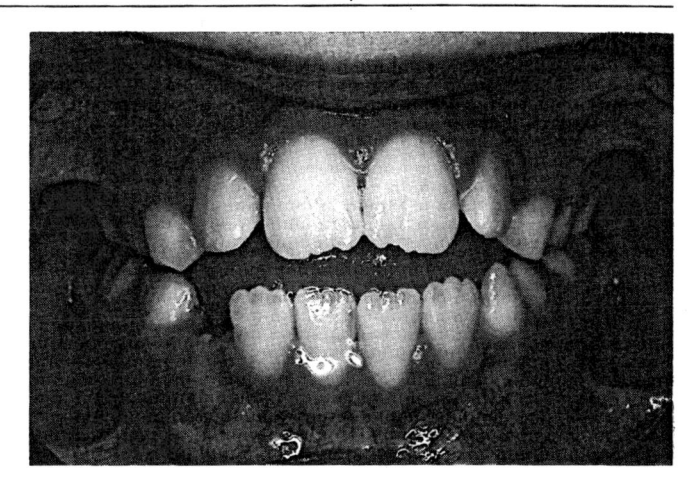

Fig. 4-1 This patient had a blanket-sucking habit until age 7 years. The bite was opened 4 mm.

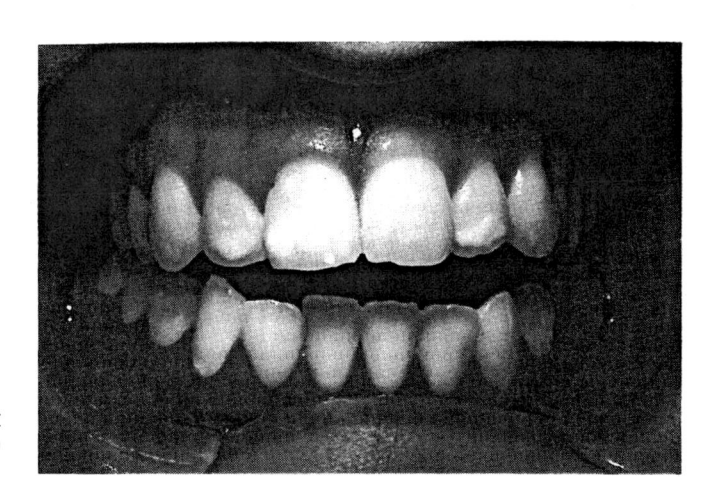

Fig. 4-2 The orthopedic result of a prolonged digit-sucking habit in an adolescent.

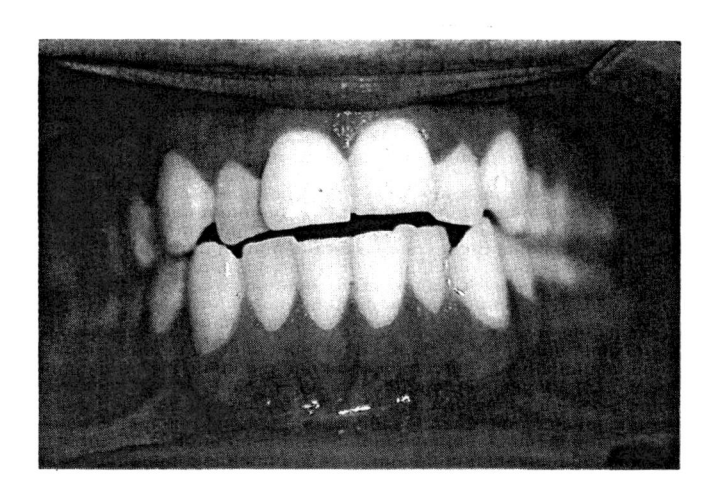

Fig. 4-3 Open bite resulting from an early thumb-sucking habit.

Examination and Diagnosis for Malocclusion

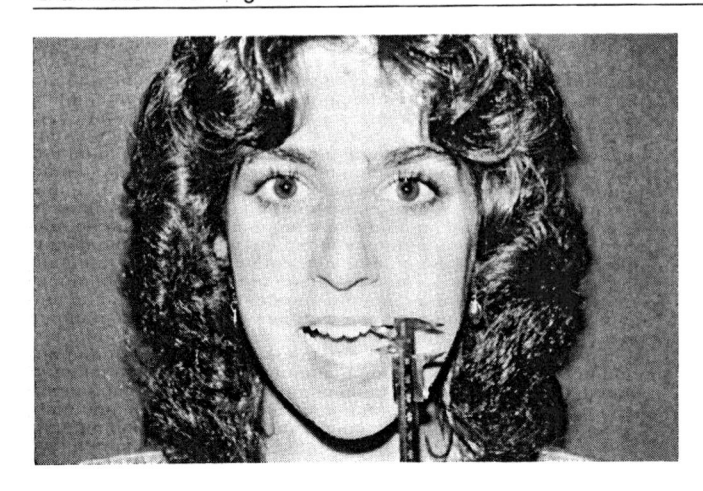

Fig. 4-4 Painful limited mouth opening may indicate anterior disc displacement. This is as wide as this patient can open.

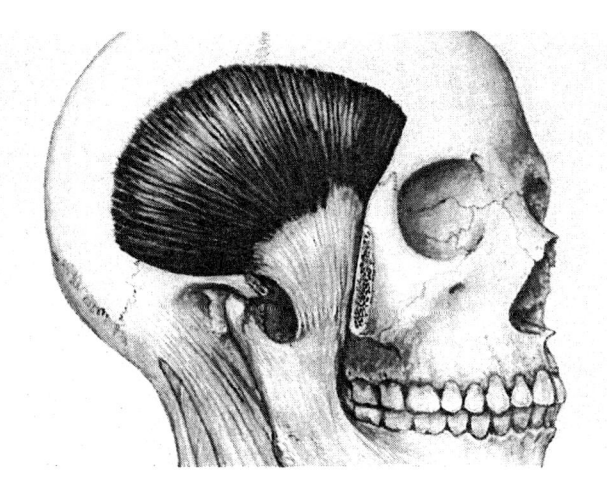

Fig. 4-5 The anatomical location of the origin and insertion of the temporalis muscle.

and temporomandibular joint is initiated by asking the patient to open the mouth as wide as possible and noting deviations from the smooth opening pathway. An S-curve of the midline opening path or a "ragged" opening can mean condylar abnormality. Measurement of the interincisal maximum opening (Fig. 4-4) is accomplished with a Boley gauge. The maximum adult opening should be at least 35 mm; less may indicate a closed lock condition with anterior disc displacement (see Chapter 10). Midline discrepancies are noted from an imaginary vertical line centered between the eyes, through the tip of the nose, to the midlines of the central incisors, and symphysis of the chin. A mandibular, deviation from the midline could mean pathology in the dental or condylar component. Unilateral loss of dental tissue or a hyperocclusion from a dental restoration may lead to symptoms of craniomandibular joint disorder.

It is of utmost importance that a *past history* of craniomandibular joint symptoms be noted in the dental record. For patients undergoing treatment for malocclusion, these records are critical. It would be ethically incorrect and legally unwise to institute treatment without a thorough history of pre-

Examination of the Occlusion

vious craniomandibular joint symptoms.[13] The patient is questioned as follows:

1. Have you ever had any clicking, popping, or cracking of the joint in front of your ears? The patient is instructed to open and close the mouth while the clinician palpates the temporomandibular joint.
2. Have you ever had head, neck, or back pain?
3. Do you ever get a feeling of "stuffiness" or "ringing" in your ears?

Answers to these questions contribute to a complete evaluation of the craniomandibular articulation.

Clicking or popping in the joint is caused by the interaction of the head of the condyle, the disc, and the articular eminence of the zygomatic portion of the temporal bone. Treatment of capsular dysfunction with orthopedic appliances is discussed in Chapter 10.

Head, neck, and back pain are frequent symptoms of craniomandibular joint disorder. The anterior fibers of the temporalis muscle arise from the anterior temporal fossa. This anatomical position can cause muscular pain to imitate eye ache. Many patients with craniomandibular disorders have consultations with optometrists or ophthalmologists (Fig. 4-5).

Muscular evaluation

Muscular evaluation includes firm palpation of the anterior, medial, and posterior segments of the temporalis muscle. The following muscles are also palpated for tenderness or spasm: masseter, pterygoid, mylohyoid, digastric, sternocleidomastoid, posterior vertebral, trapezoid, pectoralis, deltoid, and levator scapulae. Additional muscular evaluation is discussed in Chapter 10.

Condylar location

The spatial relationship and location of the condyle in the glenoid fossa should be determined, particularly if there are signs of temporomandibular joint pathology. To help determine condylar location, the clinician can palpate the distal part of the condylar head from the external auditory meatus (Fig. 4-6). This procedure is best accomplished with the clinician standing in front of the patient. The fifth digits are placed in the external auditory meatus. As pressure is applied forward toward the condyle, the patient is instructed to open wide and close tightly. Increased pressure on one finger, or an elicitation of pain from either or both condyles, will aid the diagnostician in localizing condylar position. This position can be further documented, if necessary, via transcranial radiographs (Fig. 4-7). Signs found through examination and symptoms of craniomandibular joint disorders are evaluated in Chapter 10.

Head posture is important for good occlusion. Head and pelvic tilt may yield further information about malocclusion. Note the orbicularis oris muscle and lip seal. Lip competence and seal are criteria for judging necessity of treatment. Poor lip seal and hypotonic lip musculature can result from loss of vertical dimension, excessive overjet, or a lack of midface or mandibular development.

Considerable data have been assembled at this point in the examination: a visual inspection, patient perception of the problem, patient and family history, and muscular and condylar evaluation.

Examination of the occlusion

The molar and canine relationships are noted, along with any abnormalities of overjet, overbite, and anterior or posterior crossbite. If posterior crossbite exists, a note is

Examination and Diagnosis for Malocclusion

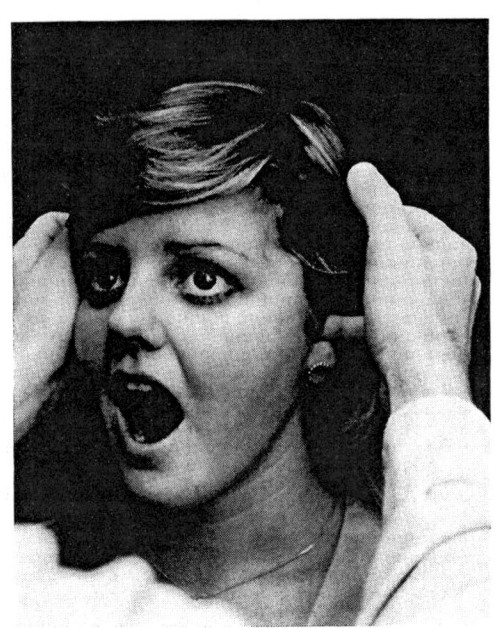

Fig. 4-6 Pain on palpation of the distal aspect of the condylar head through the external auditory meatus may indicate a distally displaced mandibular condyle with joint disorder.

recorded indicating unilateral or bilateral crossbite. Anterior or posterior dental crowding or spacing is also determined. Deviation or shift of the midline on opening or closing is noted. Lateral mandibular excursions should have a smooth-flowing movement.

Examination of the intraoral soft tissues

Color and texture variations of the intraoral soft tissues are documented with color photography. Lip form and fullness are examined. The intraoral soft tissues are visually inspected and palpated for oral lesions. Variations in tonsillar and adenoidal tissue and in tongue size are noted. Check for ankyloglossia. If the lingual frenum is thick and short, the tongue mobility can be compromised. Restricted tongue mobility may interfere with patient adaptation to an orthopedic appliance.

Assessment of oral hygiene and examination of the dentition

The patient's oral hygiene is also evaluated. Only under unusual circumstances (e.g., painful temporomandibular joint dysfunction) should any orthopedic therapy begin before scrupulous oral hygiene techniques are observed. Gingival tissues that hemorrhage on gentle probing will not satisfy even the most basic criteria for appliance insertion. An oral environment showing calculus or plaque accumulations will not be improved by the insertion of fixed *or* removable appliances. Attention to oral hygiene with a mouth free from plaque should be assured before treatment is instituted.

The teeth are evaluated for caries and the need for occlusal sealants. Missing teeth, ankylosed teeth, abnormalities in eruption time or sequence, rotated teeth, and areas of unusual occlusal wear are charted. Variations from the normal in tooth size and shape are noted. Flattened cusps may indicate bruxism. A narrowed or "peg" lateral, a supernumerary incisor, or a site of previous infection (Turner's tooth) may influence the final treatment plan.

Preliminary diagnosis

During record gathering, a list of possible diagnoses—the differential diagnosis—is compiled. A final diagnosis will be made after necessary radiographs, dental study models, and photographic records have been taken. Consultation with the patient and parent is necessary to discuss the pre-

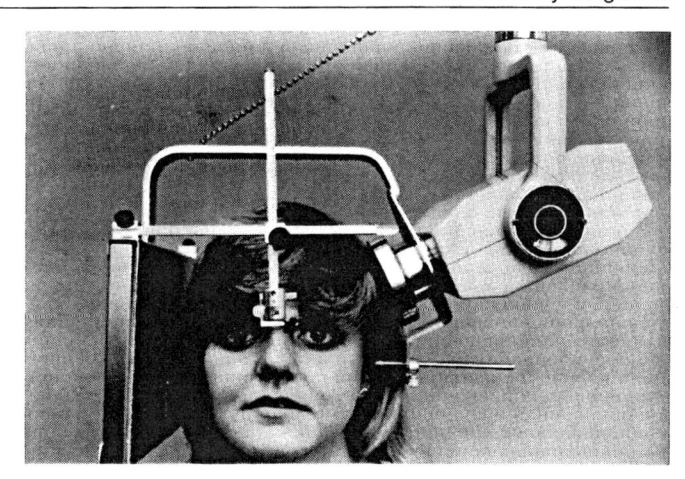

Fig. 4-7 The transcranial radiograph is useful for viewing the lateral aspect of the hard tissue components of the temporomandibular joint.

liminary findings of the visual, auditory, muscular, and oral examinations. A coordination of the patient and family history with the current condition of the patient would include a discussion of how some abnormalities could be inherited and how others might result from oral habits or trauma. A tentative diagnosis and prognosis can now be provided.

Assuming that the parental response to a tentative diagnosis and prognosis is positive, it is still important to determine if the patient is positively motivated. The prognosis should be kept realistic and based on a completion of orthopedic records and full cooperation of the patient and parent throughout the course of treatment.

If either parental or patient response is negative, then treatment should be delayed or a second opinion suggested. The patient and parent should be informed of the best dental age for treatment and the individual is placed on a recall schedule. When the parents want to delay treatment in the presence of severe mandibular retrusion, maxillary protrusion or other occlusal disharmony, a note of this desire to wait is made in the dental record. In addition, a statement of the correct dental age to begin treatment and a clarification of the professional opinion should follow: "Mrs. Smith, waiting a few months will probably not hinder treatment for your son/daughter; however, please be careful that the protruding incisors do not become fractured." This statement emphasizes a multifaceted concern for total health.

If the clinician wants the patient/parent to have another consultation, the suggestion for a second opinion should be made in a friendly, positive manner: "Mrs. Smith, we realize that Susan is very precious to you. We want the treatment that is best for Susan. You are not going to hurt our feelings if you would like to get a second opinion. We encourage it. Our treatment involves a financial commitment on your part and a considerable time involvement from both of us. It would be best for you to feel comfortable with our opinion."

Educational aids can help a parent or patient see the results of treatment. Photographs, color transparencies, and study models of completed cases are excellent for showing what can be accomplished with maxillofacial orthopedic techniques. Take-home pamphlets can be educational and motivational for new patients.

A proposed fee range based on the tentative diagnosis should be given to the parent or patient before extensive record gathering is accomplished. A definitive fee and an approximate time commitment is given after the final diagnosis. Once the clinician has a pledge of cooperation from the patient and parent, a radiographic examination can begin.

Radiographic examination

Current radiobiological concern for radiation dosage requires a brief discussion of the value of a radiographic examination.

Four points should be made to the parent:

1. Radiographs aid in arriving at a correct diagnosis.
2. The radiographs can disclose undiagnosed pathology.
3. Radiographs monitor treatment progress.
4. Radiographs will be limited to necessary documentation.

If the parent and patient are going to be 100% cooperative, they need a full understanding of the care that will be undertaken to minimize radiation dosage. A discussion of minimal dosage and proper lead apron shielding for the neck and body may be helpful. Parents' reactions to the clinician's suggestion of radiographic examination can be generalized as follows:

1. Parents who do not want any radiographs. Have this fact initialed in the dental record after an explanation that only limited treatment may be possible without radiographs.
2. Parents who want only the minimal or absolutely necessary radiographs.
3. Parents who say, "Take whatever films you want," and show lack of concern about radiographic procedures. This type of parental attitude may be cause for concern. Chapter 6 contains a discussion of parental remarks and patient behavior that can compromise even the most carefully thought-out treatment plan.

Which radiographic survey is best for the individual? There are many criteria: age, treatment timing, and patient/parent acceptance. Each patient requires a careful examination to arrive at a correct diagnosis. Full documentation is needed for ethical and legal purposes. *The determining criterion is: what films are necessary for the overall health of the patient?*

Health professionals and the public are becoming increasingly concerned about the potential hazards of low-level ionizing radiation. There is evidence that even small doses of radiation involve some risk to the patient. Children and young adults—the group treated most frequently for malocclusion—are the most susceptible to radiation-induced carcinogenesis.[14] Fabrikant[15] has indicated that solid cancers of the breast (female) and of the thyroid gland (young children and females) are the most important late somatic effects of low-dose ionizing radiation. Although the risk is small, the diagnostic regime should include every available method to reduce exposure to radiation. The most effective method is to limit the number of dental films to those that have a direct benefit to the dental health of the patient. *Concern for malpractice litigation or complete record documentation for case history presentation to specialty board reviewers is not justification for radiation overexposure of the individual.*[16] Other unacceptable reasons for exposing a patient to dental radiation have been summarized by Taylor:[17]

1. to impress patients
2. as a source of extra income
3. as proof of dental treatment for insurance carriers

Valachovic and Lurie[14] and others[18-22] have several recommendations that can

Radiographic Examination

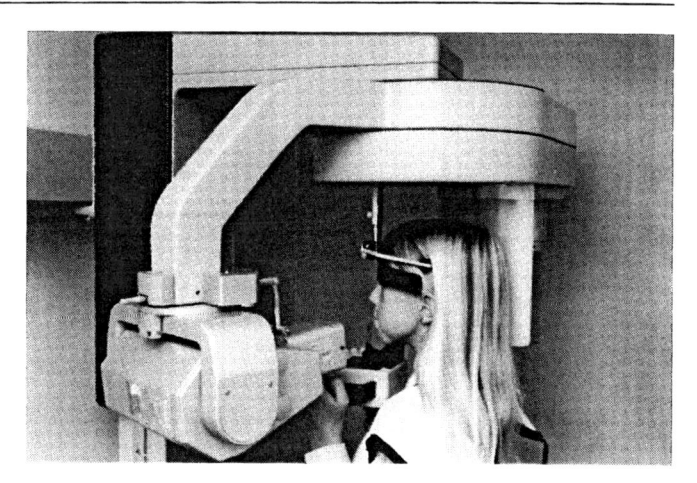

Fig. 4-8 Panoramic radiography is useful for diagnosing gross pathology of the maxilla and mandible, and for determining relative tooth development and position.

significantly reduce risk to the patient from diagnostic radiation without compromising diagnostic benefit:

1. routine use of protective shielding (e.g., lead apron and neck collar)
2. use of film-size beam guiding collimation devices
3. use of 16-inch long cone with high-KVP and short-exposure-time equipment
4. use of high-speed film
5. use of modern equipment that has undergone recent or routine monitoring and inspection

If the patient has a low caries incidence and no clinical dental abnormalities, periapical films may be postponed. Transillumination with a fiber optics system can aid in diagnosing interproximal caries. Developing premolars are often visible with large bitewing radiographs in children.

Panoramic radiography

A well-developed, centrally positioned panoramic radiograph for diagnosis and treatment of malocclusion is worth the initial expense for the equipment or the inconvenience of an outside referral. The radiograph is quick and comfortable for the patient and easy for the assistant to take (Fig. 4-8). It exposes the patient to less total body radiation than a full-mouth intraoral series of 14 separate films. This film gives a clear view of the specific anatomical region of the maxillofacial structures to be treated. The maxillary and mandibular dentitions are easily viewed for abnormal eruption sequence, crowding, congenitally missing teeth, malpositioned unerupted teeth (e.g., maxillary permanent canines), and third-molar position and development. Gross pathology of the maxilla and mandible (e.g., neoplasms, odontogenic tumors, cysts, and traumatic injuries) can be identified. The condyle and temporomandibular joint are visible. (Temporomandibular joint symptoms coincident with a diagnosed malocclusion may require further radiographic investigation. Radiographic diagnosis of TMJ pathology is discussed in Chapter 10.)

The panoramic radiograph may also aid the patient and parent in a visual understanding of the cause of the malocclusion during presentation of the treatment plan. Lead collar shielding will help protect the thyroid gland.

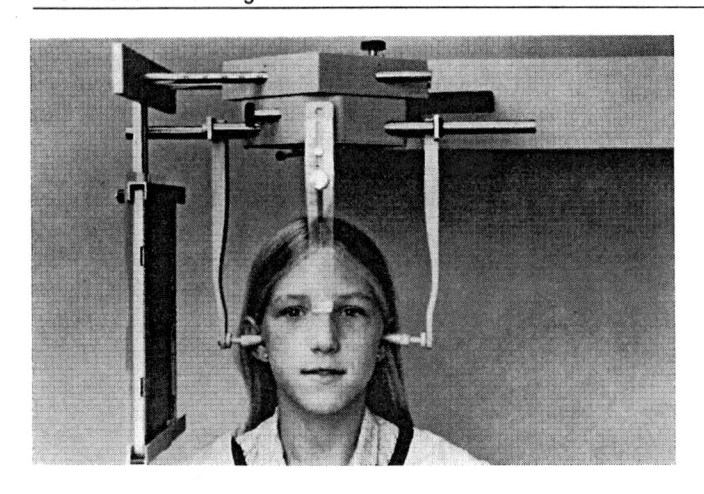

Fig. 4-9 A standard head fixation device allows for three-point stabilization. A reproducible head position during treatment will demonstrate the direction of facial growth.

Cephalometric radiography

A comprehensive knowledge of cephalometric radiography is necessary for a basic understanding of craniofacial growth and development. The mechanics of a cephalometric radiographic headholder are standardized and pictured in Fig. 4-9. This standardization is done for two reasons:

1. A set 60-inch distance between beam source and film allows for a standard, repeatable degree of magnification from the diverging central ray.
2. A set film- and head-tracing size and method of head fixation allow for standard reproducible serial films for growth and treatment documentation.

The value and hazards of cephalometric radiography for children and adolescents have been discussed in the literature.[16,23-31] Radiobiological awareness has helped health professionals develop a concept of risk versus benefit, as discussed earlier. Concern for thyroid protection from radiation has led to the usage of a lead-impregnated shielding collar.[32] The most effective method of reducing cephalometric radiation is to reduce the number of cephalometric radiographs whenever possible. Silling et al.[33] have shown that the more experienced the clinician, the less reliance is placed on the cephalometric radiograph. In one study the majority of board-certified diplomats of the American Board of Orthodontics, and those board-eligible "felt that they could arrive at a satisfactory treatment plan in all cases [presented] whether or not they had a cephalogram." Tenti[34] suggests that a distinction be made between the clinical and research use of cephalometrics. The contention is that an excess of lines and angles may be a handicap—not an advantage—in treatment planning. On the other hand, Fields et al.[35] have attempted to show the importance of cephalometric analysis by demonstrating that a soft tissue analysis is unreliable. Since lip and head posture, all facial features, and dental occlusion are correlated to arrive at a diagnosis, it is not essential to rely on any one diagnostic aid. However, a cephalometric analysis may improve the accuracy of the diagnosis and helps to ensure a complete plan of treatment.

Diagnostic errors are possible because of the variation in cephalometric reference lines. Intracranial reference lines help to reduce errors in positioning the head in the cephalostat. Foster et al.[36] have shown considerable variation in intracranial refer-

Standard Cephalometric Landmarks

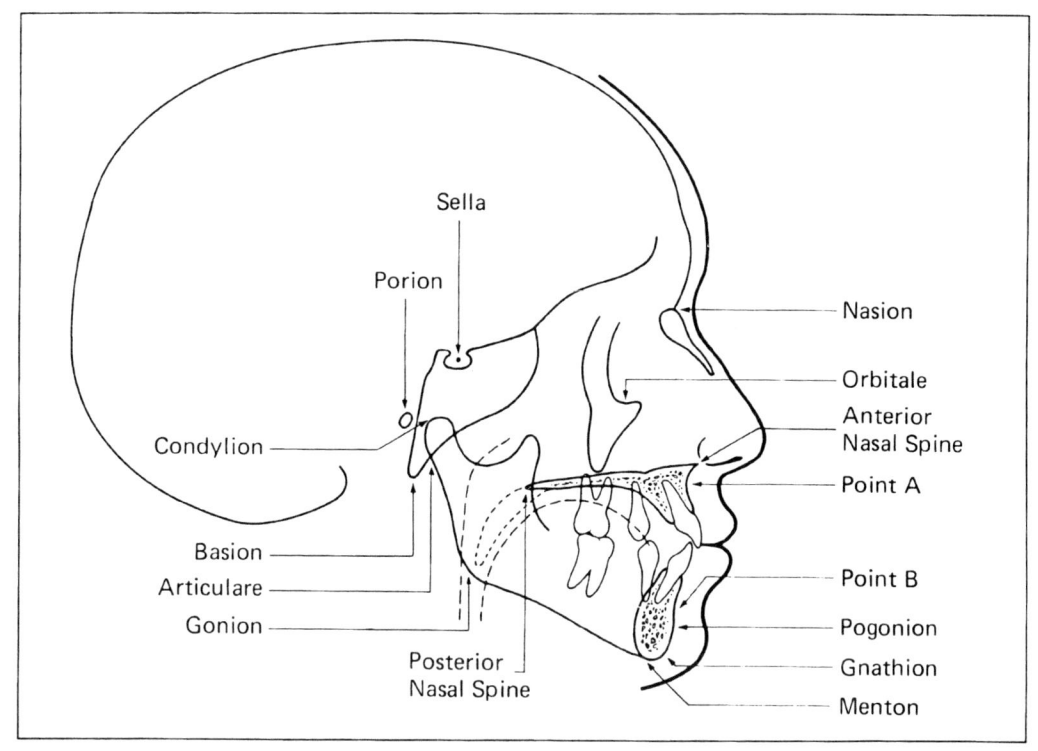

Fig. 4-10 Basic cephalometric landmarks. Sixteen of the most frequently used cephalometric landmarks are labeled and defined in this chapter. (Courtesy of H. Loevy.[41])

ence lines, both to each other and to a true horizontal. This study contends that the variation is so great that "strict adherence" to precise reference lines in cephalometric evaluation is to be questioned. Moorrees et al.[37] state that intracranial reference lines lack stability because of biological variation:

> Clinical judgment may be a better guide than reliance on cephalometric analyses, unless compensation is made for variation in the inclination of the intracranial reference line.

Although cephalometric norms can aid in making a differential diagnosis, treatment planning should not be dictated by cephalometric interpretation alone.

Moyers and Bookstein[38] contend that conventional cephalometrics misrepresents growth. Instead of portraying a generalized enlargement in many directions, cephalometric technique delineates growth as a vector displacement.

A rational view is presented by Watson:[39]

> Cephalometrics is a tool for a frame of reference for increased understanding of growth, treatment responses, and therefore planning of treatment.

Standard cephalometric landmarks

Figure 4-10 shows the standard cephalometric landmarks on a lateral skull tracing. The landmark abbreviations are identified as follows:

Examination and Diagnosis for Malocclusion

Ba	**Basion:** The midline point of the inferior border of the anterior portion of the foramen magnum.		sects the posterior angle of the mandible.
P	**Porion:** "Machine porion" is the uppermost point in the center of the metal ear rod of the cephalostat. The anatomical porion represents the most superior point of the skeletal external auditory meatus.	Po	**Pogonion:** The most anterior point of the mandibular symphysis.
		Gn	**Gnathion:** The point that bisects the anterior angle of the mandible. The anatomical midpoint between pogonion and menton.
		Me	**Menton:** The most inferior point of the symphysis as seen radiographically.
S	**Sella:** The radiographic center of the pituitary fossa (sella turcica).		
N	**Nasion:** The most anterior junction of the nasal bone and frontal bone suture viewed from the lateral cephalogram.		
Or	**Orbitale:** The midpoint between the two radiographic projections of the orbits.		
Ar	**Articulare:** The intersection of the contour of the sphenoid bone and the posterior contour of the condylar process.		
Cd	**Condylion:** The most superior point of the condylar head as seen on the cephalogram.		
ANS	**Anterior Nasal Spine:** The most anterior radiographic projection of the nasal spine.		
PNS	**Posterior Nasal Spine:** The posterior spine of the palatine bone. The most distal projection of the hard palate.		
A	**Subspinale:** The most distal point of the premaxilla.		
B	**Supramentale:** The most distal point of the anterior mandibular alveolar process.		
Go	**Gonion:** The point that bi-		

Additional information can be gained from studying longitudinal tracings of the lateral skull radiographs:[40]

1. prediction of growth changes in the craniofacial complex
2. evaluation of craniofacial abnormalities
3. aid in treatment planning of malocclusion
4. evaluation of the success of maxillofacial appliance treatment

The cephalometric radiograph predicts anterior-posterior and vertical growth relationships.

1. The chin can be related to the cranial base.
2. The maxilla and mandible can be related to each other.
3. The teeth, particularly the incisors, can be related to each other.
4. Tooth position can be evaluated in the supporting structures.

Each anatomical landmark and cephalometric landmark is used to gain a specific piece of information for growth and treatment prediction. No attempt has been made to include all the cephalometric landmarks and measurements. A few of the more common assessments are shown graphically (Figs. 4-11 to 4-27).

Standard Cephalometric Landmarks

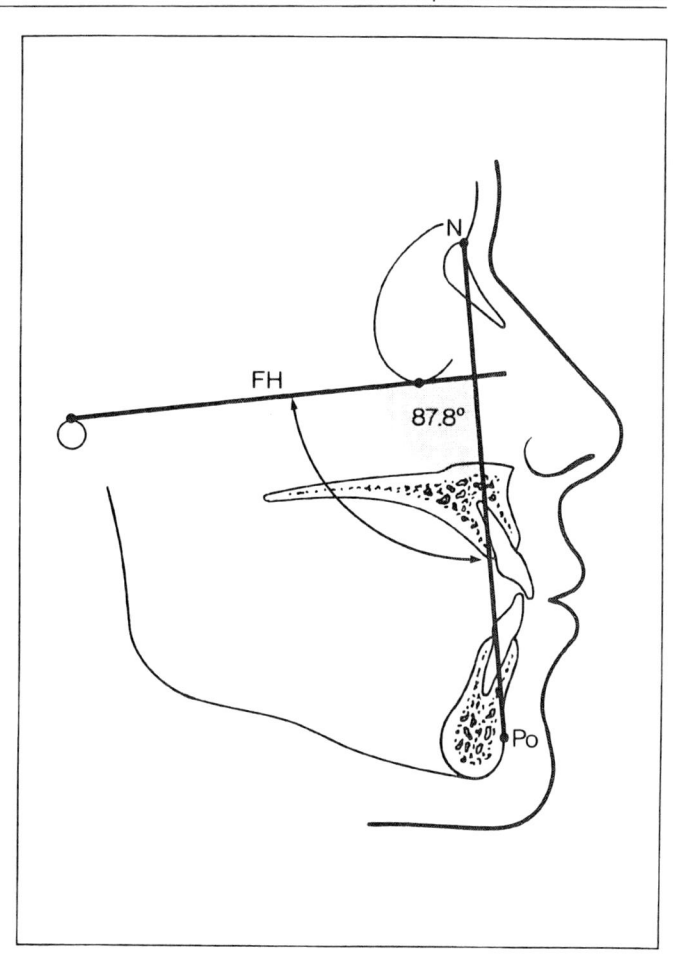

Fig. 4-11 Facial Angle Assessment. The average facial angle in Caucasians is 87.8°. Facial angles greater than 87.8° indicate a tendency toward mandibular prognathism. Facial angles less than 87.8° indicate a tendency toward mandibular retrognathism. Facial angle assessment allows the clinician to assess skeletally the anterior-posterior relationship of the chin to the cranial base.

The cephalometric film is also a lateral skull radiograph. In addition to the standard cephalometric landmarks, bone anomalies, such as fractures, and pathologic osseous changes should be noted.

Cephalometric analysis

Several researchers have developed their own cephalometric analyses. Some of the more popular are those by Bimler, Björk, Downs, Enlow, Moorrees, Ricketts, Sassouni, Steiner, Tweed, and Witts. Most of these researchers include many more measurements than have been presented here.

It is not the intention to develop a complete text of the available analysis. This section presents a guide to some of the more widely used cephalometric measurements for detection of sagittal, vertical, and dental discrepancies. The clinician should keep in mind that although these analyses are acceptable, they still contain sources of potential errors: errors in tracing, image conversion from a three-dimensional body to a two-dimensional radiograph, variation in

Examination and Diagnosis for Malocclusion

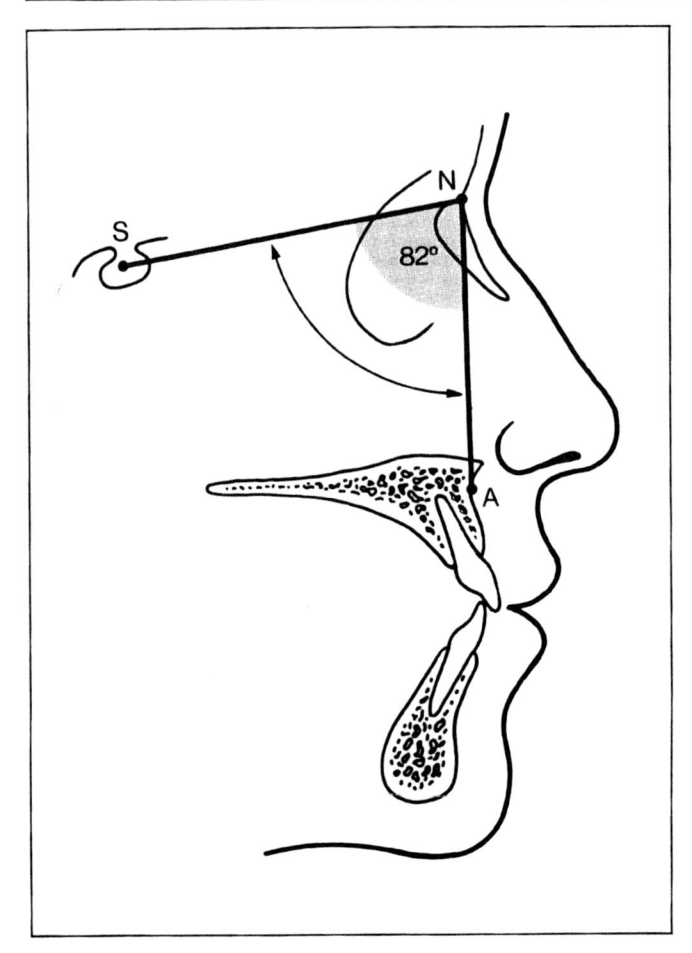

Maxillary sagittal skeletal relationships

Fig. 4-12 A normal maxillary skeletal and dentoalveolar relationship. The normal SNA is 82°. Notice the lip fullness and normal profile.

relative head position, and distortion and positional changes in equipment (x-ray source and film).[41]

Growth changes are generally studied and diagnoses or predictions made using several anatomical or external landmarks. Some of these lie on a curve (gonion) or two curves (menton) or none (porion). Some are at the intersection of two structures (articulare) (Fig. 4-10). Several authors have shown errors in tracing and variability of landmark location.[42,43] Baumrind et al.[44] have shown that a rotational error of one degree in the mandible from a landmark placed 100 mm away can produce a displacement in the observed portion of 1.74 mm. Moyers and Bookstein[38] have shown how several shapes were drawn through three points without changing the angle measurement.

The cephalogram

The cephalogram is meant to be used as a guideline. It is one of several diagnostic criteria available. Reliance on any one diagnostic aid may lead to an unbalanced diagnosis and a flawed treatment plan. For example, if the computer printout from an

Standard Cephalometric Landmarks

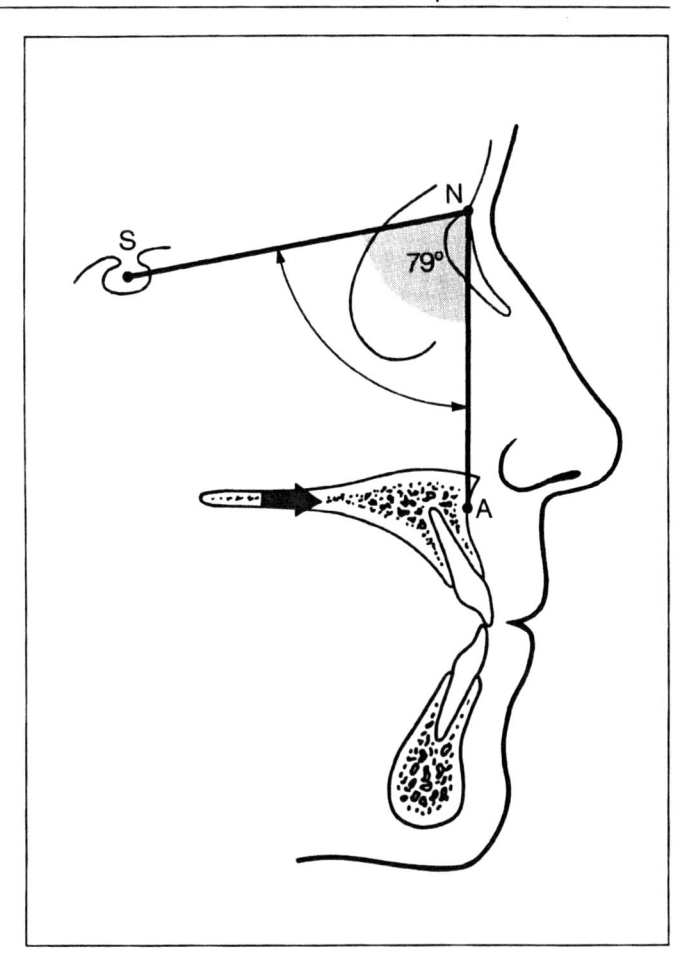

Fig. 4-13 A slight skeletal maxillary retrusion. Treatment can include maxillofacial orthopedic therapy to induce maxillary growth; a maxillary sagittal appliance is used such that the acrylic will not touch the anterior teeth. In severe cases, a Delaire's Face Mask or surgical maxillary advancement may be required. Note the flat upper lip.

analysis advises four premolar extractions, a careful evaluation of the face is needed. Are fuller lips needed? Would the facial esthetics and facial musculature benefit from a reduction of tooth structure and possible loss of alveolar supporting structure? Peck and Peck[45] have demonstrated that the public may prefer a slightly more protrusive dentoalveolar profile than current cephalometric standards permit. Would the temporomandibular joint function as well with a reduction of vertical dimension? Extraction of teeth anterior to the first molar may reduce the vertical dimension.[46]

Holdaway[47] has emphasized the use of a soft tissue cephalometric analysis as a way of obtaining more meaningful diagnostic information than by sole reliance on a hard tissue cephalometric analysis. Emphasis is needed for facial esthetics and balance, in addition to excellence of occlusion.

The goal is to guide growth and development. The parent or patient is informed that the cephalogram is an aid to establishing a starting point for treatment. Problems with developing malocclusion will be interpreted and intercepted before development. Early prevention is usually easier than treatment later. Good records are essential. (Chapter 14 will delineate some of the newer meth-

97

Examination and Diagnosis for Malocclusion

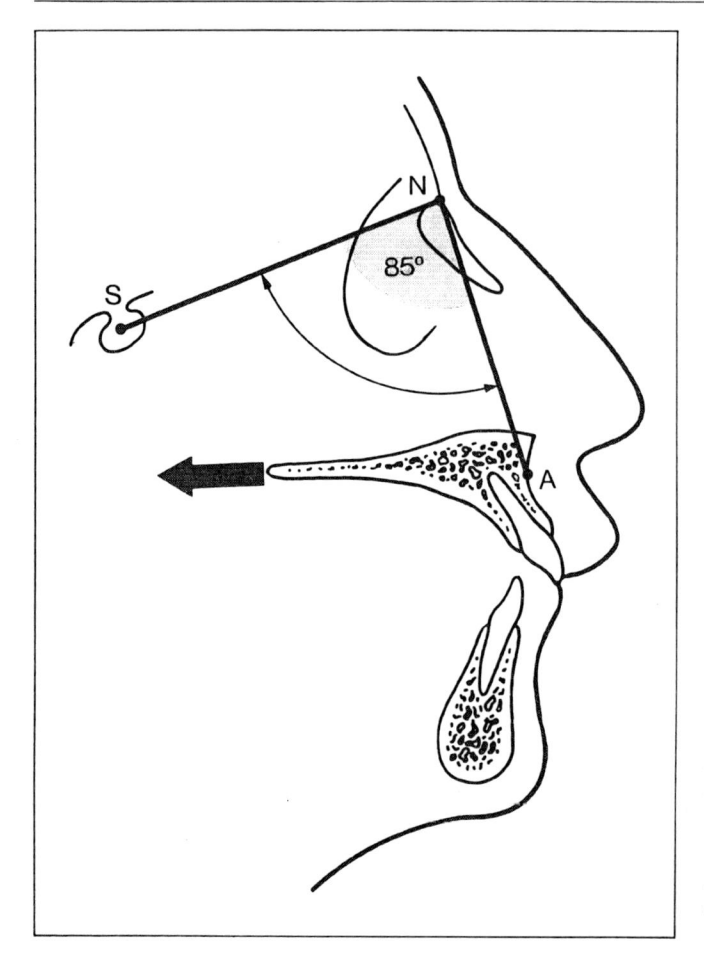

Fig. 4-14 Maxillary skeletal protrusion. Treatment can include early maxillary retraction with headgear or surgical repositioning of the maxilla. If maxillary premolar extraction is contemplated, care must be taken to avoid occlusal, facial, or condylar disharmony.

ods to study shape changes and the future of craniofacial growth prediction.)

Photographic examination and records

There are four primary reasons for a complete photographic examination. First, full face, profile, and intraoral color slides are excellent for documenting a starting point for treatment. Second, photographs permit harmless treatment progress records to be taken at regular intervals. Third, start-to-finish treatment photographs can easily be reproduced from transparencies for a posttreatment report for the patient and parent. Fourth, consultation with colleagues and legal documentation is more precise with good-quality photographs.

The photographic equipment does not have to be elaborate; a standard 35 mm SLR camera with a 50–90 mm adjustable macro 1:3.5 lens will prove very practical for dental photography. A point source attached variable-intensity flash unit will ensure the proper light requirement. Bellows and ring-light attachments can be utilized for additional versatility.

Photographic Examination and Records

Figs. 4-15a to c Care must be taken to use more than one reference source for diagnosis.

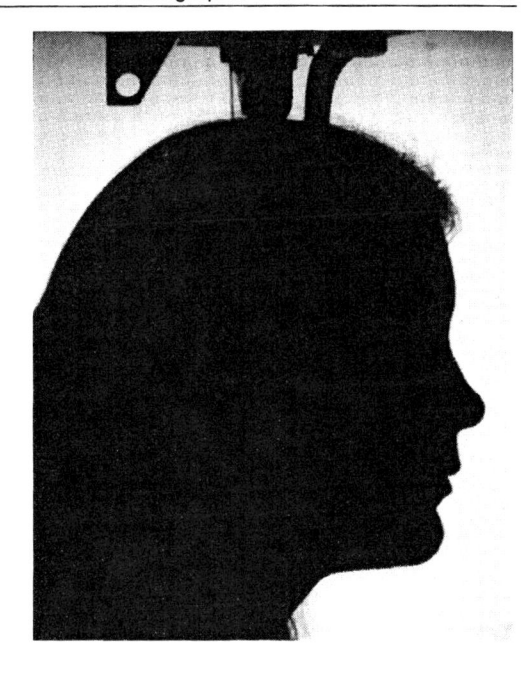

Fig. 4-15a Shows a patient with an acceptable facial profile.

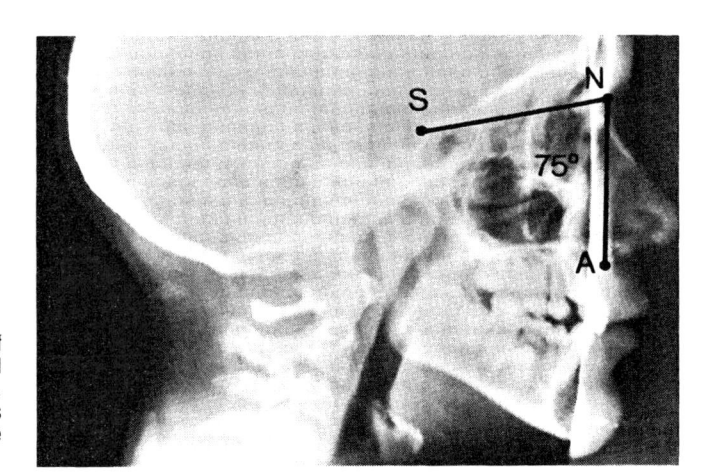

Fig. 4-15b Shows an SNA of 75°, which could be associated with skeletal maxillary retrusion. In this case, the patient presents an inclination of the cranial base (low sella).

There are several excellent guides to intraoral photography.[48] Repeated photographic exposures at different light and f-stop settings will provide a range of exposures. Selection of the best exposure settings for the camera and light source can be marked for future reference. If office space permits, a tripod or other camera fixation device can be utilized to standardize the camera-subject focal distance.

Patient photographs are limited only by the expertise, experience, and time of the photographer. Training ancillary personnel will maximize efficiency.

99

Examination and Diagnosis for Malocclusion

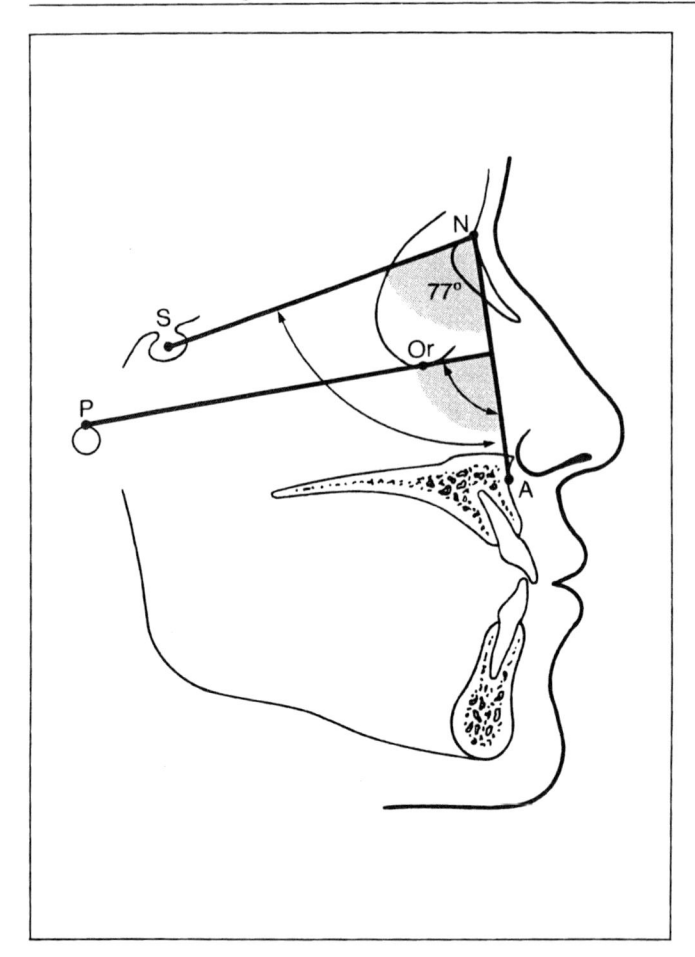

Fig. 4-15c Detailed diagnostic records can be obtained from more than one reference source. For example, the Frankfort Horizontal (porion-orbitale) to NA can be used. The numbers vary depending on the age and gender of the individual.

Photographic views

The following four photographic views are standard:

1. Full face The face and head of the patient should fill the camera field except for a 5 to 10 cm border of contrasting background. Use a dark background for light-complexioned individuals; a contrasting background for dark-complexioned patients. A deep blue felt background shows well in color transparencies and minimizes shadows.

2. Profile view This photograph is taken at a 90° angle from the frontal view. The patient should be in a comfortable standing position with the head in a natural rest position. Attempting to make the mandible parallel with the floor may distort the posture of the patient. The facial profile should fill the viewing field except for the 5 to 10 cm border of contrasting background.

3. Frontal view with teeth in natural occlusion Cheek retractors are necessary for maximum visualization of the occlusion. A printed sticky label on the cheek retractors should contain the following information: name of the patient, age in years and months, current date, and problem. In addition, the patient's complaint, type of appli-

Photographic Examination and Records

Mandibular skeletal sagittal relationships

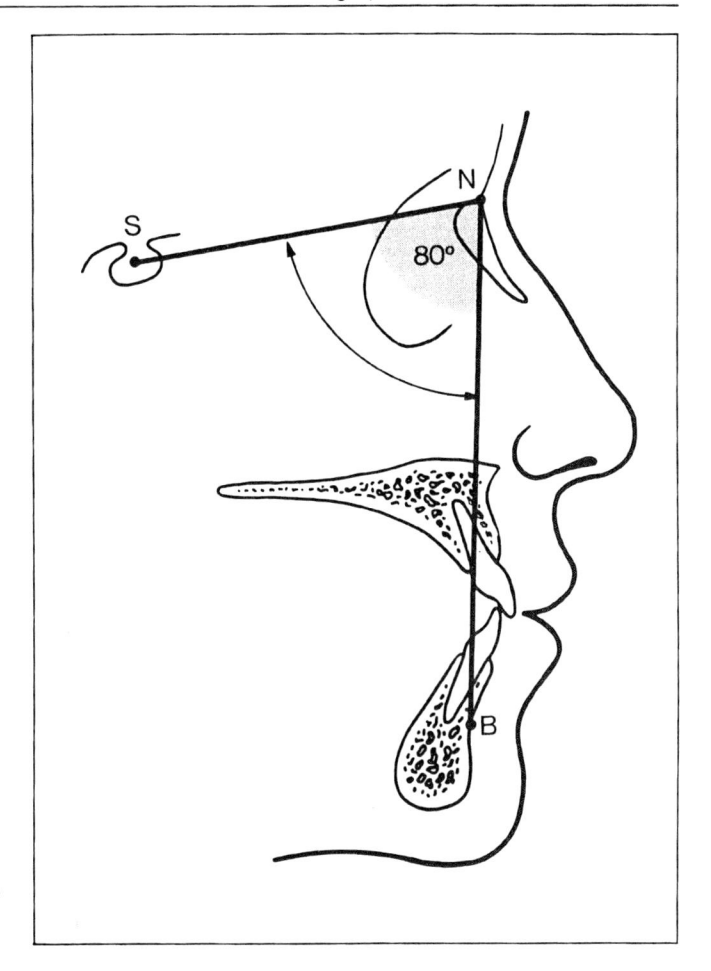

Fig. 4-16 A normal SNB angle of 80°, associated with normal craniofacial development.

ance, length of time the appliance has been worn, and other information is included as space permits. The view should have the occlusion centered but include the printed label in the field. A 12 to 14 cm focal length is suggested.

4. Frontal and lateral close-up views with teeth in natural occlusion The incisors should be centered in the frontal view with the teeth filling the view. The canines are centered in the lateral view. A 6 to 8 cm focal length is suggested.

These photographs will satisfy the minimal requirements for documentation.

Additional views are desirable and dic- tated by signs and symptoms of the patient, or need for documentation for presentation. Buccal views taken with a mirror show the posterior dental occlusion. Maxillary and mandibular mirror views allow occlusal visualization of the dental arches. Occasionally, views of the teeth in maximum lateral and anteroposterior excursion are useful for documentation. If the patient has temporomandibular joint pathology and concomitant postural complications, full frontal and lateral body photographs are useful documentation. Posttreatment photographs frequently reveal postural correction.

Photographs of the study models can be

Examination and Diagnosis for Malocclusion

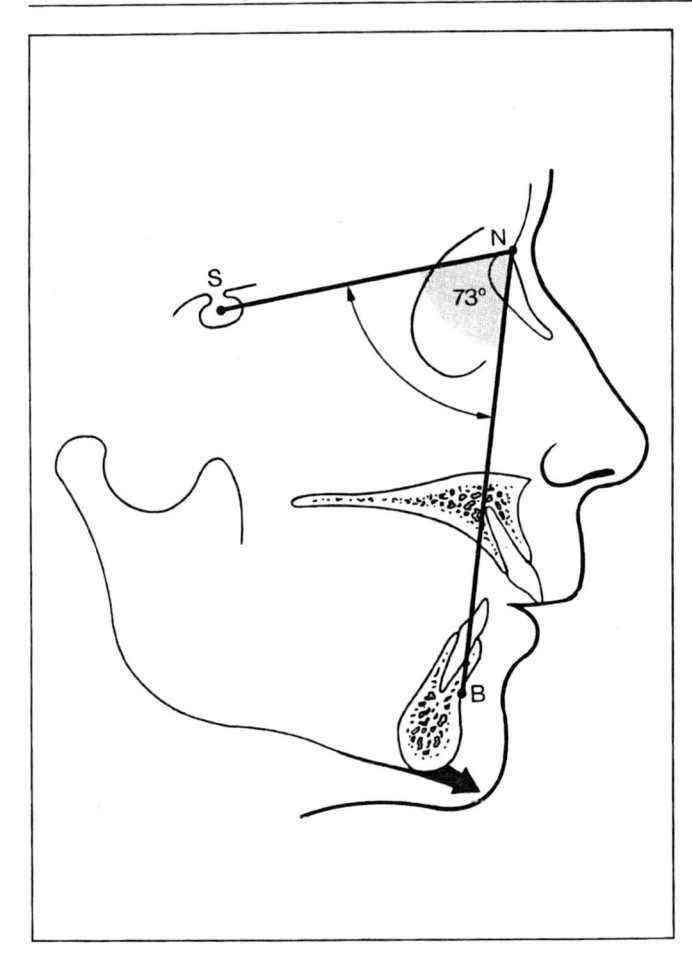

Fig. 4-17 Mandibular skeletal retrusion. Treatment includes forward repositioning of the mandible with a maxillofacial orthopedic appliance.

prepared for group presentation. A mirror angled view of study models can show both buccal views and frontal view on the same slide. Facial and profile views of the patient with the appliance in the mouth can demonstrate some of the facial changes that occur with good patient cooperation. These photographs can help motivate patients during treatment. A photograph of the appliance worn during treatment on a contrasting background can demonstrate appliance type and construction to curious patients and parents. Serial photographs are useful for evaluating periodic changes in occlusal relationships, the level of dental hygiene, health of the gingival tissue, and arch development.[49]

Consulting with colleagues is much easier with color photography. Before, during, and after photographic treatment records can be an inexpensive method of ensuring legal documentation. Posttreatment litigation is very unusual with photographic evidence of the preexisting dental condition.[50] Gholston[51] has shown the reliability and accuracy of intraoral photography. This study demonstrates the precision of recording defined anatomic occlusal landmarks for electronic reduction and computer analysis.

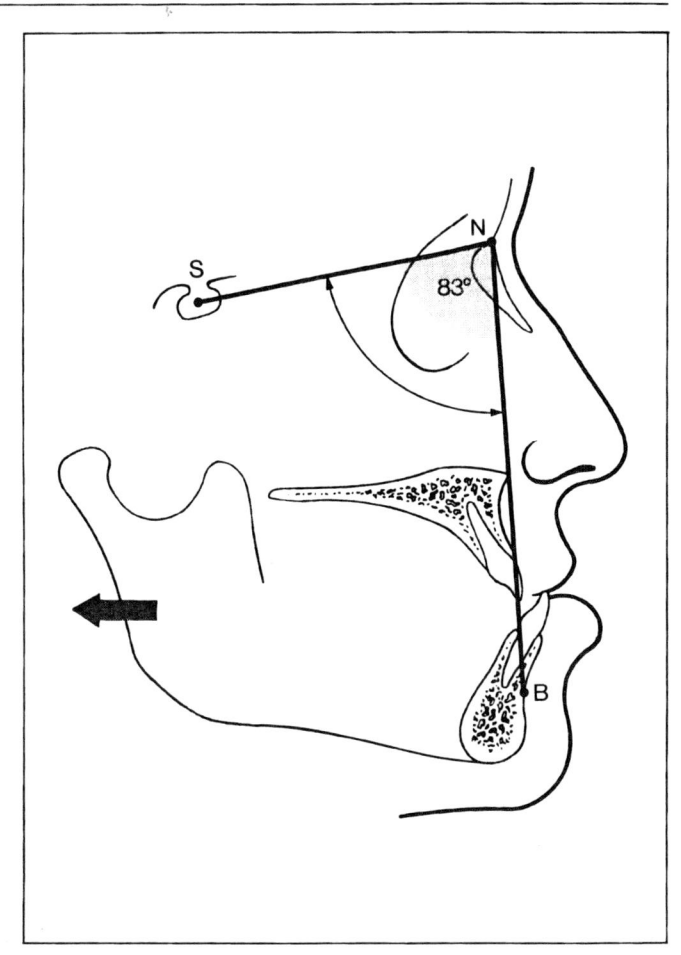

Fig. 4-18 Mandibular skeletal protrusion. Treatment may include chin-cap therapy in the primary or early mixed dentition or mandibular surgical repositioning in the adult.

It would be a mistake to underestimate the value of a posttreatment photographic report. The cost of having colored prints made from the transparencies is minimal as compared with the gratitude and satisfaction expressed by the patient, and additional referrals from that patient. Regardless of age, the patient is a dynamic source of referrals. The individual will have a sense of accomplishment and well-being, which is part of the treatment goal: to make the patient feel special.

Examination of study models

Properly finished and occluded study models of the dental arches complete the examination process and aid treatment planning and documentation (Fig. 4-28). The impressions can be taken with a carefully selected perforated stock tray. Any tray excess is trimmed and the tray is muscle-bordered with a soft-beading wax. A high-grade alginate or rubber base impression is taken of each dental arch. The alginate impressions require proper protection with damp towels, and are sealed in a plastic bag along with the occlusal wax indication of the maximum

Examination and Diagnosis for Malocclusion

ANB angle assessment

The ANB angle is the difference between the SNA angle and SNB angle. A normal reading for ANB would be 2°. Since SNA and SNB establish the anterior-posterior relation of the maxilla and mandible to each other and to the cranial base, an ANB angle significantly higher than 2° would indicate maxillary protrusion, mandibular retrusion, or a combination of both. A negative ANB angle would indicate a concave facial profile and possible lack of midface development, or mandibular prognathism.

Maxillofacial orthopedic appliances can be very useful in correcting large deviations from the norm in the ANB angle. For very severe ANB discrepancies, one or more surgical procedures may be needed for correction. Tooth movement alone in large ANB discrepancies (without concomitant skeletal development) is subject to relapse.

Vertical relationships

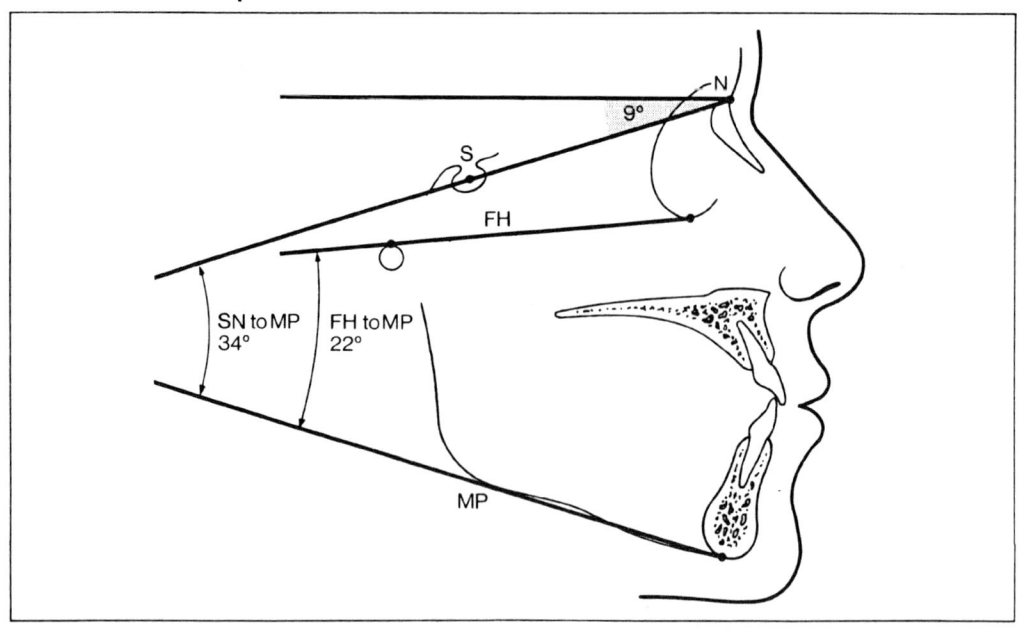

Fig. 4-19 The normal vertical dimension. The Angle SN to mandibular plane averages 34° and can be supplemented with the Frankfort Horizontal to Mandibular Plane Angle in patients with a steep inclination of the cranial base angle. Moorrees has suggested that an SN-True Horizontal angle greater than 9° indicates a greater-than-normal cranial base inclination. The FH-Mandibular Plane Angle is suggested for SN-True Horizontal angles greater than 9°.

Examination of Study Models

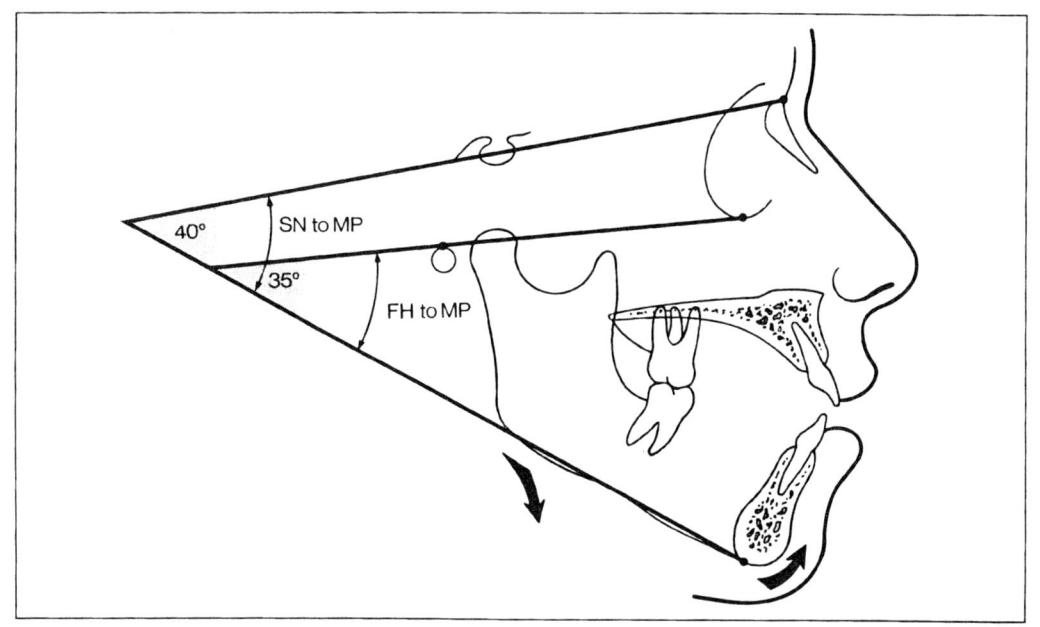

Fig. 4-20 A patient with a high mandibular plane angle and anterior open bite. Treatment should be directed at rotating the mandible anteriorly, which will reduce the vertical dimension and correct the lip incompetence.

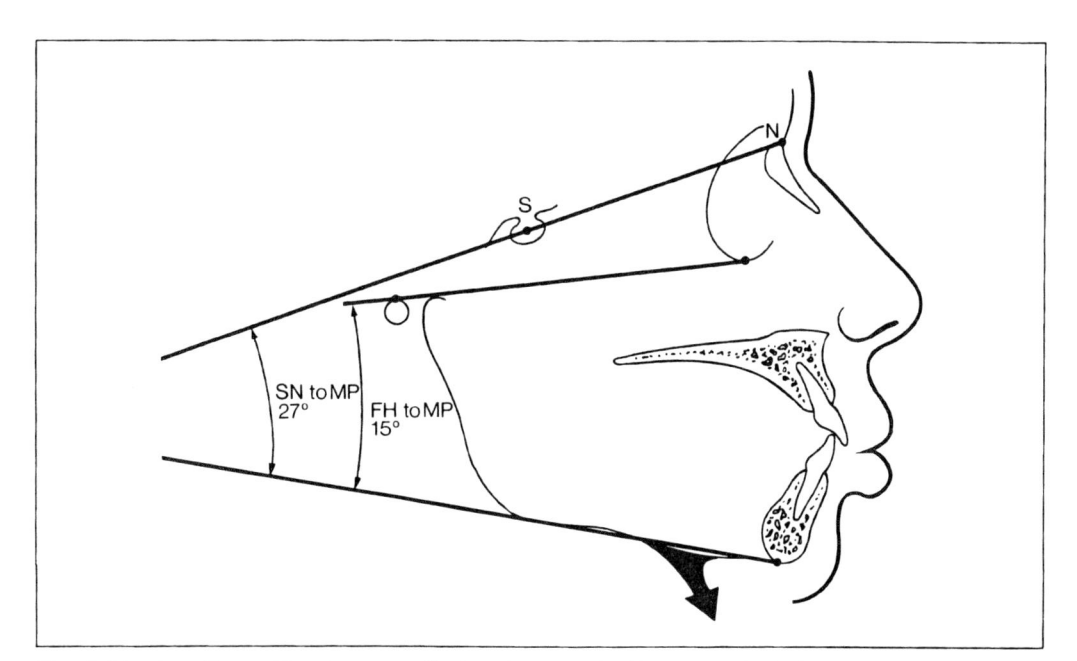

Fig. 4-21 A patient with a low mandibular plane angle. Treatment includes opening the vertical dimension and forward mandibular repositioning. Correction of the skeletal components will improve the facial profile.

Examination and Diagnosis for Malocclusion

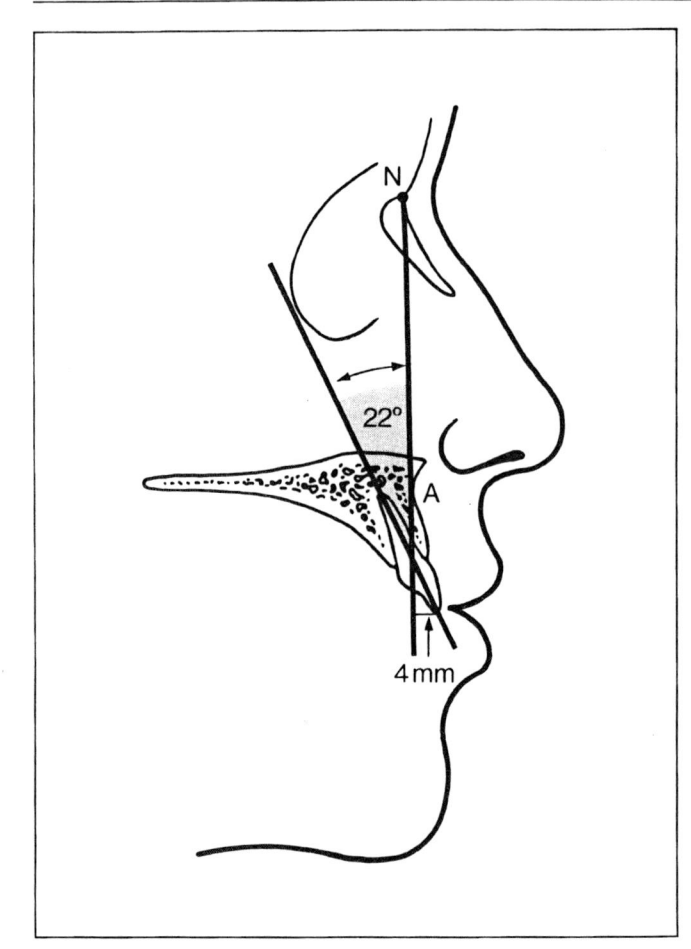

Anterior dental relationships

Fig. 4-22 A normal maxillary incisor inclination. Tooth position and inclination are important to esthetics and to the stability of the dental and skeletal component. A change of inclination of the maxillary anterior teeth can affect condylar position as well as the position of the mandibular incisors.

intercuspation. These impressions can be sent to a laboratory that specializes in fabricating dental models. The laboratory is instructed to pour, trim, polish, and label the dental study models. The label is etched into each cast and includes the patient's full name, age in years and months, and the current date.

Another impression is taken of the arch or arches after a final diagnosis has been made. These impressions are poured into a high-grade bubble-free dental stone and sent to the laboratory along with complete instructions for fabrication of the appliance. This stone model or set of models should be trimmed (to eliminate bulkiness for shipping), labeled with the name of the patient and doctor, and dated. Closely trimmed working models are easier for the technician to handle and, being lighter, less expensive to mail. Writing on the stone model is done with a waterproof pen. If wax-construction bites are necessary, at least two are included for the laboratory technician. The working models or duplicate working models should be returned to the clinician in case of changes or fracture of the appliance.

Finished, properly occluded study models are used for completing the diagnosis

Examination of Study Models

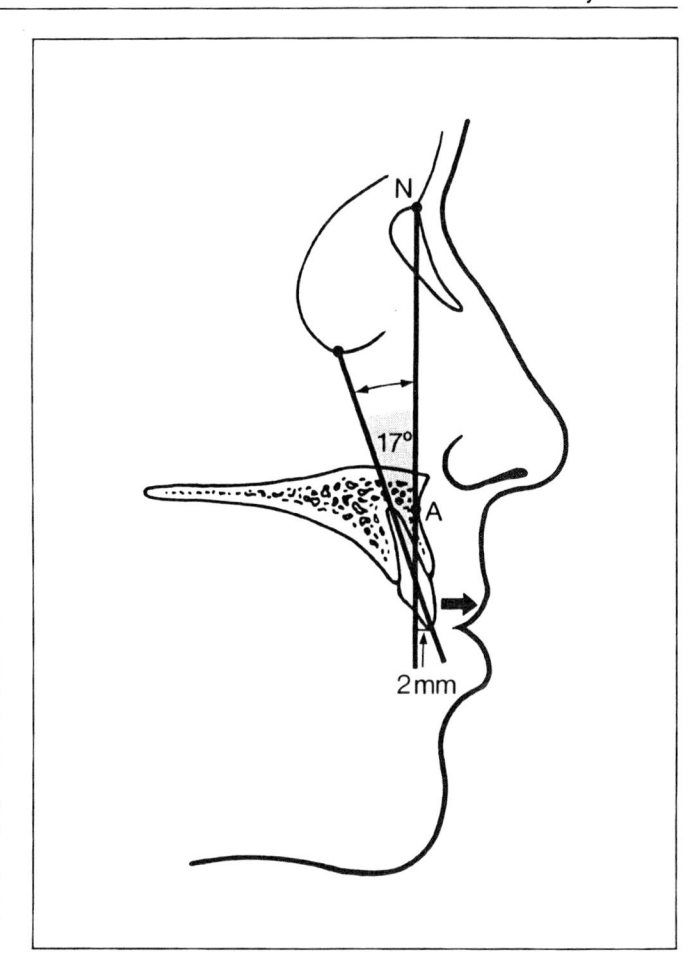

Fig. 4-23 A normal upright maxillary incisor. Notice the flatness of the upper lip. Treatment can include flaring the maxillary incisors with fixed or removable appliances. If the upright maxillary incisors are associated with a maxillary skeletal retrusion, then a sagittal appliance can be used with the acrylic touching the lingual anterior tooth surfaces. Labialization of the maxillary incisors can increase the arch circumference and aid in the correction of dental crowding.

and plan for treatment of the malocclusion, and for case presentation to the patient or parent. Some clinicians, however, are finding that a precise photographic documentation of the existing malocclusion can reduce the expense and space needed for storage of the dental study models.

Space analysis

If there is dental crowding in the mixed dentition, then a space analysis is completed from the working stone models. Several different space prediction analyses are available: direct measurement from the radiograph, Tanaka and Johnson,[52] Pont,[53] and Schwarz.[54] The clinician should use the analysis that is best suited for that particular patient and practice.

Tanaka and Johnson's analysis

An analysis of the mixed dentition provides a method of estimating the amount of space available in the arch for the succeeding permanent dentition. To complete the analysis, three major factors must be known:

1. The mesiodistal widths of the mandibular incisors. This is done by measur-

Examination and Diagnosis for Malocclusion

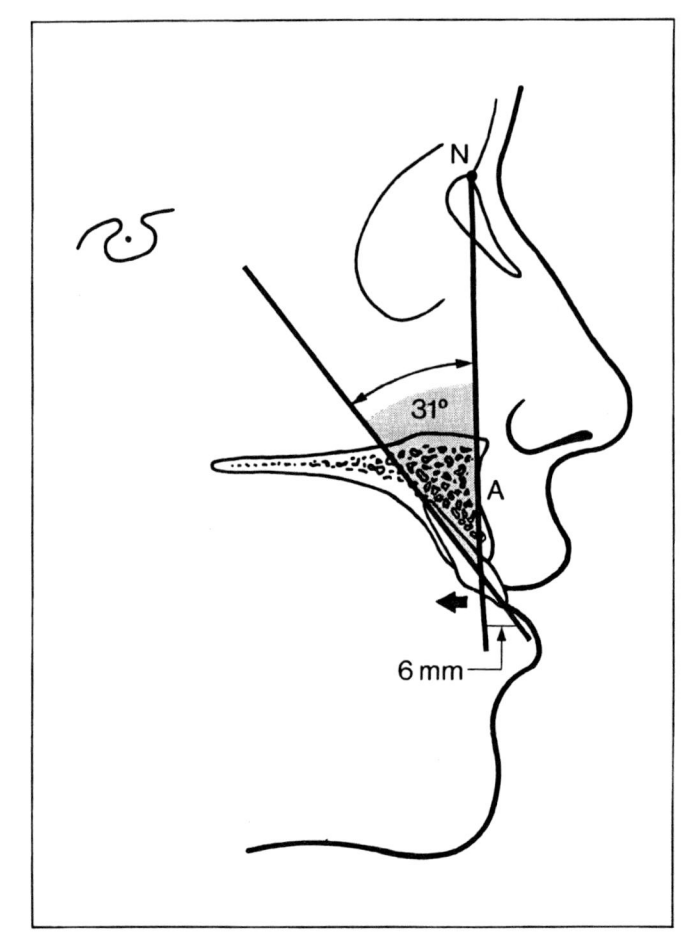

Fig. 4-24 Excessive labial tipping. Treatment includes uprighting the incisors. Care must be taken not to lock the mandible in a retruded position. (See Chapter 10.)

ing the greatest mesiodistal dimension of each mandibular incisor with a pointed Boley gauge.

2. Prediction of the size of the permanent canines and premolars. This is done by taking one-half of the sum of *all* the mandibular incisors and adding 10.5 mm for the mandibular arch and 11.0 mm for the maxilla. For example:

lower right lateral	6.5 mm
lower right central	5.9
lower left central	6.1
lower left lateral	6.5
	25.0 mm

Mandibular

$X = \frac{Y}{2} + 10.5$

$X = \frac{25}{2} + 10.5$

$X = 12.5 + 10.5$

$X = 23.0$ mm

Maxillary

$X = \frac{Y}{2} + 11.0$

$X = \frac{25}{2} + 11.0$

$X = 12.5 + 11.0$

$X = 23.5$ mm

Examination of Study Models

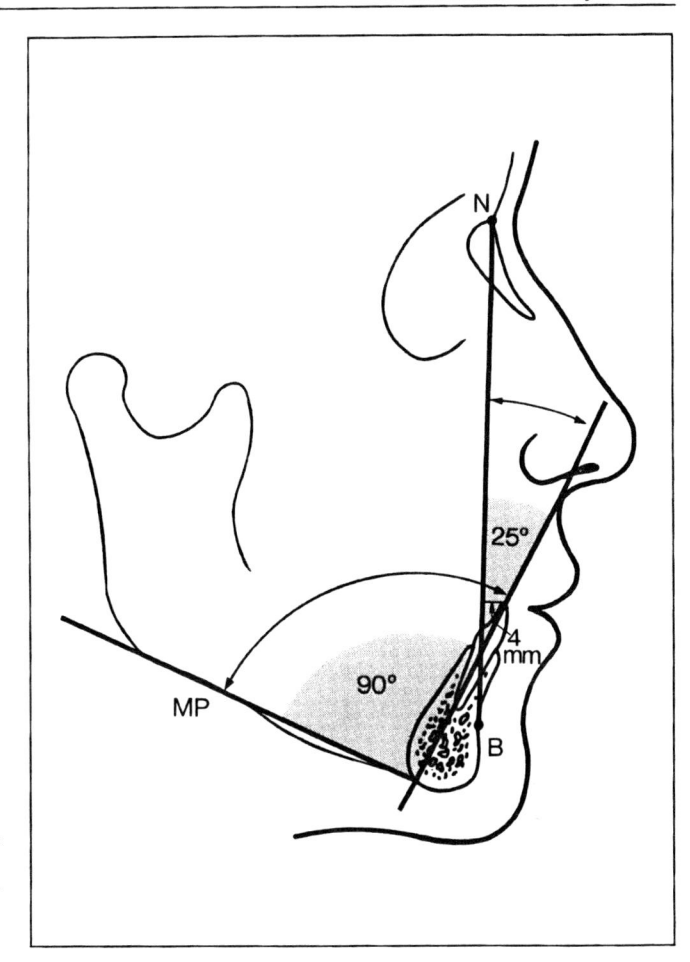

Fig. 4-25 Normal inclination of the lower incisors. In this case, the inclination of the mandibular incisor is related to NB (25°) and to the mandibular plane (90°).

X = predicted arch length necessary per quadrant for the permanent canines and premolars; Y = size of the four permanent mandibular incisors.

3. The space available after the incisors are correctly aligned. If the incisors are not correctly aligned, mark the cast where the incisors should lie. This is done by marking one-half the sum of Y from the midline. Measure from the mesial of the first permanent molar to this mark. This is the available space *(Z)* (Fig. 4-29).

Pont analysis

In the early 1900s, Pont developed an index for relating the sum of the maxillary incisors to the anterior and posterior dental arch width. The analysis can be used for both arches, but it is not totally reliable because it utilizes the maxillary incisors, which are more variable in size than the mandibular incisors. Mathematically, it is expressed as follows:

$$A = \frac{(SI) \times 100}{80},$$

where A is the distance necessary for cross

Examination and Diagnosis for Malocclusion

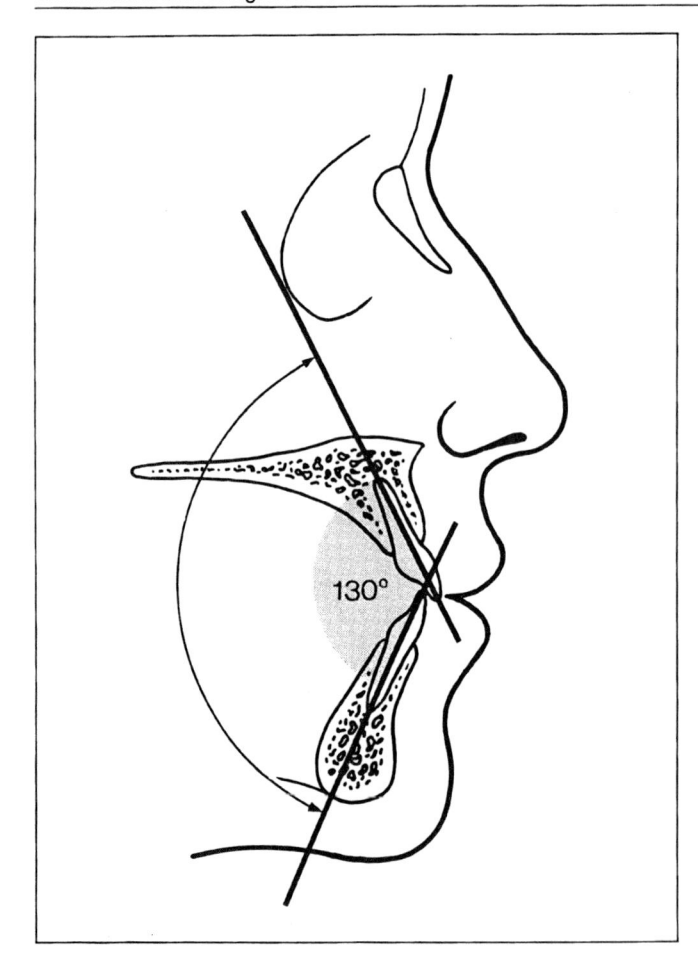

Fig. 4-26 The angle formed by the long axis plane of the maxillary to mandibular incisor determines the interincisal angle. An average angle would be 130°. (This angle varies greatly in different racial groups.) A lower-than-average interincisal angle would indicate a tendency toward dental protrusion. If the angle is significantly higher than 130°, then the incisors would be too upright. Large interincisal angles are often associated with deep overbite and/or Class II, Division 2 malocclusion. At the completion of treatment, the proper interincisal angle is important to the stability of the dental component.

arch width at the maxillary first premolar measured at the distal pit of each first premolar, and SI is the sum of the incisors in millimeters.

For example, if the incisor prediction shows that 42 mm are needed at the premolar area and the pit-to-distal distance is only 39 mm, then the arch must be developed 3 mm in the premolar area to accommodate all the anterior teeth.

The posterior arch width is determined by another formula:

$$B = \frac{(SI) \times 100}{64},$$

where B is the distance necessary for cross arch width at the maxillary first molar measured from central fossa to central fossa of the first molar.

In the lower arch the cross arch measurements are made from the buccal interproximal embrasure of the mandibular first and second premolars and the middle buccal cusp tips of the mandibular first molars.

Schwarz analysis

Schwarz devised a simplified method of predicting the anterior arch development at the distal fossa of the maxillary first premo-

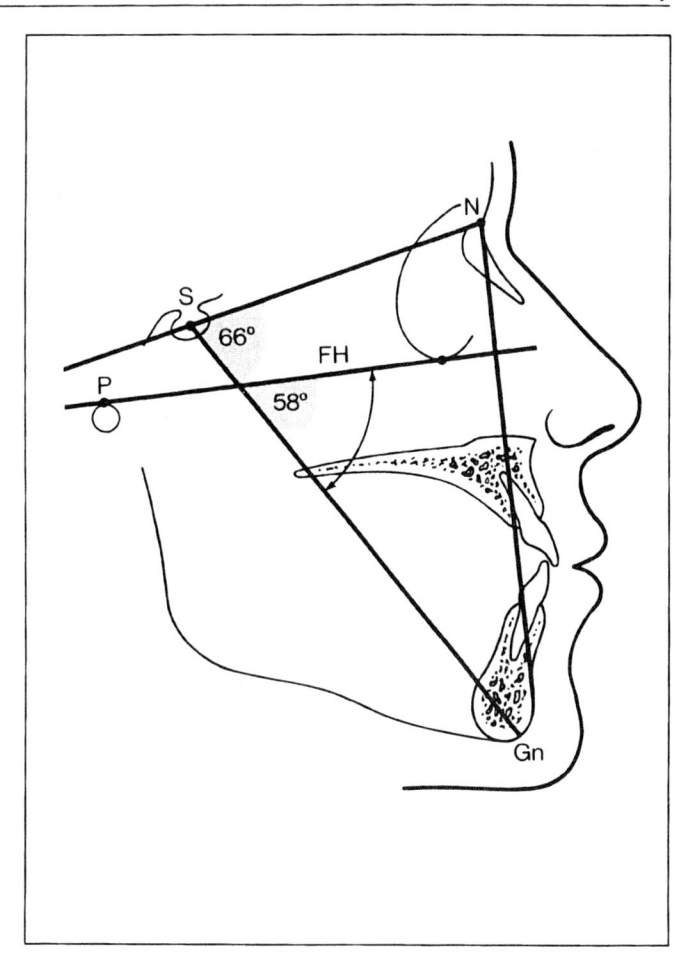

Fig. 4-27 Y-Axis Angle Assessment. An assessment of the angle formed between the Y-Axis and the Frankfort Horizontal or Sella-Nasion Line indicates the future direction of lower facial growth. The average value of the Y-Axis–Frankfort Horizontal Angle is 58°; the Y-Axis–Sella-Nasion Angle averages 66°. Angles larger than average show a tendency toward downward and backward growth. Angles smaller than average show a trend toward more forward or horizontal growth in the lower face.

lars. The prediction is expressed mathematically:

$Sl + 8$ = Anterior arch width necessary.

The sum of the incisors, measured in millimeters, plus 8 mm equals the anterior arch width necessary for full development and proper arch length of the anterior segment. By adding another 8 mm, the same formula can be used for posterior arch development at the maxillary first molar as measured from the central fossa. The mandibular arch development can be predicted using the same formula and measuring from the buccal cusp tip of the first premolar for anterior arch width development. The mid-buccal cusp tip of the mandibular first molar is used for analysis of posterior arch width development (Fig. 4-30).

Summary

The examination of the study models completes the record-gathering process. A diagnosis is formulated from the data collected. Information has been evaluated from the following: medical and dental history for parents and patient, posture, atti-

Examination and Diagnosis for Malocclusion

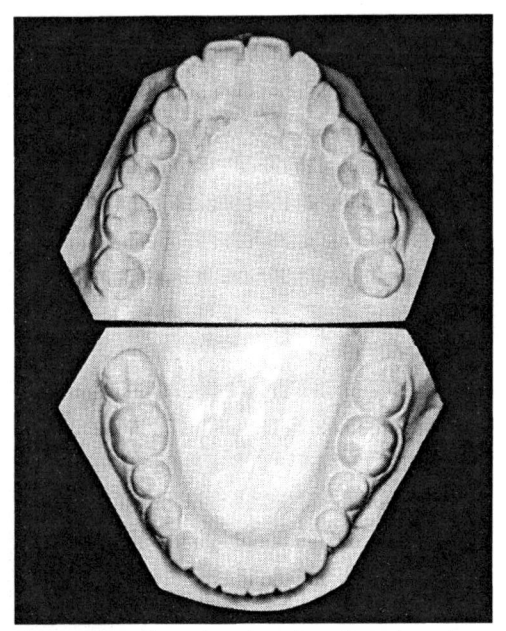

Fig. 4-28a Two dental arches that do not require dentoalveolar correction.

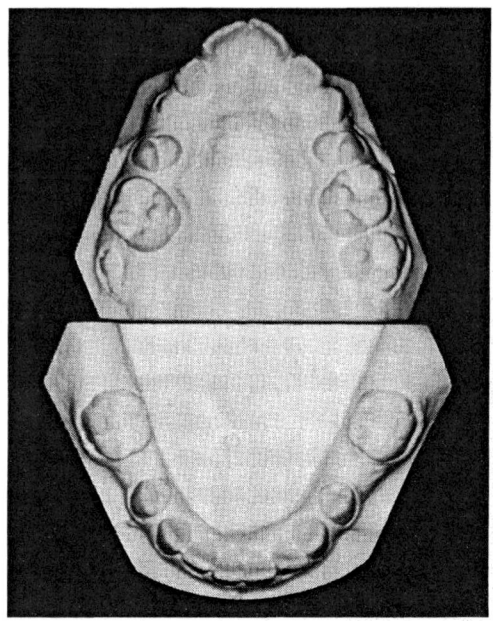

Fig. 4-28b A constricted maxillary arch that appears to need lateral expansion.

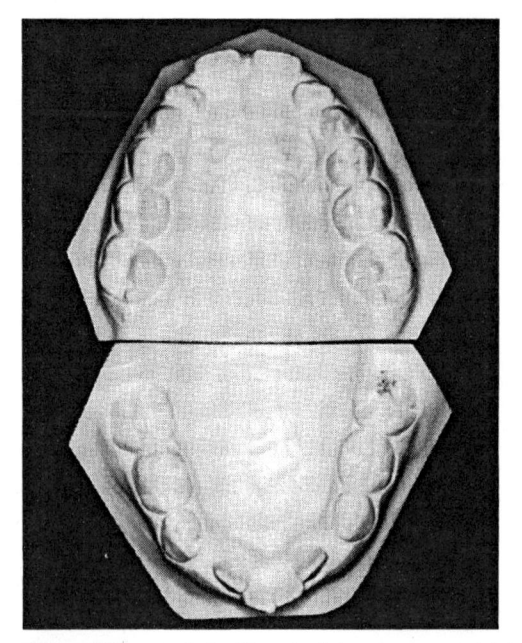

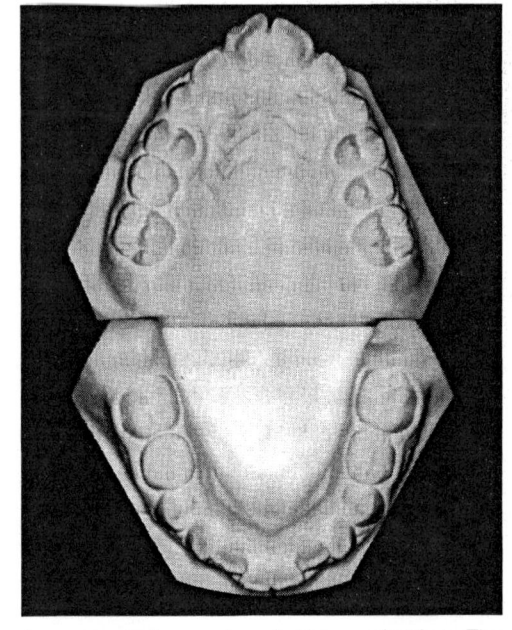

Figs. 4-28c and d The decision to expand laterally or sagittally requires further evaluation. The Schwarz and Pont analyses provide methods for width analyses in the permanent dentition.

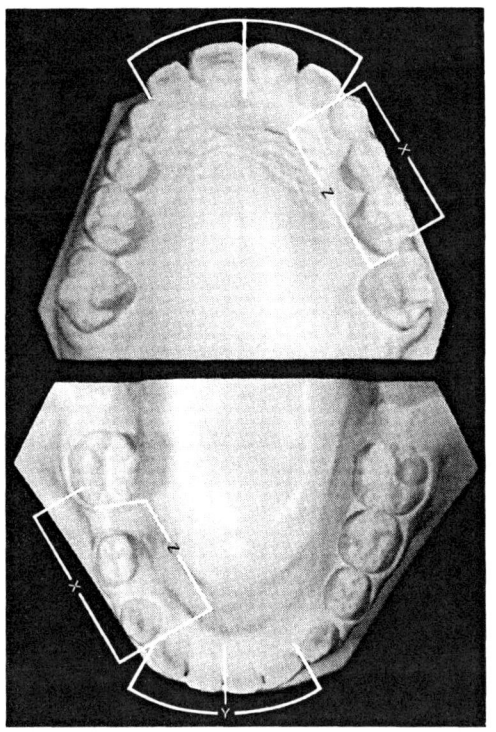

Fig. 4-29 Tanaka and Johnson mixed-dentition analysis. The analysis is done bilaterally. In this example, space is lacking in the mandibular right quadrant.

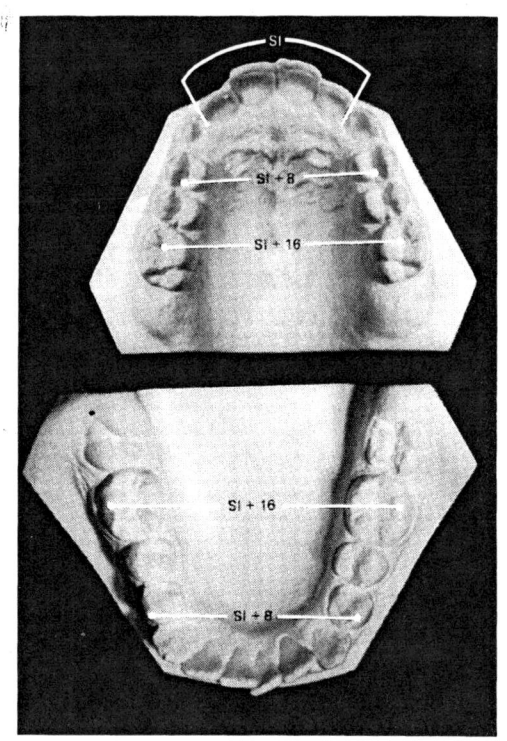

Fig. 4-30 Schwarz's analysis.

tude, muscle tone and tenderness, temporomandibular joint function, radiographic and photographic examination, and an analysis of the study models.

Some of the examination procedures may seem trivial or unimportant for arriving at a diagnosis. However, the experienced clinician will evaluate all the information gathered, achieve a personal rapport with the patient and parent, establish the diagnosis, and direct a successful treatment plan to completion.

If the records have been collected in an orderly and sequential manner, a diagnosis will be evident.

References

1. El-Mangoury, N. H. Orthodontic cooperation. Am. J. Orthod. 80:604–622, 1981.
2. Berg, R. Post-retention analysis of treatment problems and failures in 264 consecutively treated cases. Eur. J. Orthod. 1:55–68, 1979.
3. Melsen, B., Stensgaard, K., and Pedersen, J. Sucking habits and their influence on swallowing pattern and prevalence of malocclusion. Eur. J. Orthod. 1:271–280, 1979.
4. Larsson, E. Dummy- and finger-sucking habits with special attention to their significance for facial growth and occlusion. Swed. Dent. J. 64:667–672, 1971.
5. Larsson, E. Dummy- and finger-sucking habits with special attention to their significance for facial growth and occlusion. Swed. Dent. J. 68:55–59, 1975.

6. Larsson, E. Dummy- and finger-sucking habits with special attention to their significance for facial growth and occlusion. Swed. Dent. J. 1:23–33, 1978.
7. Subtelny, J. D., and Subtelny, J. D. Oral habits—studies in form, function, and therapy. Angle Orthod. 43:347–383, 1973.
8. Engelman, J. A. Measurement of perioral pressures during the playing of musical wind instruments. Am. J. Orthod. 51:856, 1965.
9. Herman, E. Dental consideration in the playing of musical instruments. J. Am. Dent. Assoc. 89:611–619, 1974.
10. Herman, E. Orthodontic aspects of musical instrument selection. Am. J. Orthod. 65:519–530, 1974.
11. Gualtieri, P. A. May Johnny or Janie play the clarinet? Am. J. Orthod. 76:260–275, 1979.
12. Herman, E. Influence of musical instruments on tooth positions. Am. J. Orthod. 80:145–155, 1981.
13. Leib, M. M. A cloud—larger than a man's hand. Int. J. Orthod. 18:17–19, 1980.
14. Valachovic, R. W., and Lurie, A. G. Risk-benefit considerations in pedodontic radiology. Pediatr. Dent. 2:128–146, 1980.
15. Fabrikant, J. I. Risk estimation and decision making: the health effects on populations of exposure to low levels of ionizing radiation. Pediatr. Dent. 3:400–413, 1982.
16. Lurie, A. G., and Brandt, S. Risk/benefit considerations in orthodontic radiology. J. Clin. Orthod. 15:469–475; 478–484, 1981.
17. Taylor, L. S. Dental radiology, trends, issues and problems. J. Am. Coll. Dent. 49:14–20, 1982.
18. Darzenta, N. C., and Tsamtsouris, A. Radiography in pedodontics. J. Pedod. 2:228–236, 1978.
19. Santangelo, M. V. Dental radiology: focus for the eighties. Pediatr. Dent. 3:385–392, 1982.
20. Barnett, M. Reducing unnecessary radiation exposure from x-rays: the role of the Bureau of Radiological Health. Pediatr. Dent. 3:393–395, 1982.
21. White, S. C. Radiation in pediatric dentistry: current standards in pedodontic radiology with suggestions for alternatives. Pediatr. Dent. 3:441–447, 1982.
22. Nowak, A. J. Radiation exposure in pediatric dentistry: an introduction. Pediatr. Dent. 3:380–384, 1982.
23. Cohen, M. Reduced radiation for an orthodontic survey. Am. J. Orthod. 44:513–517, 1958.
24. Cohen, M., and Hammond, E. Cephalometrics in the atomic age. Am. J. Orthod. 43:592–597, 1957.
25. Paden, W. W. A survey of radiation hazards in orthodontics. Am. J. Orthod. 46:575–587, 1960.
26. Franklin, J. B. Radiation hazards in cephalometric roentgenography. Angle Orthod. 23:222–228, 1953.
27. Franklin, J. B. Radiographic phenomena in cephalometric roentgenology. Angle Orthod. 27:162–170, 1957.
28. Franklin, J. B. The effect of aluminum filter disks in roentgenographic cephalometry. Angle Orthod. 32:252–269, 1962.
29. Franklin, J. B. Newer studies of radiation exposure in cephalometric roentgenography utilizing the Rando head phantom. Angle Orthod. 43:53–64, 1973.
30. Hamplemann, L. Risk of thyroid neoplasms after irradiation in childhood. Science 160:159–163, 1968.
31. Clark, D. E. Association of irradiation with cancer of the thyroid in children and adolescents. JAMA 159:1007–1009, 1955.
32. Block, A. J., Goepp, R. A., and Mason, B. S. Thyroid radiation dose during panoramic and cephalometric dental x-ray examination. Angle Orthod. 47:17–24, 1977.
33. Silling, G., et al. The significance of cephalometrics in treatment planning. Angle Orthod. 49:259–262, 1979.
34. Tenti, F. V. Cephalometric analysis as a tool for treatment planning and evaluation. Eur. J. Orthod. 3:241–245, 1981.
35. Fields, H. W., Vann, W. F., Jr., and Vig, K. W. L. Reliability of soft tissue profile analysis in children. Angle Orthod. 52:159–165, 1982.
36. Foster, T. D., Howat, A. P., and Naish, P. J. Variation in cephalometric reference lines. Br. J. Orthod. 8:183–187, 1981.
37. Moorrees, C. F. A., et al. New norms for the mesh diagram analysis. Am. J. Orthod. 69:57–71, 1976.
38. Moyers, R. E., and Bookstein, F. L. The inappropriateness of conventional cephalometrics. Am. J. Orthod. 75:599–617, 1981.
39. Watson, W. G. Your frame of reference. Am. J. Orthod. 81:250–252, 1982.
40. Hunter, W. S. A study of inheritance of craniofacial characteristics as seen in lateral cephalograms of 72 like sexed twins. Trans. Eur. Orthod. Soc. 41:41–59, 1965.
41. Loevy, H. T. Dental Management of the Child Patient. Chicago: Quintessence Publ. Co., 1981.
42. Baumrind, S., and Frantz, R. C. The reliability of head film measurements. Am. J. Orthod. 60:111–127, 1971.
43. Baumrind, S., and Frantz, R. C. The reliability of head film measurements. Am. J. Orthod. 60:505–517, 1971.
44. Baumrind, S., Miller, D., and Molthen, R. The reliability of head film measurements. Am. J. Orthod. 70:617–644, 1976.
45. Peck, H., and Peck, S. A concept of facial esthetics. Angle Orthod. 40:284–318, 1970.
46. Wilson, W. L. The development of a treatment plan in the light of one's concept of treatment objectives. Am. J. Orthod. 45:561–573, 1959.
47. Holdaway, R. A. A soft-tissue cephalometric analysis and its use in orthodontic treatment planning. Part I. Am. J. Orthod. 84:1–28, 1983.
48. Freehe, C. L. (consulting ed.) Photography, Dental Clinics of America. Philadelphia: W. B. Saunders Co., 1968.
49. Jarabak, J. R., and Fizzell, J. A. Technique and

References

Treatment with Light-wire Edgewise Appliances. 2nd ed. St. Louis: The C. V. Mosby Co., 1972.
50. Gehrman, R. E. Dental Photography: Today's Camera and the Growing Practice. Tulsa: PennWell Publishing Co., 1982.
51. Gholston, L. R. Reliability of an intraoral camera: utility for clinical dentistry and research. Am. J. Orthod. 85:89–93, 1984.
52. Tanaka, M. M., and Johnson, L. E. The prediction of the size of unerupted canines and premolars in a contemporary orthodontic population. J. Am. Dent. Assoc. 88:798–801, 1974.
53. Bimler, H. P. The Bimler appliance. p. 357. In T. M. Graber and B. Neumann (eds.) Removable Orthodontic Appliances. Philadelphia: W. B. Saunders Co., 1979.
54. Schwartz, A. M. Lehrgang der Gebissregelung. 2nd ed. Vol. 1. Vienna: Urban and Schwarzenberg, 1956.

Chapter 5

Postural and Nutritional Considerations

Head and body posture are important for a correct diagnosis and treatment result. Side bending of the head or winging of the scapulae are classic signs of possible postural complications of malocclusion or disorders of the craniomandibular articulation (Chapter 10).

The examination and diagnostic process (Chapter 4) also requires the integration of adequate patient nutritional information in order to achieve the optimal end result of treatment. It makes little sense to correct a malocclusion and ignore a potential periodontal or dental caries problem. Correcting a malocclusion for an individual who is nutritionally out of control will rarely enhance overall health.

The primary goal of optimal nutrition for treating malocclusion is early prevention of occlusal and facial growth discrepancies (caries or early tooth loss). An excellent nutritional status may shorten treatment time and help the appliances function better. If the nutritional status of the patient is questionable, a method of discovery is suggested with a health quiz, diet experiment, and proposed schedule of vitamin and mineral supplementation, all of which are explained later in this chapter.

Postural considerations

A diagnosis is made after careful consideration of all possibilities from the data. If the examination has been accomplished carefully, the diagnosis and treatment will enhance the health of the individual. The overall treatment goal is to bring the patient closer to a state of optimal health. Since heredity is an important predisposition for malocclusion,[1,2] observation of parental facial form, posture, and occlusion may aid in arriving at a diagnosis.

If the patient's postural position on entering the examination room shows the shoulders rolled inward, cervical spine curved forward, and the head in extension (Fig. 5-1), this could indicate cranial or cervical discomfort. Some research indicates that patients with an Angle Class II malocclusion tip the head upward to compensate for the retruded mandible.[3] The relationship of the head in extension on the atlas (Fig. 5-2) can compress neurovascular bundles that traverse to the external musculature of the cranium.[4] This compression may cause peripheral nerve entrapment, neuropathy, and muscle pain.[5] Figures 5-3 and 5-4 show abnormal and normal occiput-atlas relationships.

The patient is questioned about the location of any possible head pain. Since there is a strong correlation among facial pain, temporomandibular joint pain, and cervical

Postural and Nutritional Considerations

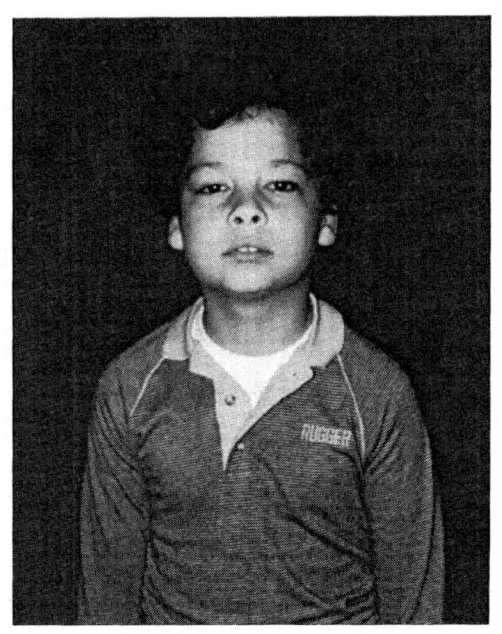

Fig. 5-1 R. T. as he presented for treatment with a chief complaint of severe headache several times each week.

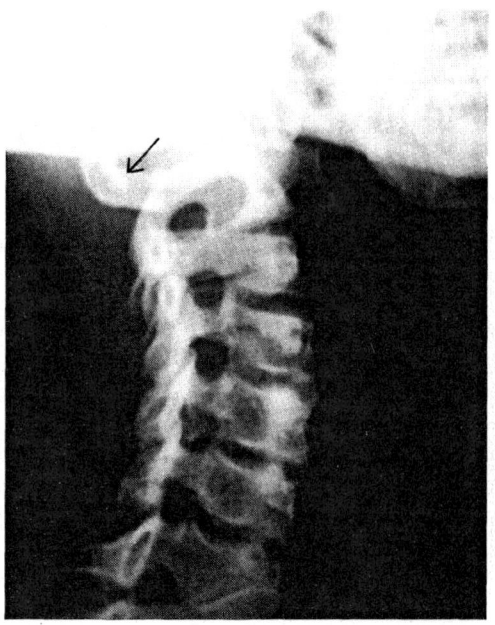

Fig. 5-2 This head position presents the possibility of nerve compression pathology. Note the position of the occiput of the cranium and the atlas or C-1 vertebrae. Osseous projection is from the occiput. (Courtesy of Ira M. Yerkes, D.M.D.)

spinal pathology,[6] it is important that the source of the pain be located. Once area localization has occurred, the proper health professional can be called in for consultation and treatment planning. Figure 5-5 diagrammatically shows the craniocervical areas that are affected by upper cervical nerve irritations.

Head posture

The position of the head or the orthostatic stability of the cranium over the cervical spine is important in diagnosing pain and dysfunction in the craniomandibular region.[7] Kapandji[8] considers the head in equilibrium when the eyes can look ahead horizontally. In this position, the occlusal plane and the auriculonasal plane (AN) (which passes through the nasal spine and the superior border of the external auditory meatus) are also horizontal.

The head and neck resemble a lever system (Fig. 5-6) with the fulcrum 0 at the level of the occipital condyles. A force is produced by the weight of the head (G) applied through its center of gravity lying near the sella turcica. A force is produced by the posterior neck muscles (F), which constantly counterbalance the weight of the head. The strength of the posterior neck muscles determines the extent to which this weight is properly counterbalanced. The constant tone of the posterior neck muscles prevents the head from tilting forward. An awareness of correct head position with respect to the observed head position can suggest the possibility of malocclusion before direct examination of the dentition. Fig-

Postural Considerations

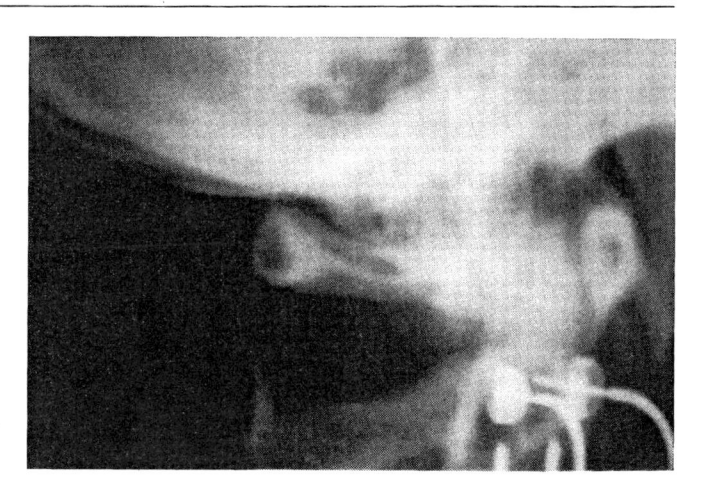

Fig. 5-3 Close approximation of occiput and atlas.

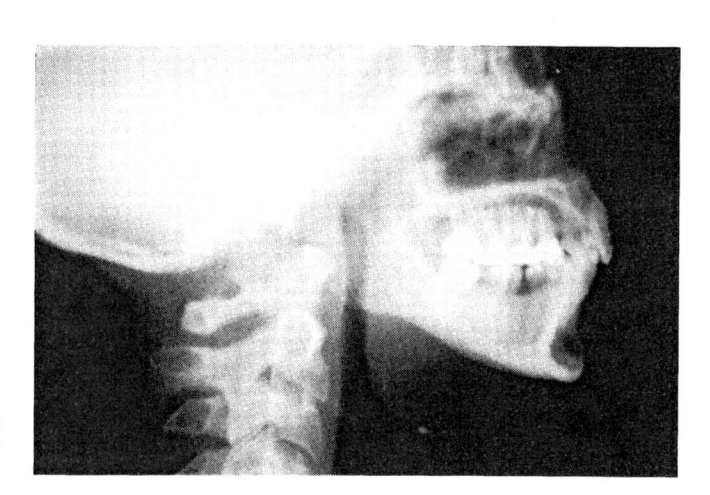

Fig. 5-4 Normal radiographic space between atlas and occiput.

ure 5-6 shows the relationship of the center of gravity of the cranium to the spinal column.

The strong posterior neck muscles help to balance the head in the correct postural position (Fig. 5-7). If strong, bulging sternocleidomastoid muscles are evident, as in Fig. 5-8, then a possible postural complication of a malocclusion could be suspected.

Other criteria for determining the correct head position are the bipupilar, otic, and transverse occlusal planes (Fig. 5-9).[9]

The dental occlusion, muscles of mastication, and craniocervical muscles are interrelated. In the presence of a malocclusion, the musculature will try to "unbalance" the mandible and cranium to one side or backward to compensate for the dysfunction. However, bioreceptors in the middle ear and tooth proprioception reposition the head to keep the bipupilar, otic, and transverse occlusal planes parallel to the horizon. Most often, the head will adopt a more forward position on the cervical spine. As the head repositions forward, the sternocleidomastoid muscles contract, bulge, and become more prominent as they try to keep the head in extension and the three planes parallel to the horizon.

Postural and Nutritional Considerations

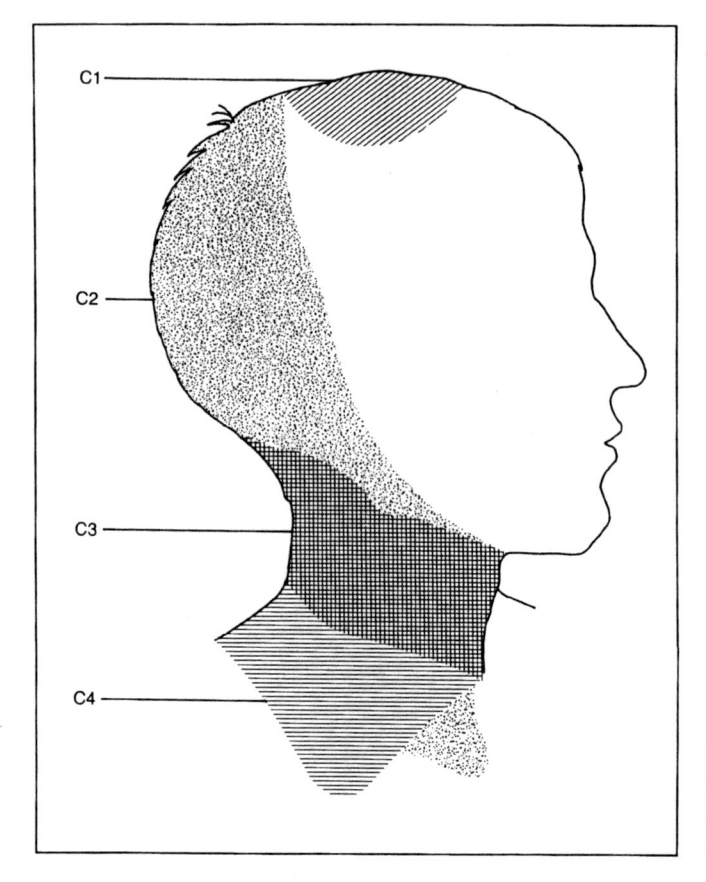

Fig. 5-5 An irritation or lesion in C-1 through C-4 can affect specific areas of the head and neck, with painful hyperesthesia or even anesthesia.[7]

Correlation of body posture and facial form

It is important to correlate body posture and facial form with other diagnostic data. An everted lower lip and deep mentonian groove can be the result of a reduced vertical dimension, or lack of vertical growth of the face (Figs. 5-10a to c). Cephalometric radiography can confirm vertical growth discrepancies and guide treatment. For example, a patient with a well-proportioned maxilla, a smaller-than-normal mandibular plane angle, and no mandibular incisor tooth structure visible in maximum intercuspation may require a treatment plan that redirects or stimulates mandibular growth and vertical development.

A patient with a shortened upper lip, an ANB angle lower than average, and anterior crossbite should be evaluated to assess whether the problem is mandibular prognathism, hypotonic maxillary development, or both. (Occasionally these patients are nicknamed by unkind classmates because of the flattened facial appearance.) If the malocclusion is the result of a lack of midface development, treatment should be directed at stimulating maxillary growth and horizontal development. Mandibular prognathism may be treated with chin-cup external retraction. The best results are obtained when treatment is initiated early, by age 6.[10] If mandibular prognathism is excessive, with an anterior crossbite of more than 6 mm and the maxilla is within normal cephalo-

Postural Considerations

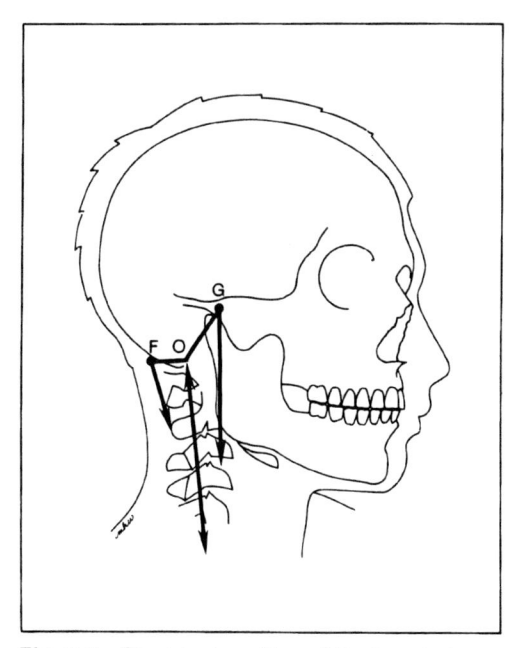

Fig. 5-6 The ideal position of the head places the center of gravity slightly forward of the cervical spine. (Modified from Kapandji.)

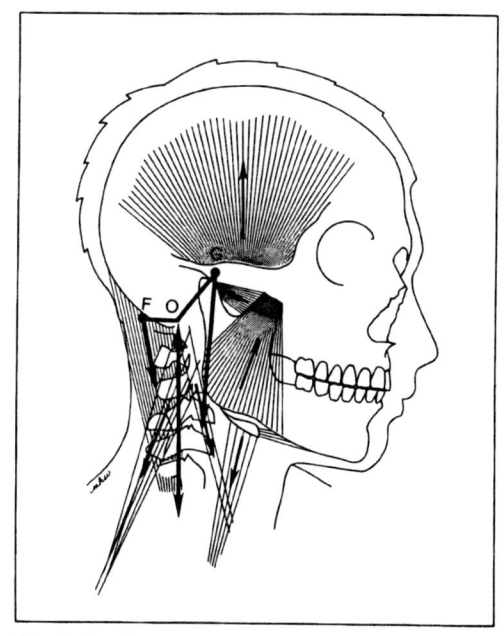

Fig. 5-7 With the cranium balanced in this orthostatic position, there is little need for strong anterior cervical musculature.

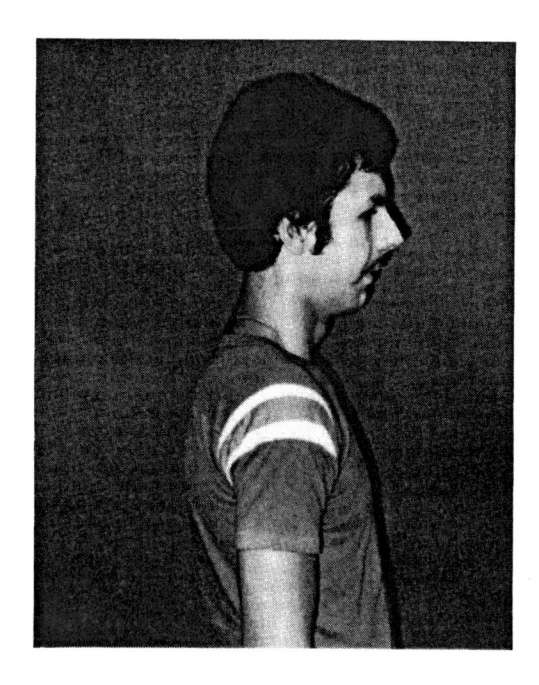

Fig. 5-8 The well-developed sternocleidomastoid muscles are evident. This patient had been previously treated with four premolar extractions for dental crowding. The posture and facial profile are unacceptable; head, neck, and back pain were not evident before treatment.

Postural and Nutritional Considerations

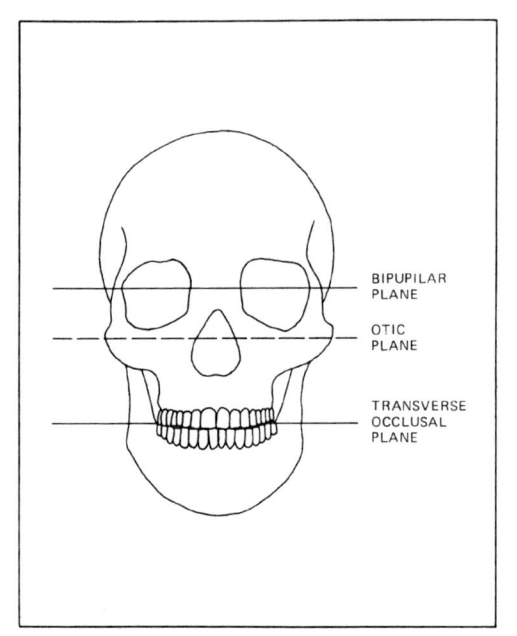

Fig. 5-9 In a normal postural position, these three planes are parallel to each other and to the floor.

metric limits, then surgical reduction of the size of the mandible may be a consideration after the patient has matured and mandibular growth is near completion. The reduction osteotomy can be suggested earlier, if the size of the mandible interferes with the psychosocial development of the patient. However, the patient and family should be informed that further surgical intervention might be necessary if there is further disproportionate mandibular growth.[11] McNamara[12] has discussed the relationship between impaired and obstructed breathing and changes in mandibular posture and function. Significant improvement in facial growth patterns were observed after upper airway obstructions were removed. Mitani[13] has shown that the fundamental growth components of mandibular prognathism are established early in life. Once the mandibular growth components were established as excessive in this study, the growth rate was seen to be similar to that of the normal face before puberty.

Nutritional considerations

When the stomatognathic system fails because of dental stress (e.g., tooth loss, dental caries, or craniomandibular disorder), a common cause is a modern "civilized" lifestyle. Of particular significance in lifestyle errors is improper nutrition.[14]

> The food we find in supermarkets, restaurants, and cafeterias is so familiar to us, so completely intermeshed with almost every aspect of our lives, that it is difficult to come to the realization that some of it eaten in the quantities now generally consumed, may be debilitating or deadly.
>
> Nevertheless, a growing number of studies suggest that that is exactly the case. The amounts of fat, saturated fat, cholesterol, sugar, and salt being consumed in the United States may be major factors in the incidence of heart disease, bowel, breast, and colon cancer, diabetes and stroke, to name some of the most widespread diseases that have been related to diet. These dietary elements, like other substances having an adverse cumulative effect on the body, appear innocuous, even appealing, in individual portions. However, their impact may be devastating.
>
> Sen. George McGovern[15]

The nutritional status of the patient is evaluated to ensure a proper diagnosis and facilitate treatment planning. The requirements of certain nutrients can be expected to be elevated for an individual who is subjected to the demands of rapid growth, biomechanical oral intrusion of an appliance, and almost continual fast-food advertising.

Postural Considerations

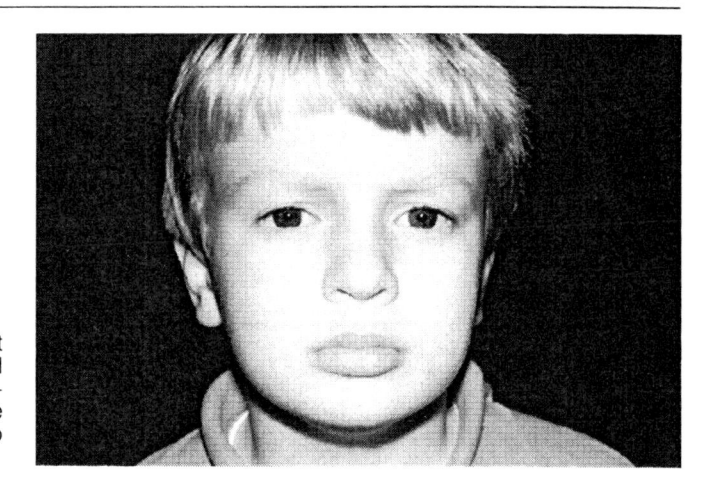

Figs. 5-10a to c This patient demonstrates a lack of vertical development and a Class II malocclusion (overjet 7 mm). Notice the everted lower lip and deep mentonian groove.

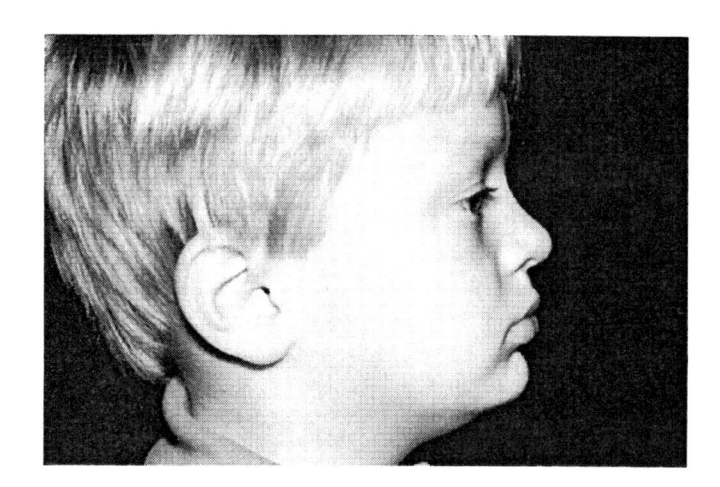

Fig. 5-10b

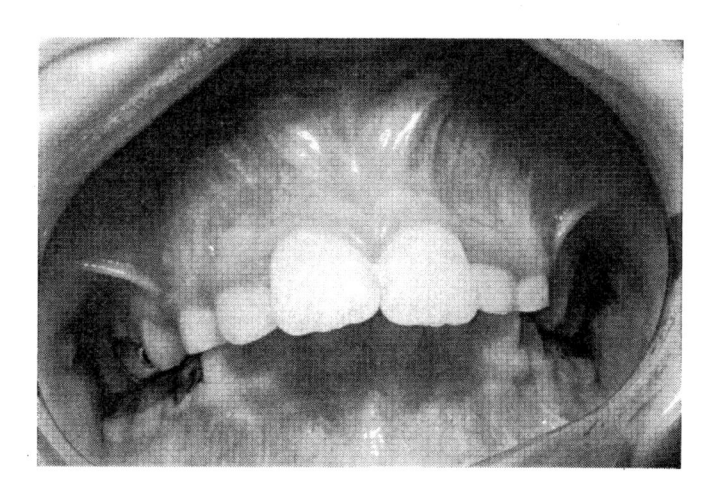

Fig. 5-10c

Factors that influence the nutritional status of the rapidly growing child are a nonnutritious diet, emotional stress, and a high level of physical activity.[16]

Nutritional considerations are most critical during growth and development, especially amidst environmental challenges. Such challenges act on the growing patient, particularly the adolescent facing the physiological and psychological stresses of puberty. The nutritional status of the patient with a malocclusion can affect the biological response of the periodontal ligament and bone to orthopedic forces, and the response of the periodontium to orthodontic bands and brackets.[16]

Influence of ascorbic acid on maxillofacial orthopedics

Many nutrients influence the biological response to orthopedic forces on the dentition and craniofacial skeletal tissues; ascorbic acid is a classic example. Cheraskin and Ringsdorf[17] have studied the effects of ascorbic acid levels during treatment for malocclusion. It has been shown that patients receiving treatment for malocclusion may benefit from ascorbic acid supplementation. Seven out of 10 patients being treated for malocclusion were found deficient in Vitamin C testing.[18] A lack of this nutrient interferes with collagen synthesis by preventing the hydroxylation of proline to hydroxyproline. This interference of hydroxylation affects the health of the periodontal ligament by causing edematous spaces and histologic disorientation of fibroblasts and collagen fibers while the teeth are undergoing orthodontic forces. The formation of osteoid tissue is also adversely affected. Animal studies have shown untoward histologic alterations to the periodontium as forces were applied to the teeth when the diet was deficient in ascorbic acid. These animals demonstrated enlarged endosteal spaces with osteoclasts, an uneven periosteal surface with osteoclastic activity, and periosteal hemorrhages.[19]

McCanlies et al.[20] have shown that ascorbic acid may have an effect on the stability and posttreatment retention time of animals that have undergone orthodontic forces. Vitamin C supplementation may benefit patients during and after treatment.

Nutrition is also an important factor in plaque control for the patient being treated for malocclusion. Although most orthopedic forces do not utilize a banded technique, the status of the periodontium must be monitored throughout treatment. Dusterwinkle et al.[21] have shown that patients with banded orthodontic treatment and multivitamin-trace mineral supplementation had a more favorable gingival condition than patients subjected to orthodontic banding and a placebo supplement. A bonded technique may cause less stress to the periodontal membrane because of less chance for plaque accumulation and little or no interference with the periodontal ligament space. The foreign body effect of an appliance in the mouth (fixed or removable) will cause an increased amount of dental plaque. If a plaque-free dentition cannot be maintained, a delay in treatment until oral hygiene is improved is preferable to iatrogenic gingival pathology.

There is evidence that the use or abuse of alcohol or drugs may increase nutritional requirements. A nutritional deficiency in the mother may result in cleft lip or cleft palate in the offspring. This phenomenon has been shown in laboratory animals.[22] The administration of vitamin and mineral supplements to pregnant women may lessen the chance of nutritionally induced cleft lip or cleft palate.[23]

Health varies with level of nutrition

Improper nutrition leads to poor health and possibly death (Fig. 5-11). Conversely, optimal health can be achieved when optimal

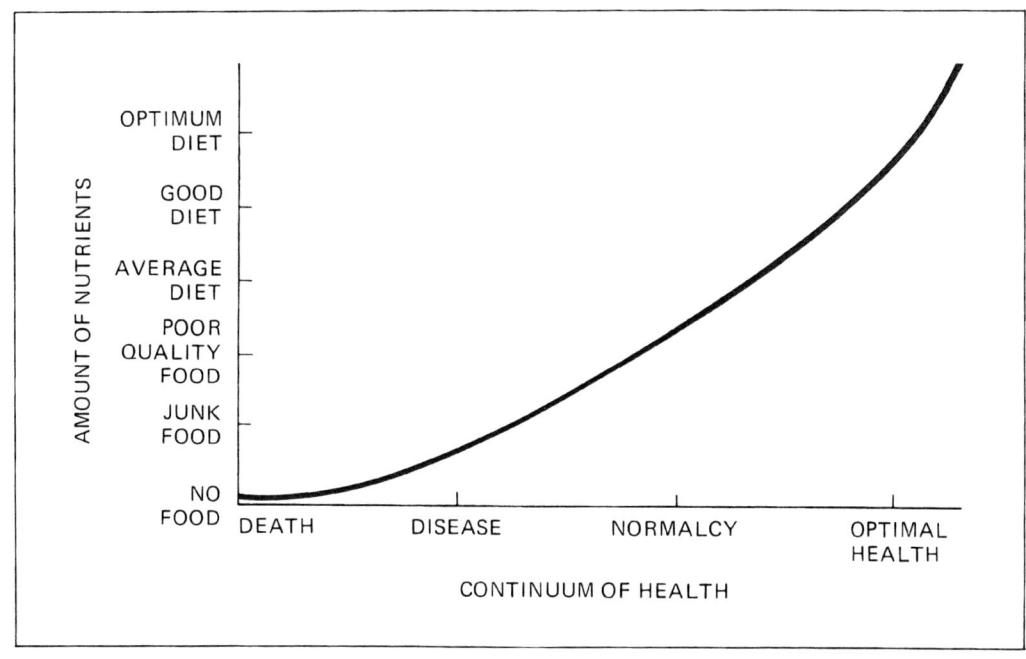

Fig. 5-11 Continuum of health.

nutrition for the individual is combined with other positive health habits (e.g., exercise, proper sleep, and abstinence from smoking). The current nutritional status of most developed countries is far less than optimal. What can be done to bring about optimal nutrition on an individual basis in the dental office when treating malocclusion?

RDA and nutrition

Many people feel that when the RDA requirements (recommended dietary allowance), have been met, *all* nutritional requirements have been satisfied. In reality, meeting the RDA or MDR (minimum daily requirements) will prevent gross forms of disease, but the necessary nutrients to approach optimal health may still be lacking.

The RDA is formulated by a committee: The Food and Nutrition Board of the National Academy of Sciences. The purpose is to determine the amount of nutrients that would prevent death or serious illness from an overt deficiency in most people. These are by no means the amounts that lead to the best possible health! The optimal daily intake may be two to five times the RDA. For vitamin C, the optimal amount may be five to 100 times the RDA for a given individual.

Even with the RDA as a minimum nutritional requirement, a surprising number of people have historically been malnourished in the United States. In 1942, only one person in 1,000 escaped malnutrition in some form.[24] While many nutrients were not studied, the most deficient nutrients were vitamins A and D and the minerals calcium and phosphorus.

U.S. national statistics

In 1955, the U.S. Department of Agriculture (USDA) found that only 6% of Americans'

125

diets met the RDA standards.[25] In 1959, the USDA showed that 75% of American women had less than 66% of the RDA of calcium and 40% were low in vitamins B and C. In 1969, the U.S. Public Health Service released figures from a 12,000-person, 10-state study of people from all walks of life. They based their study on written surveys and blood and urine samples. The study showed the following:[26]

- 20% had one or more essential nutrients below the minimum acceptable levels
- 19% were deficient in vitamin B_2
- 15% were deficient in vitamin C
- 13% were deficient in vitamin A
- 33% of children under 6 years of age had iron-deficiency anemia
- 5% had protein or calorie shortages severe enough to cause a pot belly and winged scapula
- 5% had iodine deficiency severe enough to cause enlarged thyroids

In summing up our nutritional status, Mayer stated (as chairman of the 1969 White House Nutrition Conference): "Malnutrition, whether caused by poverty or improper diet, contributes to the alarming health situation in the United States today."[26]

Dr. Edith Weir of the USDA reported in 1971 that if we all met the minimal RDA levels, about 300,000 deaths a year from heart disease and stroke and 150,000 deaths from cancer could be prevented.[25]

The changing American diet

From a nutritional point of view, the most significant changes in the American diet in the last 65 years have been:[27]

Increase in fat consumption. Fat provided 42% of our calories in 1976, *31% more* than the 32% of our calories that fat supplied in 1910.

Decrease in complex carbohydrates. Complex carbohydrates (basically starch) accounted for only 21% of our calories in 1976, *43% less* than the 37% of calories that complex carbohydrates provided in 1910.

Increase in sweetener consumption. Refined sugar, corn syrup, and other calorie sweeteners supplied 18% of our calories in 1976, a full *50% more* than the 12% caloric intake that sweeteners furnished our grandparents in 1910.

These changes would be of only academic interest if they were not linked to important changes in the public health. In January 1977, the Senate Select Committee on Nutrition and Human Needs published a study that recapped dietary changes. The report noted that six of the 10 leading causes of death in the United States are linked to diet: heart attack, stroke, arteriosclerosis, cancer, cirrhosis of the liver, and diabetes. The Senate committee called for seven specific changes in the current American diet:[15]

1. Increase the consumption of complex carbohydrates and naturally occurring sugars from about 28% of energy or calorie intake to 48%.
2. Reduce overall fat consumption from approximately 40% to 30% of energy intake.
3. Reduce saturated fat consumption to account for about 10% of total energy intake; and balance that with polyunsaturated and monounsaturated fats, which should each account for about 10% of energy intake.
4. Reduce cholesterol consumption to about 300 mg a day.
5. Reduce the consumption of refined sugars by about 45% to account for about 10% of total energy intake.
6. Reduce salt consumption by 15 to 70% to approximately 5 grams a day.
7. To avoid becoming overweight, consume only as much energy or calories as is expended; if overweight, decrease

energy intake and increase energy expenditure.

Toward optimal nutrition

Unhealthy habits detract from good nutrition. Breslow in 1974 reported a five- and one-half-year study of 7,000 Californians at the University of California. They found that those who do the following are rewarded with good health:[26]

- have adequate sleep
- eat breakfast
- stay lean
- avoid empty-calorie foods
- not smoke
- exercise regularly
- abstain from or only moderately consume alcohol

The study found that men in their mid-50s who followed six or seven of the wise health practices were equal in health to men 20 years younger who followed three or less. For men 65 to 74 years who followed all seven of the practices the likelihood of dying was the same as men who were 45 to 54 years of age who ignored the practices. Passwater estimates that if supernutrition were part of the American diet, 500,000 to 1 million lives could be saved each year.[26] A lifestyle devoted to health and nutrition leads to better health and longevity.

The quest for adequate nutrition

One of the reasons that the nation is having so many health problems is that the food *appears* to be nutritious when in fact it is not. There are two basic problems: *(1)* nonnutritious foods; *(2)* nonfoods as a large portion of the diet. In 1940, processed foods represented 10% of the American diet. In 1970, processed foods composed 50% of the diet; in 1980, they composed 60% of the American diet.[26]

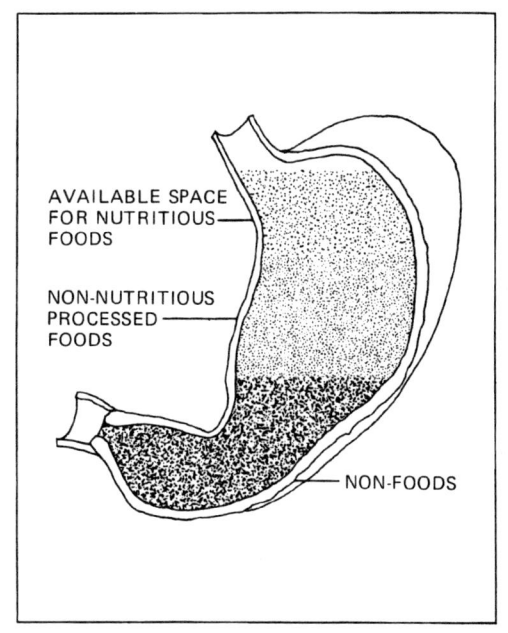

Fig. 5-12 The dietary content of a typical American stomach.

Foods rapidly lose nutrients from prolonged storage, processing, and cooking. If you eat garden-fresh peas they will lose 56% of the vitamins by the time they are cooked and served; frozen peas lose 83% and canned peas lose 94% of their nutritional value by the time they are prepared and served.

It is evident that people subsisting on refined, processed, and canned foods will not be provided with adequate nutrients. The 1969 nutrition survey has confirmed that the additional problem of nonfoods in the diet has become increasingly important.[26] Nonfoods have become part of every processed food; examples are found in colas, pastries, candy, and condiments. The amount of nonessential foods has been estimated to be 50% of the American diet (Fig. 5-12).

Brewster and Jacobson[27] have demonstrated and summarized the need for nutritional supplementation:

Postural and Nutritional Considerations

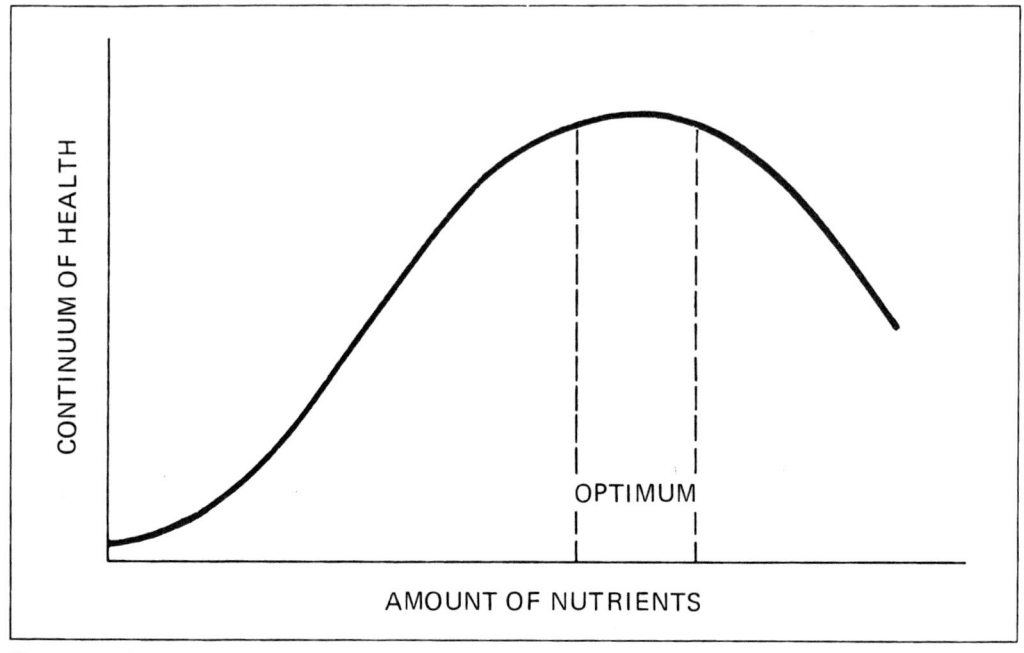

Fig. 5-13 Proper nutrition means moderation and balance. An excessive amount of any one nutrient can be deleterious to health.

1. Much of the food available for consumption is not fresh. Food loses much of its nutritional value unless consumed soon after it is harvested.
2. Commercially grown food products are grown in soil that may lack proper mineral balance. Although fertilizer supplements are added to the soil, the mineral content of commercially grown foods may be inadequate for proper nutrition.
3. Overcooking food to make it tender and easily chewed can destroy much of the nutritional value.
4. Much of the nutrient value of food is lost between harvesting and consumption. Food is chopped, husked, curried, colored, blanched, boiled, smoked, canned, and frozen before it is consumed. Many of the essential vitamins and minerals are lost in these refining processes.
5. A modern industrialized society makes many demands on the time of an individual, promoting irregular eating habits. Often, time is just not available for the purchase, preparation, and consumption of a nutritionally adequate diet.

Supernutrition

Farmers know the value of nutrition in crop production. Fryer[28] has stated that if a crop is farmed at 1 Baule (nitrogen fertilizer) unit, it will yield about 50% of its potential maximum yield. When farmed at 2 Baule units, a crop can be expected to produce 75% of its potential yield. Applying fertilizer at the rate of 3 Baule units would increase yield to 88% of maximum potential. These curves for farmers are similar to the supernutrition curves of Passwater, i.e., the greater the amount of nutrient (fertilizer), the greater the yield in health (crop). However, if too much of a nutrient is given it can become deleterious and the level of health will decrease (Fig. 5-13).

The old concept of disease prevention has related to correcting a lack of proper nutrition (e.g., vitamin C deficiency) or avoiding nonnutritious substances (e.g., sucrose); the new concept of supernutrition seeks to optimize health with the correct levels of nutrients.

Biochemical needs for supernutrition

No two people are exactly alike in height, weight, physiological, biochemical, or psychological composition. This uniqueness includes individual nutritional requirements for optimal health. Williams defined biochemical individuality in 1956:[29]

> The cumulative evidence that each individual . . . has a distinctive pattern of enzyme efficiency is hard to refute.
> . . . [I]ndividual variations in enzyme efficiency in normal individuals . . . are not of the order of 20 to 50%, but are more often at least 300 to 400%.

Definitive information is available regarding the variation in adult human needs for nine of the nearly 40 nutrients needed in the nutritional environment. The data from Williams are tabulated in Table 5-1.[30]

These limited data in Table 5-1 demonstrate wide variation in daily needs for nutrients. Nutritional requirements cannot be determined by committee for each individual. The patient should be compared with himself, not an arbitrary RDA standard. An objective method of nutritional evaluation would compare the individual with himself over a set period of time.

Individual monitoring of supernutrition

This nutritional plan has three components: the basic diet experiment, a health quiz, and a proposed schedule.

Because of the large amounts of nonfoods in the American diet and the poor nutrition available from processed foods, the basic diet experiment is used to separate the patient from nonfoods and to move toward realistic RDA levels.

The proposed dietary method to achieve optimal nutrition consists of two steps. The first step is to eliminate poor-quality foods from the diet. This is accomplished by using the "Basic Diet Experiment."[31] The second step adds nutrients like vitamins in optimal amounts. This is monitored by using the proposed "Health Quiz." These two steps can help lead to optimal health.

The Health Quiz, modified from Passwater, is used for adolescents and is constructed to arrive at a score. The quiz is largely subjective in nature, but since mea-

Table 5-1 Daily range of adult nutrient needs

Nutrient	Daily range	Number of subjects
Tryptophan	82–250 mg (3-fold)	50
Valine	375–800 mg (2.1-fold)	48
Phenylalanine	420–1,100 mg (2.6-fold)	38
Leucine	170–1,100 mg (6.4-fold)	31
Lysine	400–2,800 mg (7-fold)	55
Isoleucine	250–700 mg (2.8-fold)	24
Methionine	800–3,000 mg (3.7-fold)	29
Threonine	103–500 mg (4.8-fold)	50
Calcium	222–1,018 mg (4.6-fold)	19

surement is subclinical, the score is useful for comparative purposes. The scores are recorded and plotted.

The basic diet experiment

The diet experiment, modified from Eversaul,[31] gives suggestions for foods to increase and foods to minimize for optimal nutrition.

Foods to increase

Fresh fruits and fresh vegetables. At least one fresh vegetable and one fresh fruit should be eaten each day. Frozen products are generally acceptable, but they should be consumed in addition to the fresh foods recommended. Canned vegetables and fruits should be avoided; these processed foods may have large amounts of refined sugar or corn sweeteners, which may hinder treatment objectives.

At least one green salad should be consumed each day. Oil and apple cider vinegar dressing rather than commercially prepared dressings, which can contain large amounts of sweeteners, are preferred.

Intake of fish and seafood should also be increased. Finally, eight glasses of water and unsweetened fruit and vegetable juices—low-salt tomato, orange, low-salt V-8, carrot, pineapple, unsweetened cran-apple, or grapefruit—are advised.

Foods to decrease

For one week, the following foods are avoided: refined sugars, processed carbohydrates, artificial sweeteners, *all* forms of coffee, all colas, white flour products, salt, and alcohol.

Optional foods

Herbal teas, Pero, or Postum can be substituted for coffee. For a sweetener, up to 2 tablespoons of *unprocessed* honey can be used daily. (Read the label to make sure that no refined sugar has been added.)

Health quiz

The following quiz (modified from Passwater[26]) is scored with 5 points for each *a* answer, 4 points for each *b* answer, 3 points for each *c* answer, 2 points for each *d* answer, and 1 point for each *e* answer. The total score reflects the relative health and the likely nutritional status of the patient, and is important only as a means of periodic nutritional evaluation.

Choose only one letter for each question.

1. Blood pressure (normal from 90/60 to 140/90).
   Is blood pressure:
   a. 120/80 or less
   b. between 121/80 and 125/85
   c. between 126/85 and 140/90
   d. between 141/90 and 165/95
   e. above 165/95

2. Energy level
   Do you normally feel:
   a. peppy, zesty
   b. alert
   c. average
   d. tired, sluggish
   e. exhausted

3. Mood
   Are you:
   a. thrilled with life
   b. happy
   c. average, OK
   d. blah
   e. depressed, moody

4. Stamina
   Is your endurance:
   a. excellent
   b. good
   c. average
   d. fair
   e. poor

5. Bowel regularity
   Are your bowels:
   a. very regular
   b. mostly regular
   c. almost regular
   d. poorly regular
   e. constipated

6. Headaches
   Do you have headaches:
   a. no more than once or twice a year and mild
   b. seldom
   c. occasionally
   d. often
   e. often and severe

7. Pulse rate (after 15 minutes of rest; normals 65 to 90, average 75)
   My pulse rate is:
   a. below 65
   b. between 65 and 70
   c. between 71 and 75
   d. between 76 and 85
   e. above 85

8. Obesity
   My body weight is:
   a. less or the same as "ideal" weight (according to height/weight table, Figs. 5-14a and b)
   b. less than 10% above "ideal"
   c. between 11 and 15% above "ideal"
   d. between 16 and 20% above "ideal"
   e. more than 20% above "ideal"

9. Skin, hair, and nails
   (Improved refers to the time since you last answered the question.)

Characteristic	Condition a	b	c
skin	smooth	improved	rough
veins showing in face	none	reduced	yes
veins showing in legs	none	reduced	yes
nails, color	normal (pinkish)	—	discolored or pale
hair, condition	glossy	—	dry and brittle
hair, amount	normal or regrowing	—	balding
hair, color	normal or returning	—	graying
eyes	bright and clear	—	dull or red (blood vessels)
circles under eyes	none	reduced	yes
bruise easily	no	—	yes

Give 1 point for each answer in column a.

10. Oral

Characteristic	Condition a	Condition b	Condition c
gums	healthy	improved	diseased
tongue, color	normal	—	pale or red
tongue, surface	normal	—	rough or swollen
breath	odorless	—	halitosis
mouth sores	none	—	yes

Give 1 point for each answer in column a.

11. Miscellaneous

Condition	a	b
dizziness or fainting spells	yes	no
buzzing or ringing in ears	yes	no
allergy	yes	no
cough (chronic)	yes	no
indigestion or heartburn	yes	no
weakness if meals delayed	yes	no
hard stools	yes	no
poor appetite	yes	no
nausea	yes	no
trouble sleeping	yes	no
stiff joints	yes	no
hemorrhoids	yes	no
transparency of urine	cloudy	clear

Give 1 point for each column b answer.

Schedule for optimum vitamin supplementation

Week 1
 a. Take the Health Quiz and plot the score.
 b. Follow the Basic Diet Experiment for 10 days.

Weeks 2 and 3
 a. Take the Health Quiz and plot the score.
 b. Follow the Supernutrition Plan part one (Passwater):
  1. one high-potency vitamin and mineral pill immediately after breakfast
  2. two B-Complex tablets (50 mg each), one before or with breakfast and the other with dinner
  3. three vitamin C tablets (250 mg each), one with each meal

4. one vitamin E (200 IU) at bedtime

Weeks 4 and 5
a. Take the Health Quiz and plot the score.
b. Follow the Supernutrition Plan part two (Passwater):
  1. one high potency vitamin and mineral pill immediately after breakfast
  2. three B complex tablets (50 mg each), one at breakfast, one at dinner, and one at bedtime
  3. four vitamin C tablets (250 mg each), one at each meal and one at bedtime
  4. one vitamin E (200 IU) at bedtime

Summary

Several researchers have studied the relationship of craniofacial morphology to head and body posture. Vig et al.[32] have shown predictable jaw separation during nasal obstruction. Solow and Tallgren[33] have studied head posture and craniofacial form and the relationship of dentoalveolar morphology to craniocervical posture.[34] These studies indicate that head posture is influenced by respiration, deglutition, balance, sight, and hearing, in addition to the force of gravity. Daly and co-workers[35] have studied the effects of a standard mechanically created open bite. An 8 mm open bite resulted in extension of the neck for most of the experimental subjects. The study by Von Treuenfels[3] and reports from Harvold et al.[36] and McNamara[37] indicate that altered function may influence osseous morphology. The long-term results of treatment are dependent on physiologically compatible facial muscle balance. Although head posture and general body posture are important for diagnostic considerations, cervicospinal posture is also important for assessing the final treatment results.

A treatment regime that results in a forward head position or a dentition compromised by caries, poor coronal contact, or periodontal problems cannot be considered optimal. Orthopedic appliances stimulate and redirect bone and cartilage growth in the condylar head region, posterior border of the ramus, maxillary sutural areas, and throughout the craniofacial skeleton. A nutritionally compromised diet may result in less than optimal growth. An excess of highly refined carbohydrates combined with appliance wear may be deleterious for the dentition.

Ringsdorf and Cheraskin have demonstrated other sucrose induced defects in metabolism and suggest careful scrutiny of the label on all packaged foods. If the word sugar or other terms signifying sugar content (e.g., sucrose, invert sugar, turbinado sugar, brown sugar, dextrose, glucose, corn syrup, or corn sweeteners) are used, then be wary of the sugar content. If several of these terms are used, the food can be predominately sugar[38] (Table 5-2).

Biological individuality and flexibility must be considered when implementing changes in nutrition. The overall goal is to reduce or eliminate the intake of nonfoods, increase the intake of whole foods, and to supplement, where necessary, as determined by the score of the Health Quiz.

Even though the diagnosis is made early—based on facts from the data collected—the treatment plan occasionally must wait for the patient to mature. If an individual is not mature enough to be conscientious about wearing an orthopedic appliance or maintaining a good nutritional regime, the correct diagnosis and a well-implemented treatment plan may bring only partial success. Delayed treatment is more successful than early treatment prematurely terminated.

Postural and Nutritional Considerations

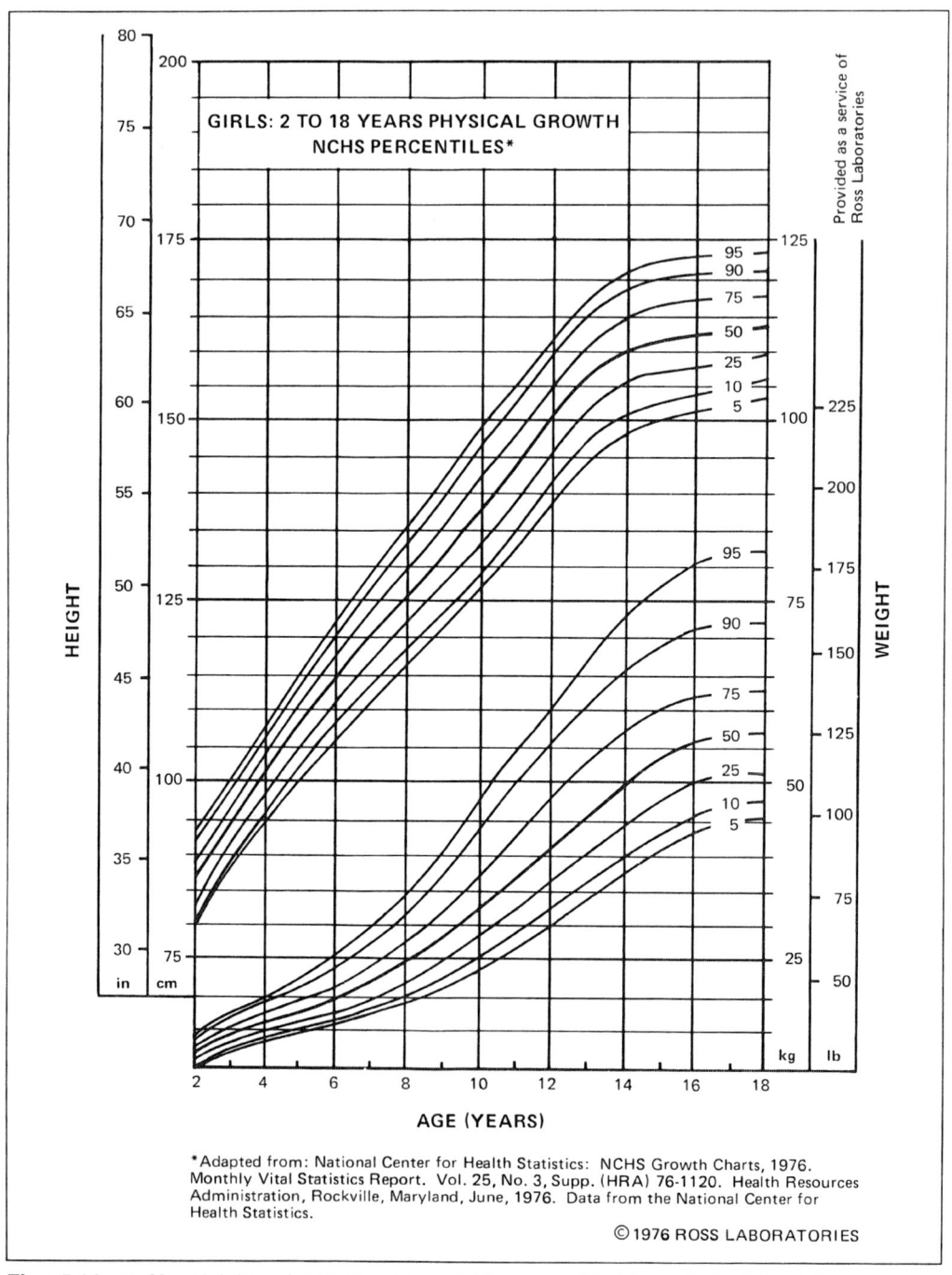

Figs. 5-14a and b Height-weight tables. The height and weight of the individual should be monitored throughout treatment. Aberrations in growth, nutrition, and health should be noted and corrected. The plotted chart can be used as a guideline for monitoring patient development.

134

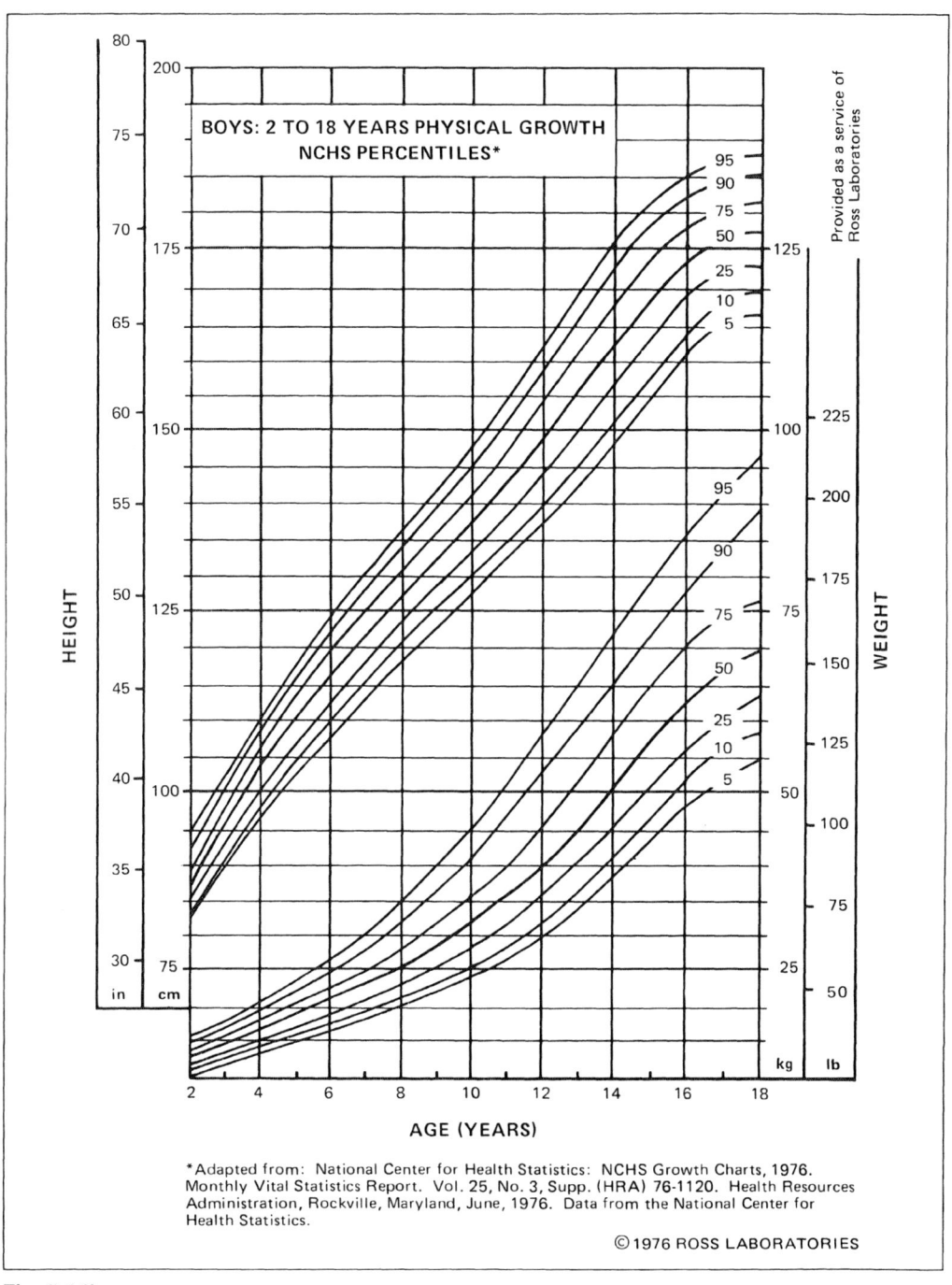

Fig. 5-14b

Table 5-2 Sucrose induced defects in metabolism*

Metabolic defects induced by dietary sucrose	Disorders influenced by metabolic defect
Increases dental plaque	Caries, periodontal disease
Increases *Candida albicans*	Oral and vaginal moniliasis
Decreases phagocytosis	All infectious disorders
Increases blood uric acid	Gout, diabetes, cardiovascular disease
Increases blood cholesterol	Cardiovascular disease
Increases bile cholesterol	Gallstones
Increases blood triglycerides	Cardiovascular disease, gout, diabetes
Increases platelet stickiness	Cardiovascular disease
Increases blood sugar	Diabetes, cardiovascular disease, periodontal disease, gout, others
Increases blood insulin	Reactive hypoglycemia, diabetes, periodontal disease
Increases body fat synthesis and storage	Obesity, diabetes, cardiovascular disease, gout, others
Limits ability of bombesin and cholecystokinin to induce satiety and inhibit eating	Obesity, bulimia, anorexia nervosa
Increases intestinal transit	Disorders of colon and rectum, varicose veins, hemorrhoids, cancer of colon and rectum, constipation
Increases urinary calcium excretion	Urinary lithiasis, osteoporosis (including alveolar bone loss)
Increases urine ph	Urinary lithiasis, genitourinary infections
Increases gastric acidity	Indigestion, peptic ulcer
Encourages malnutrition	All diseases
Increases blood pressure	Hypertension, cardiovascular diseases
Increases tissue lactic acid during circulatory arrest	Brain and CNS damage

*Reprinted with permission from J. Pedod. 8:123–137, 1984.

Concepts for early prevention of malocclusion

No age is too early to begin thinking about preventing malocclusion from occurring. Young couples contemplating a family should be counseled about the positive effects of fluoride, and the negative effects of alcohol and tobacco on the growing fetus. Some studies indicate a favorable effect of prenatal fluoride supplementation.[39-41] Other studies indicate that more research is needed to verify the immunity against dental caries in the dentition of the offspring via prenatal fluoride ingestion.[42,43]

Encourage the parent to bring the child for an oral examination before the first birthday. It is upsetting for the parent, time-consuming and stressful for the clinician, and perhaps life-threatening for the child if bottle feeding or breast feeding caries results in hospitalization and general anesthesia for treatment.

References

1. van der Linden, F. P. G. M. Genetic and environmental factors in dentofacial morphology. Am. J. Orthod. 52:576–583, 1966.
2. Nakasima, A., Ichinose, M., Nakata, S., and Takahama, Y. Heredity factors in the craniofacial morphology of Angle's Class II and Class III malocclusions. Am. J. Orthod. 82:150–156, 1982.
3. Von Treuenfels, H. Die relation der atlas position bei prognathen und progener kieferanomalie. Fortschr. Kieferorthop. 42:482–491, 1981.
4. Kopell, H. P., and Thompson, W. A. L. Peripheral Entrapment Neuropathies. Huntington, N.Y.: Robert E. Krieger Publ. Co., 1976.
5. Lance, J. W. The Mechanism and Management of Headache. 2nd ed. London: Butterworths, 1973.
6. Friedman, A. P., and Pouch, C. F. Cafeleas y Jacquecas. Buenos Aires: Universitaria, 1973, Ch. 5.
7. Rocabado, S. M. Advanced Upper Quarter Manual. Tacoma, Wash.: Rocabado Institute, 1981.
8. Kapandji, A. I. The Physiology of the Joints. 2nd ed. Edinburgh: Churchill Livingstone, 1970, p. 217.
9. Rocabado, S. M. Head, Neck, and Temporomandibular Joint Dysfunctions Manual. Tacoma, Wash.: Rocabado Institute, 1981.
10. Graber, L. W. Chin-cup therapy for mandibular prognathism. Am. J. Orthod. 72:23–41, 1977.
11. Legan, H. L., Hill, S. C., and Sinn, D. P. Surgical-orthodontic treatment of dentofacial deformities. Dent. Clin. North Am. 25:131–156, 1981.
12. McNamara, J. A., Jr. Influence of respiratory pattern on craniofacial growth. Angle Orthod. 51:269–300, 1981.
13. Mitani, H. Prepubertal growth of mandibular prognathism. Am. J. Orthod. 80:546–553, 1981.
14. Stauth, C. Applying nutritional individuality. J. Nutr. Acad. 11:14–23, 77, 1979.
15. Report of the Select Committee on Nutrition and Human Needs, U.S. Senate. Eating in America: Dietary Goals for the United States. Cambridge, Mass.: The MIT Press, 1977.
16. Hickory, W., and Nanda, R. Nutritional consideration in orthodontics. Dent. Clin. North Am. 25:195–201, 1981.
17. Cheraskin, E., and Ringsdorf, W. M., Jr. Biology of the orthodontic patient. I: Plasma ascorbic acid levels. Angle Orthod. 39:137, 1969.
18. Cheraskin, E., and Ringsdorf, W. M., Jr. Biology of the orthodontic patient. II: Lingual vitamin C test scores. Angle Orthod. 39:324, 1969.
19. Litton, S. F. Orthodontic tooth movement during an ascorbic acid deficiency. Am. J. Orthod. 65:290, 1974.
20. McCanlies, J. M., et al. Effect of vitamin C on the mobility and stability of guinea pig incisors under the influence of orthodontic force. Angle Orthod. 31:257–263, 1961.
21. Dusterwinkle, S. A., et al. Tissue tolerance to orthodontic banding: a study in multivitamin-trace mineral supplementation. J. Periodontol. 37:132–145, 1966.
22. Zawoiski, E. J. Prevention of caffeine-induced cleft palate byl-glutamic acid. Toxicol. Appl. Pharmacol. 35:123–128, 1976.
23. Peer, L. A., et al. Study of 400 pregnancies with birth of cleft lip-plate infants. Plast. Reconstr. Surg. 22:442–449, 1958.
24. The Penn State College Bulletin 36 (52), 1942.
25. Human Nutrition Research Division. USDA-ARS. Washington, D.C.: U.S. Government Printing Office, 1971.
26. Passwater, R. A. SuperNutrition. New York: Simon & Schuster, 1975.
27. Brewster, L., and Jacobson, M. The Changing American Diet. Washington, D.C.: Center for Science in the Public Interest, 1978.
28. Fryer, L. Food Supplement Dictionary. New York: Mason and Lipscomb, 1975.
29. Williams, R. J. Biochemical Individuality. New York: John Wiley & Sons, 1956.
30. Williams, R. J. Physicians Handbook of Nutritional Science. Springfield, Ill.: Charles C. Thomas, 1978.
31. Eversaul, G. Dental Kinesiology. Las Vegas, Nev.: G. Eversaul, 1980.

32. Vig, P. S., Showfety, K., and Phillips, C. Experimental manipulation of head posture. Am. J. Orthod. 77:258–268, 1980.
33. Solow, B., and Tallgren, A. Head posture and craniofacial morphology. Am. J. Phys. Anthropol. 44:417–436, 1976.
34. Solow, B., and Tallgren, A. Dento-alveolar morphology in relation to craniocervical posture. Angle Orthod. 47:157–163, 1977.
35. Daly, P., Preston, C. B., and Evans, W. G. Postural response of the head to bite opening in adult males. Am. J. Orthod. 82:157–160, 1982.
36. Harvold, E. P., Vargevik, K., and Chierici, G. Primate experiments on oral sensation and dental malocclusion. Am. J. Orthod. 63:494–508, 1973.
37. McNamara, J. A., Jr. Neuromuscular and skeletal adaptations to altered function in the orofacial region. Am. J. Orthod. 64:578–606, 1973.
38. Ringsdorf, W. M., and Cheraskin, E. Optimal nutrition: a new prescription. J. Pedod. 8:123–137, 1984.
39. Glenn, F. B. Immunity conveyed by a fluoride supplement during pregnancy. J. Dent. Child. 44:391–395, 1977.
40. Glenn, F. B. Immunity conveyed by sodium fluoride supplement during pregnancy: part II. J. Dent. Child. 46:17–24, 1979.
41. Feltman, R., and Kosel, G. Prenatal and postnatal ingestion of fluorides. J. Dent. Med. 16:190–198, 1961.
42. Thystrup, A. Is there a biological rationale for prenatal fluoride administration? J. Dent. Child. 48:103–107, 1981.
43. Driscoll, W. S. A review of clinical research on the use of prenatal fluoride administration for prevention of dental caries. J. Dent. Child. 48:109–117, 1981.

Chapter 6

Treatment Planning

Treatment planning is a step-by-step method of achieving treatment objectives. Once the goal of treatment has been established, a logical, written sequential plan of treatment can be carried out.

Treatment goals

Treatment goals should take into consideration skeletal, esthetic, and functional relationships for long-term stability. During growth, the development of the maxilla leads to mandibular maturation. Achievement of the skeletal, functional, and esthetic goals for treatment can be facilitated through the use of maxillofacial orthopedic techniques. A treatment sequence that eliminates crossbites, anterior-posterior discrepancies, and vertical dimension abnormalities helps to shorten treatment time and complicated mechanotherapy.

Meeting the dental treatment objectives[1] for molar relationships, crown angulation (tip), crown inclination (labiolingual or buccolingual inclination), rotation, tight contact, and occlusal plane may require a fixed bonded-banded technique. However, no single treatment plan is right for each patient. The overall goal for treatment is to achieve the best possible occlusion in the shortest treatment time with the smallest degree of appliance intrusion. Results are evaluated on the basis of function, esthetics, and stability.

Esthetic goals

The "esthetic" aspect of treatment refers to the achievement of harmonious sagittal, transverse, and vertical growth in the facial skeleton and to achieving proper alignment and articulation in the dentition.

Facial skeletal asymmetries can be evaluated either by measuring the full-face and lateral-face photographs or in the clinic with the patient standing in a natural posture position.[2] Discrepancies in distances of particular anatomical structures from the midline will indicate facial asymmetry (Fig. 6-1).

Lateral evaluation of facial balance is accomplished by measuring from the soft tissue glabella to subnasale (upper facial height) and from the subnasale to soft tissue gnathion (lower facial height) (Fig. 6-2). The upper facial height should equal the lower facial height. The lower facial height can be evaluated by dividing it into halves at the vermillion border of the lower lip.

The presence or absence of adequate lip seal and the relationship of the upper to the lower lip are important for treatment planning. When the lips are at rest, approximately equal amounts of vermillion border

Treatment Planning

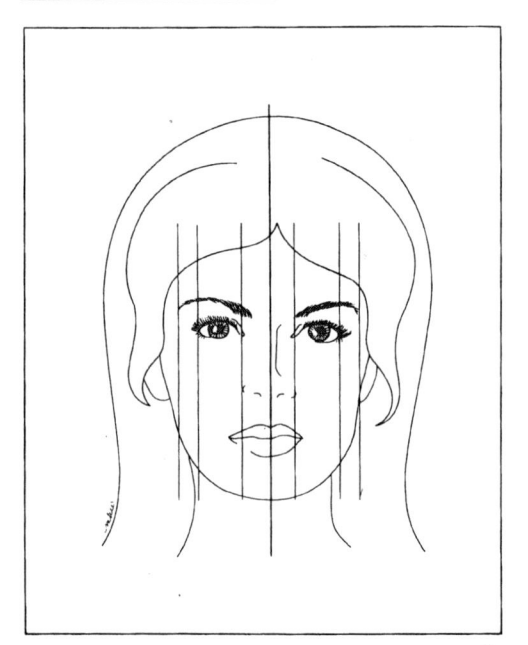

Fig. 6-1 Right and left asymmetry are easily evaluated by direct measurement from the midline.

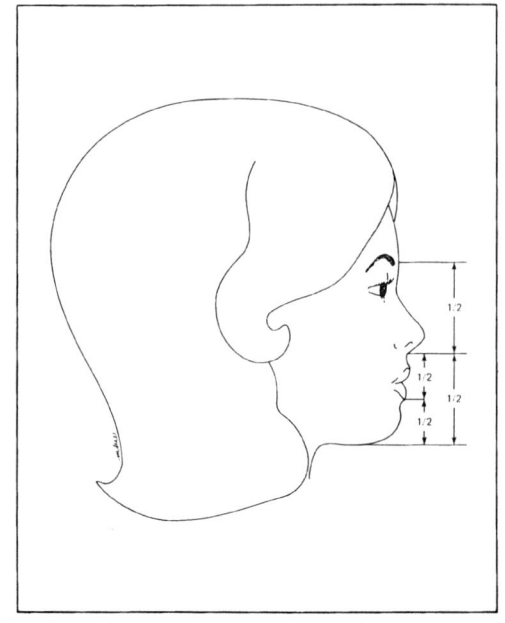

Fig. 6-2 Facial height discrepancies become evident on examination of the lateral profile.

should be visible; a small interlabial space is normal. Burstone[3] has shown that in patients with malocclusion and skeletal disharmony, the interlabial gap may be large or nonexistent. In the normal occlusal and skeletal relationship, only minimal lip contraction is needed in order to seal the lips. Facial symmetry and balance and lip posture are important concerns in setting goals for treatment planning.

Results can hardly be considered satisfactory if achievement of goals for the dental component involves a sacrifice in facial esthetics. For example, in a study of identical twin sisters, Eirew[4] has shown that extraction of premolar teeth may compromise facial esthetics. However, arch development through expansion can lead to the development of a fuller, slightly more protrusive facial profile and may help reduce dental crowding and bring about a more pleasing dental and facial appearance.

Functional goals

The functional component of treatment refers to the ability of the patient to perform mastication, deglutition, and the full range of mandibular movement without temporomandibular joint clicking or pain. One essential treatment objective is the development of a healthy, smoothly functioning temporomandibular joint articulation. The loss of tooth structure anterior to the first molar can result in a loss of vertical dimension. If the vertical dimension is reduced, the condyle may become positioned posteriorly or superiorly in the fossa. This aberrant positioning of the condyle may affect the functioning of the temporomandibular joint. Its effects can be either unilateral or bilateral and may include clicking; head, neck, or back pain; ringing in the ears; or temporomandibular joint pain.

In maximum intercuspation, the normally healthy condyle is located concentrically

Planning Treatment Sequence

within the fossa with at least 2 mm of joint space between the condyle and the temporal bone[5] (Fig. 6-3). The condyle will function smoothly in this concentric relationship to the fossa (see Chapter 10). The dental component of a normally functioning occlusion would show all teeth touching lightly at the same time in maximum intercuspation. When occlusal pressure is applied, there should be no deflection of the dental or skeletal components. The anterior guidance teeth should touch simultaneously with the posterior teeth during eccentric mandibular movements.

Stability as a treatment goal

Correction of malocclusion may take place over several years. It would be unfortunate if the treatment regime resulted in a dental component that was prone to relapse and a functional component that caused temporomandibular joint problems to develop later. If teeth are moved through the bone as a result of mechanical force, the periodontal fibers tend to bring the teeth back toward the original position. If teeth are mechanically moved from a stable position in the basal alveolar bone, a tendency to return to the original, more stable position is occasionally evident after completion of treatment. Maxillofacial orthopedic techniques guide the growth of the maxilla and mandible and counteract neuromuscular forces from the soft tissue components (tongue, cheeks, lips) (see Chapter 3). This increases the stability of the treated dentition.[6]

The stability of the periodontium is an additional consideration. The more protracted the treatment process and the more mechanotherapy that is utilized, the greater the chance of iatrogenic problems resulting from treatment (Fig. 6-4). Root resorption or elongated crowns can both result from prolonged or incorrect mechanotherapy (Fig. 6-5). If tooth movement through the bone is

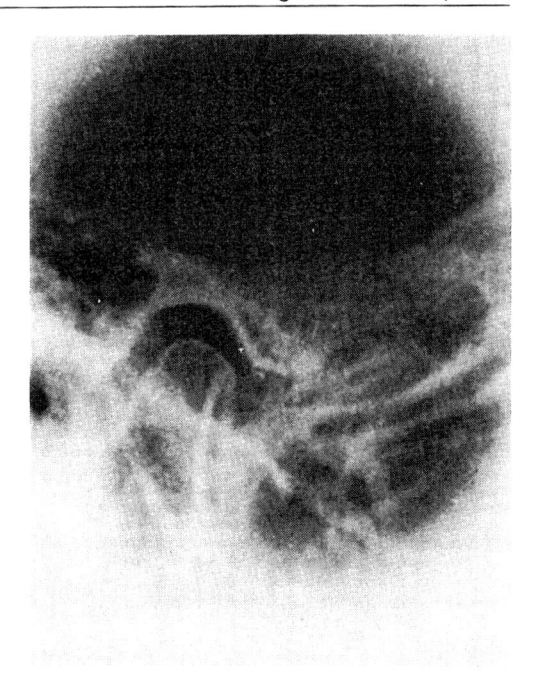

Fig. 6-3 This transcranial radiograph of a normal condyle-fossa relationship shows that the radiolucent articular disk is in its correct relationship to the mandibular condyle. Note the even amount of radiolucent joint space between the temporal bone and the condylar head. (Courtesy of Dr. William K. Solberg.)

minimized and natural development of the dentition encouraged using orthopedic forces, then the dental and temporomandibular joint components will be stable, with healthy periodontal tissues.

Planning treatment sequence

The course of treatment is to be kept basic. No one pattern of treatment can be effective for all patients. The prognosis for each patient should be viewed realistically. Realistic treatment goals can only result from objectivity in assessing the needs of each individual. A comprehensive examination and a well-delineated diagnosis are more

Treatment Planning

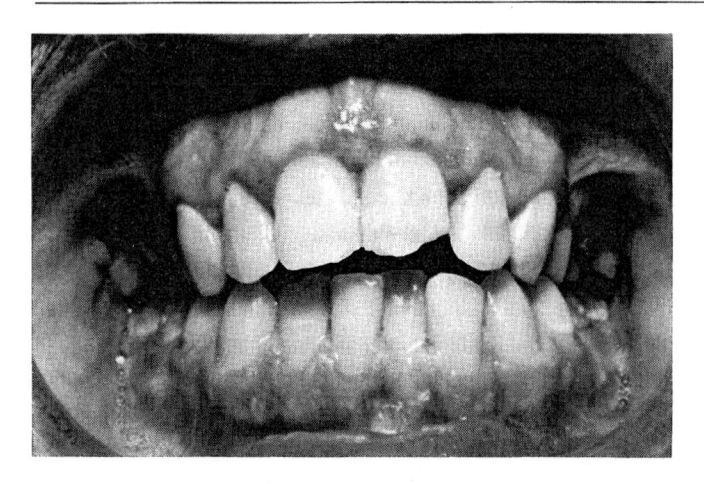

Fig. 6-4 Patient and parent are concerned about bleeding gingival tissue and dental relapse after three years of fixed therapy.

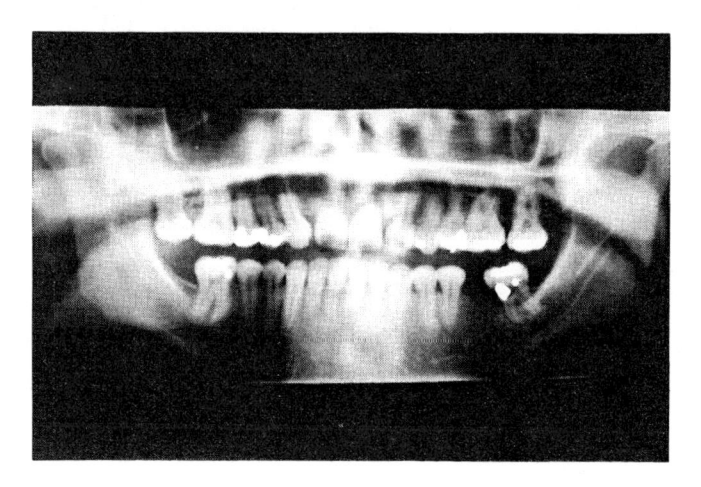

Fig. 6-5 Root resorption was so severe that endodontic therapy was attempted to halt further root loss in the left central incisor. The patient wore a fixed appliance for three years.

important than the type of appliance used. Almost any appliance method properly utilized is capable of correcting many types of malocclusion.[7]

Orthopedic appliances balance the functional and structural components of the craniofacial region. Long-term stability results from treatment that balances or counteracts facial muscular forces that act on the dentoalveolar component when appliances are removed. If compensatory muscle function has been eliminated, mechanical retention should not be necessary. It must be recognized, however, that most occlusal relationships change (if slightly) post-retention.

The treatment sequence should be appropriate to the patient's maturity and desire for correction of the malocclusion, but the following sequence is useful for the correction of many types of malocclusion.

First, correct any crossbites as early as possible. Timing for crossbite correction is often dictated by the maturity of the patient. Since there is frequently a habit involved with posterior crossbite, curbing the habit and correcting the crossbite are accomplished simultaneously between ages 5 and 9.

Second, unlock the dental crowding. If second molars are considered for extraction, the developmental morphology of the third molar is assessed on a panoramic radiograph. If the prognosis for the eruption of the third molars is favorable, the second molars are removed as soon as they erupt, or as soon as biological development is adequate (see Chapter 11). If crowding is minimal, or if early treatment will aid the treatment plan, a maxillary sagittal appliance can help uncrowd the dentition beginning as early as age 9 years.

Third, correct the jaw-to-jaw relationship. Maxillofacial orthopedic appliances are very effective in guiding and stimulating maxillary or mandibular growth. These appliances work well from the earliest point at which patient acceptance is possible (usually ages 8 to 10), and as long as the patient is still growing. Maxillofacial orthopedic appliances are most effective during the rapid growth years between ages 8 and 18.

Fourth, correct any dental rotation and level the arch. By the time the fourth phase of treatment has begun, there is adequate space for the greatest mesial-distal width of the teeth. Many minor dental rotations will have self-corrected or will have been corrected with the maxillofacial orthopedic appliance. Severely rotated teeth and arch leveling require fixed appliance therapy (Chapter 7).

Family constellation considerations

Effective treatment planning cannot overlook the patient's family constellation. The following questions should be answered before treatment commences:

1. Are the parents together and functioning as a family unit; are they separated or divorced; or is one or the other deceased? (Do not consider this question too personal.) In cases where the child is living with a single parent, consideration of the working time of the parent is essential to ensure the keeping of appointments and satisfactory completion of the treatment plan. Maxillofacial orthopedic appliances need fewer adjustments than do fixed appliances; broken maxillofacial appliances do not usually require immediate attention.
2. The family financial condition should be taken into consideration. Do other siblings require treatment? Is there a dental insurance program? A hastily thought-out treatment plan can be hindered or not brought to completion if the parent does not feel that he or she can afford to bring the patient in for adjustment visits.

Emotional age

The clinician must be aware of the emotional age of the patient. Females tend to mature emotionally more quickly than do males; a 9-year-old female may quickly adjust to an orthopedic appliance, whereas a 9-year-old male may not be mature enough. The important consideration here is the patient's desire for treatment. A strong patient desire for correction of the malocclusion will improve the chances for successful completion of the treatment plan. If the patient makes negative statements or offhand remarks that demonstrate a lack of real desire for treatment, it would be better to wait until the patient is more mature before initiating therapy.

Presentation of treatment plan

The presentation of the treatment plan does not have to be elaborate or involve expensive aids. Photographs and study models are helpful, especially if their subjects are similar to the individual presenting for treatment. The presentation of the treatment plan can begin at the chair in the treatment room; the explanation of time and fee considerations should take place in a private office (Fig. 6-6). The presentation of the

Treatment Planning

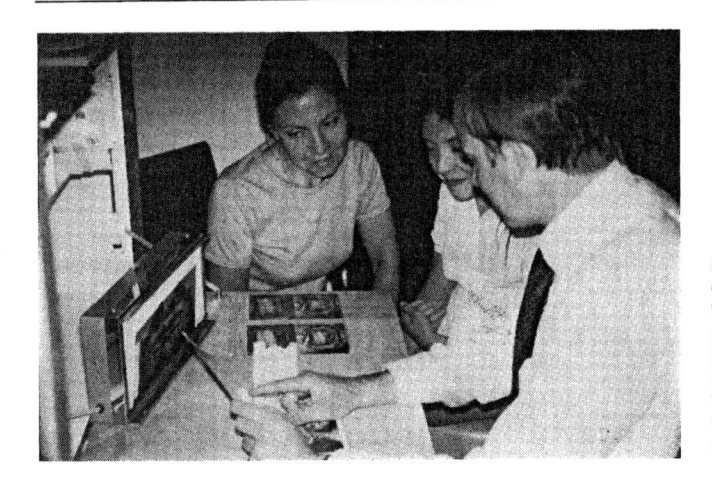

Fig. 6-6 Patient and parent discuss the child's malocclusion with the clinician. Many parents prefer to include the young patient in all discussions of treatment.[8] This may help encourage the young patient's participation, which is essential to the success of orthopedic appliance therapy.

treatment plan includes a straightforward explanation of the problem and a reasonable method for correction. As part of the presentation, the treatment goals are discussed, defined, and written down.

Specific treatment goals should be defined in advance. Adult treatment goals may be more limited than goals for a growing child. It can be beneficial to set a time and fee schedule limit for adult treatment plans. A four-month treatment plan with a limited treatment objective does not bind an adult to a treatment plan that might be too ambitious. If the four-month trial period is successful, then a more comprehensive treatment plan can be initiated. An explanation of advantages and disadvantages of orthopedic appliances are helpful for the parent or patient.

Advantages of orthopedic appliances

1. The appliances enhance facial esthetics by correcting muscle imbalance and skeletal deficiencies. Shortened lower face height, retrognathic mandibles, narrowed dental arches, and anterior-posterior growth discrepancies are readily treated.
2. Dental esthetics are preserved because the premolar teeth are usually not removed. The patient finishes treatment with a more complete dentition. The smile is fuller and more teeth are visible when the patient smiles.
3. Dental function is enhanced because there are usually four more teeth in the final result. If second molars are extracted and the third molars allowed to erupt, the dentition would contain 28 teeth. If premolars are extracted, the impacted third molars are also frequently extracted later. The patient is left with only 24 teeth.
4. The function of the temporomandibular joint is not compromised. Since premolar teeth are not removed, the vertical dimension is not reduced, nor is the condyle retro- or superiorly positioned in the glenoid fossa. Maxillofacial orthopedic appliances can aid in the treatment of some temporomandibular joint disorders (see Chapter 10). The appliances protect the integrity and smooth functioning of the temporomandibular joint.
5. Since the appliances are removable, oral hygiene is enhanced. The teeth can easily be flossed and brushed; the appliances can be cleaned with a brush or soaked in a denture-cleaning solution. Sticky foods are not trapped between

the appliance and the dentition for long periods of time. The removable appliance generally is kinder to the tooth surfaces, root integrity, and supporting alveolus.[9]
6. Emergencies usually do not have to be seen immediately. Broken or uncomfortable appliances should be corrected as soon as possible but, in the meantime, the patient does not have to suffer discomfort; the appliance is removable.
7. The dental component is stable after the appliances are removed. Functional appliances move teeth minimally through the alveolus so that periodontal fibers do not cause relapse of the final result. The teeth are guided into a stable occlusion as the individual matures.
8. The patient's self-esteem is enhanced. Maxillofacial orthopedic appliances correct facial discrepancies early. This helps the child to react more positively to his or her environment. A greater feeling of well-being results. A child's facial structure has a serious impact on his or her self-esteem. A receding lower jaw can significantly reduce a child's self-image. Individuals with balanced facial skeletal components feel good about their appearances: grooming, scholastic achievement, and self-confidence all are improved.

Disadvantages of maxillofacial orthopedic appliances

1. Since the appliances are removable, the patient can choose not to wear them. From the beginning, it should be stressed that without good patient cooperation, treatment results will be minimal.
2. The appliances can be lost or broken if not kept in the mouth or in their proper carrying case. If the appliance is not worn while eating, it must be kept in a secure case. Too frequently, appliances are lost because of improper storage.
3. Some tooth movements cannot be accomplished effectively with functional appliances. Teeth cannot be bodily moved through the alveolus. Severe rotations cannot easily be treated with orthopedic appliances. More precise finishing and leveling results are obtained with fixed appliances.
4. Some children cannot tolerate the bulkiness of a functional appliance. Physically and mentally handicapped patients might have difficulty wearing an orthopedic appliance.

Caution

Certain remarks or actions on the part of the patient or parent will alert the clinician as to the advisability of instituting or continuing treatment. The sincere desire for treatment must be present. If the parent says "Susan can't wear that appliance. She won't be able to eat, be a cheerleader, take Spanish, talk in school," etc., then the clinician has a problem. A parent who is unconcerned about radiographs, cost of treatment, or the type of appliance suggested may also be unconcerned about getting the patient to adjustment appointments on time or about the financial arrangements.

Stress teamwork. The parent, patient, and dental staff must work together for maximum treatment results. Get the patient involved with the treatment. The parent should be supportive, but the patient has to be responsible for wearing the appliance. Patient involvement is more effective in gaining cooperation than is taking the traditional authoritarian role of the dentist.

Timing the initiation of treatment

Each recall examination includes notes on the status of the occlusion. The overjet,

Treatment Planning

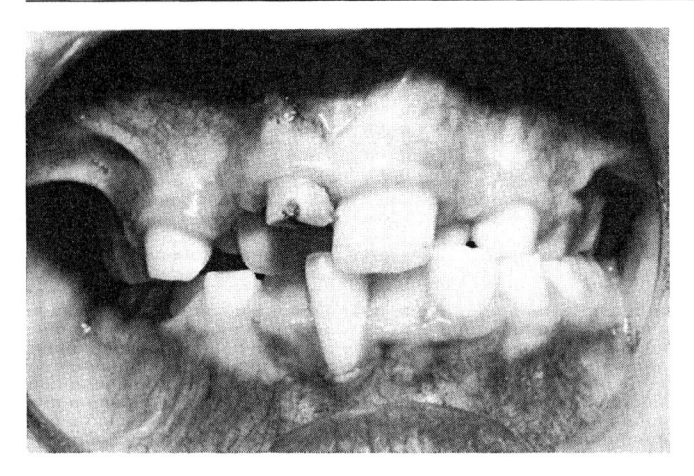

Fig. 6-7 Treatment should be initiated early in Class I crowded conditions when an improper occlusal relationship is deleterious to the periodontium. This patient presented with an abscessed, overretained primary incisor that resulted in an anterior maxillary crossbite and labial stripping of the gingival tissue from a mandibular incisor.

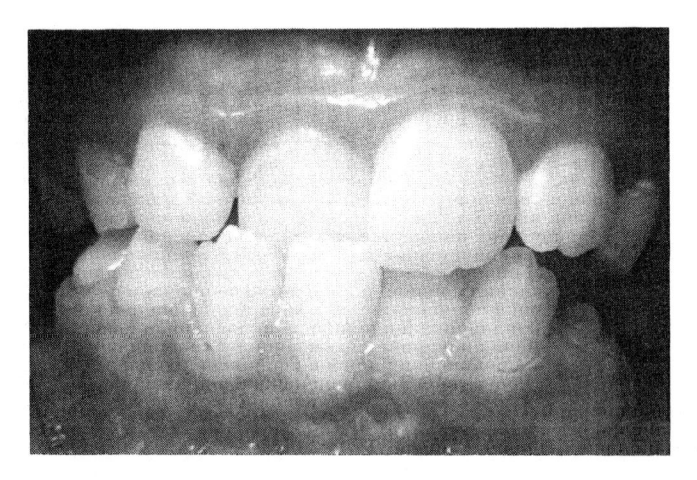

Fig. 6-8a Moderate gingival stripping from improper anterior occlusion.

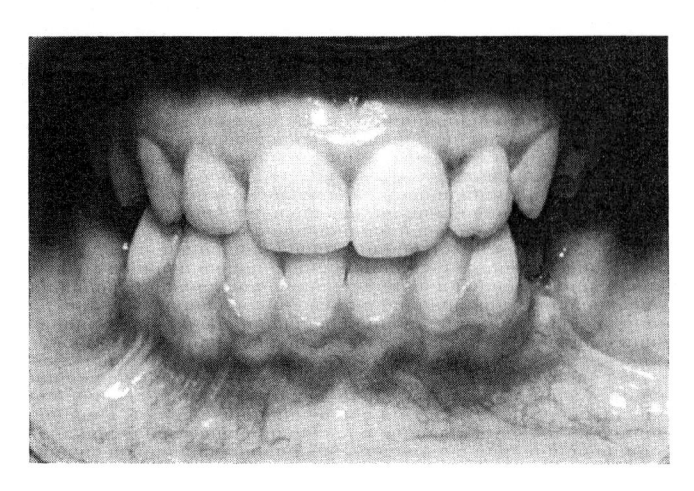

Fig. 6-8b Gingival stripping reversed with proper early treatment.

Class II Malocclusion

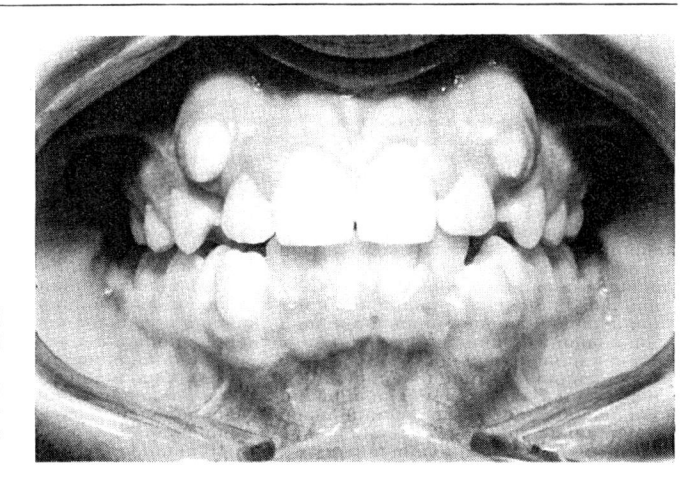

Fig. 6-9 This patient requested treatment for his Class I crowded malocclusion at age 13.1 years. Treatment would have been easier and more rapidly accomplished if initiated one to two years earlier.

overbite, or open bite are measured in millimeters; any crossbite or crowding is noted. Unusual facial growth patterns, headaches, or temporomandibular joint symptoms are also noted. Digit or blanket sucking and tongue habits are discussed and evaluated. If a developing malocclusion can be diagnosed early, treatment planning and treatment can begin at the proper time.

Treatment timing guidelines

The following guidelines suggest ages for treatment initiation. It should be stressed, however, that patient desire for treatment and emotional maturity are even more important than age in assessing treatment initiation.

Class I malocclusion

The molar and canine are in a Class I relationship, but there is dental crowding, spacing, or rotation. Think through the following questions:
1. How does the facial skeleton and orthostatic position of the head relate to the rest of the body?
2. Is any crowding per arch severe enough to consider removal of a second molar?
3. In what stage of morphological development is the third molar?
4. Is there any dysfunction of the temporomandibular joint?

If there is crowding without severe overjet or TMJ symptoms, initiation of treatment can wait until 10.5 to 12 years of age. Starting earlier may prolong the treatment time (Figs. 6-7 to 6-9). In Class I crowded dental arches where the third molars are developing normally, the second molars should be removed and third molars allowed to erupt. Second molar extraction is initiated on eruption of this tooth into the oral cavity. If third molars are absent, second molars are not extracted. A three-way expansion appliance (Fig. 6-10) will aid in uncrowding the maxillary dentition. A mandibular sagittal appliance will aid uncrowding of the mandibular arch.

Class II malocclusion

Class II, Division 1 malocclusion should be treated early if the following conditions apply:

Treatment Planning

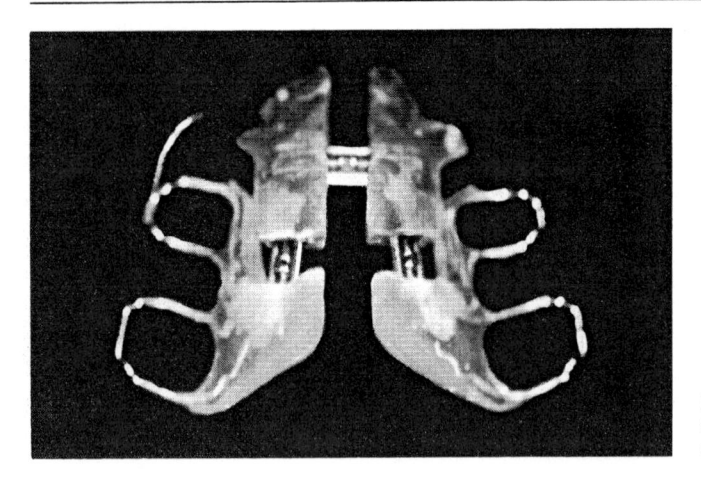

Fig. 6-10 Three-way maxillary sagittal appliance without occlusal coverage.

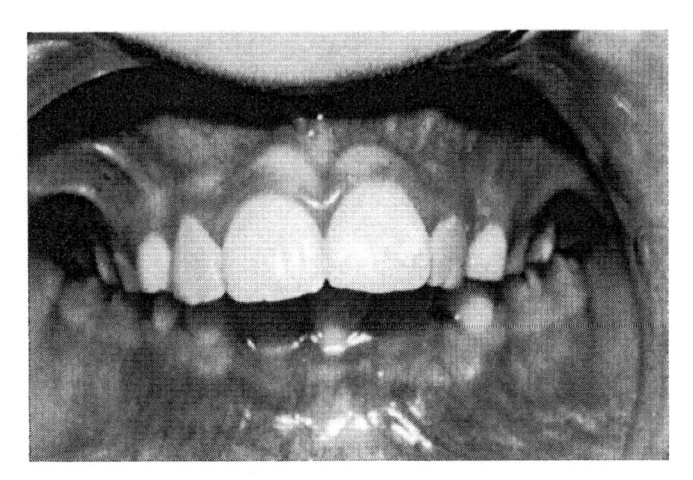

Fig. 6-11 This 8-year-old female was being teased and called "dogteeth" by some unfeeling classmates. Possible psychological effects in themselves are reason enough to begin treatment early.

1. There is overjet of 5 mm or more with labially inclined incisors.
2. The patient is mature enough to have a sincere desire for treatment.
3. TMJ symptoms are present.

Treatment can begin early (between ages 8 and 10 years) where there is severe maxillary dental protrusion or painful TMJ symptoms. Flaired central incisors are likely to fracture, particularly in males. This is reason enough to consider early treatment (Figs. 6-11 and 6-12a to d).

Class II, Division 2 malocclusion can wait for treatment until age 10 to 12 years, unless there are symptoms of temporomandibular joint disorder. If the following questions are answered affirmatively, treatment should begin as soon as possible.

1. Does the patient get headaches, particularly in the supra- or retro-orbital region?
2. Is there any neck or back pain or dysfunction associated with poor posture?

Young patients with symptoms of temporomandibular joint disorder usually are not

Class III Malocclusion

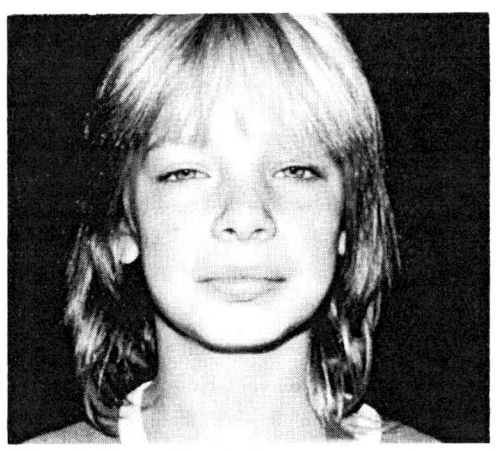

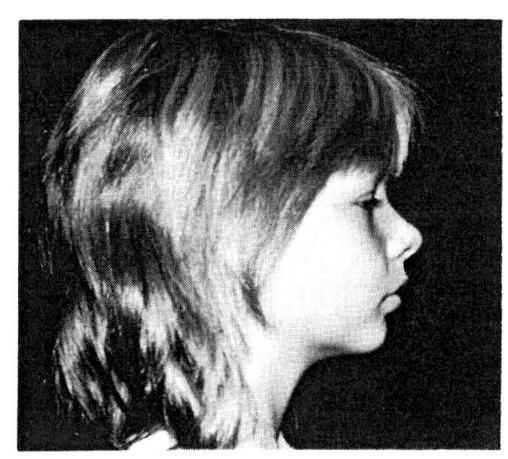

Figs. 6-12a and b Before treatment. A lack of vertical dimension can distort labial and facial contour.

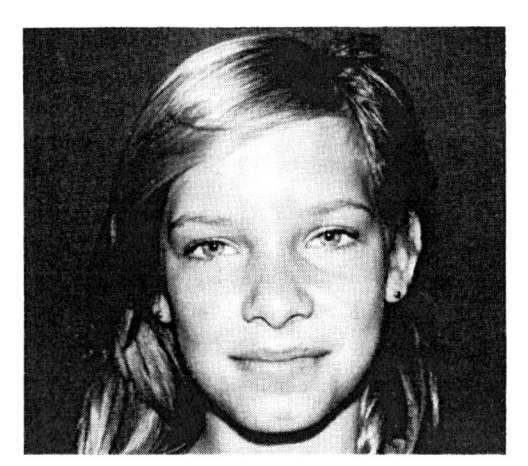

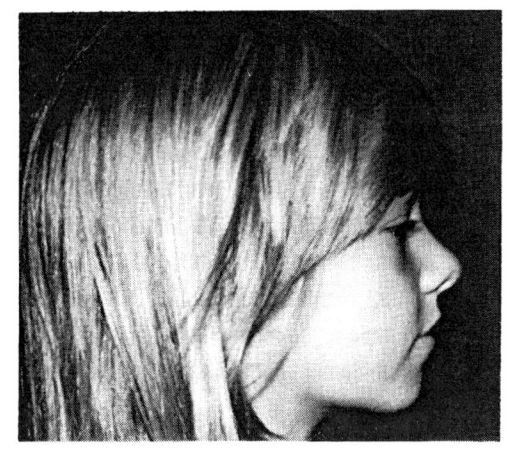

Figs. 6-12c and d Posttreatment. Maxillofacial orthopedic appliance (bionator) correction of a growth discrepancy will enhance facial beauty. Treatment time was 14 months.

mature enough to wear a mandibular repositioning appliance until age 8 (Figs. 6-13a to e).

Class III malocclusion

Class III malocclusion is treated as early as patient cooperation permits. Some investigators suggest chin-cap therapy as early as ages 5 to 6 years.[10] Others continue external restraint on the growing mandible as long as the patient will tolerate the chin straps. Answers to the following questions help determine treatment timing:

1. Is there a true skeletal mandibular pro-

Treatment Planning

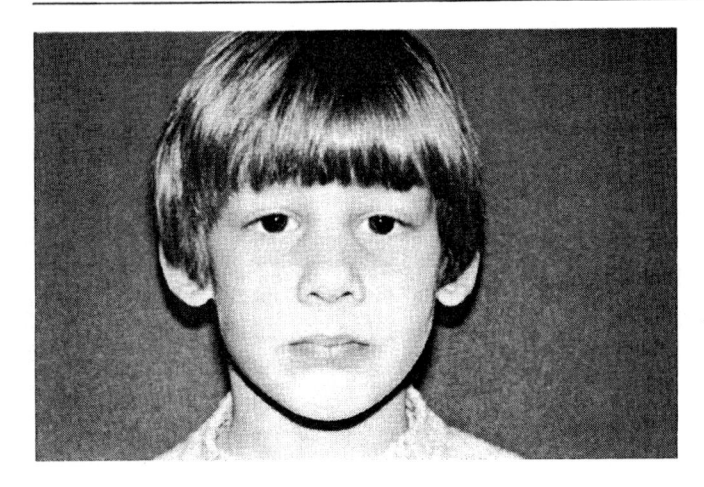

Figs. 6-13a and b This 6-year-old patient complained of a severe headache two to three times per week.

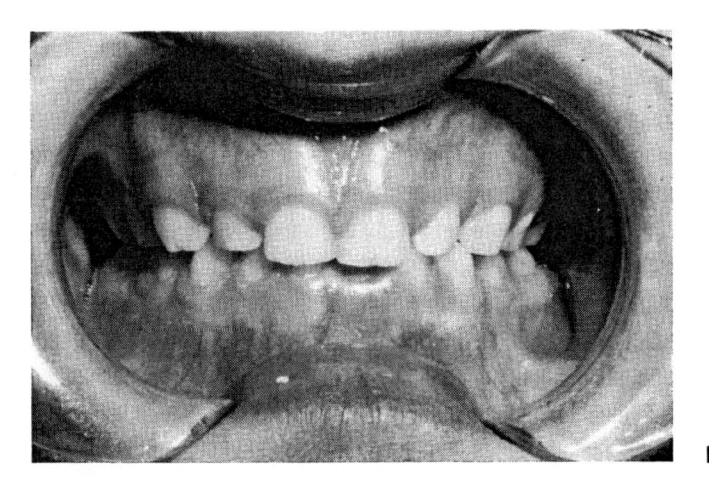

Fig. 6-13b

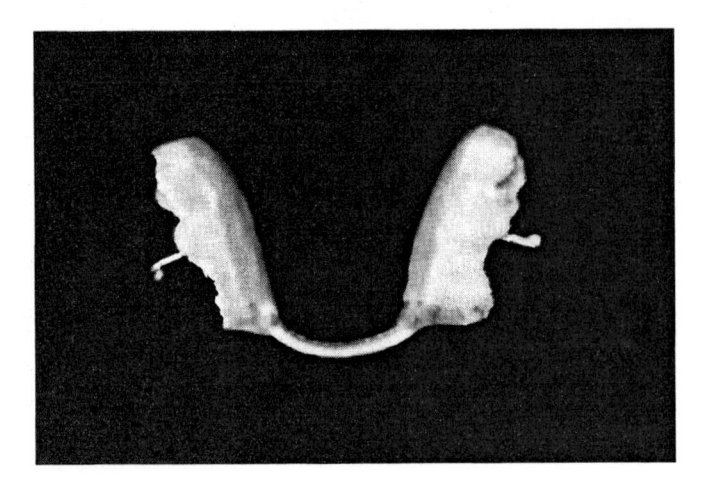

Fig. 6-13c Occlusal splint for re-establishing vertical dimension.

Class III Malocclusion

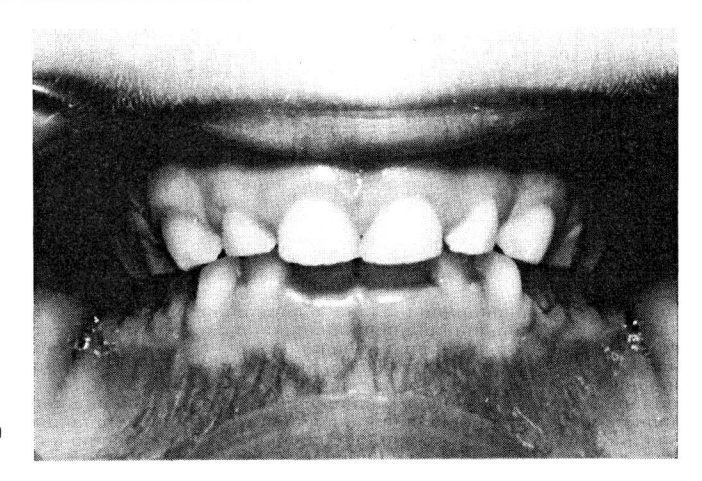

Fig. 6-13d Vertical dimension opened approximately 1.5 mm.

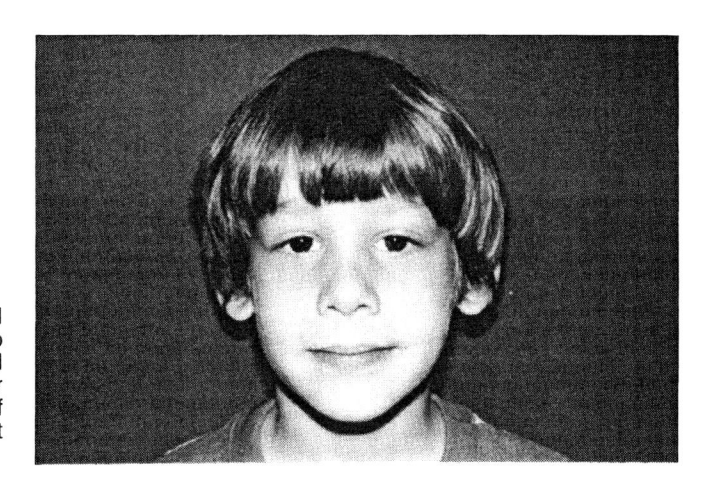

Fig. 6-13e With proper vertical dimension, headaches are no longer severe. Patient mentioned only mild headaches once or twice per month. Correction of the malocclusion can begin at age 8 to 10 years.

trusion, or is there maxillary retrusion?
2. Would the patient benefit from a more fully developed midface region?

A sagittal appliance can help in the treatment of maxillary underdevelopment and anterior crossbite.

Early evaluation

The Angle classification defines dental position in a sagittal or anterior-posterior relationship. The transverse and vertical dimension relationships also need consideration. As a general guideline, the following forms of malocclusion are treated early (usually treatment may be initiated between ages 8 to 10):

1. open bite
2. dental Class III
3. skeletal Class III
4. Class II, Division 1 patients with extreme overjet
5. dental and skeletal posterior crossbite

Treatment for deep bite malocclusion

151

can begin later (between ages 10 and 12) unless there are symptoms of temporomandibular joint dysfunction. If there is head, neck, or back pain, or if there are other temporomandibular joint disorder symptoms, then treatment should begin as early as possible. Dickson[11] found that starting treatment later (age 14) resulted in a lower failure rate. Björk,[12] however, stressed the effectiveness of early treatment. Moyers,[13] and Ahlgren and Laurin[14] have shown the value of treating the patient during a growth spurt.

Summary

Presentation of a treatment plan should be an enjoyable learning experience for parent and patient. It is a chance to get to know the clinician better. If there is resistance to a treatment plan, and this resistance is not easily overcome, then a short waiting period (six to 12 months) is suggested. If a second opinion is desired, one or two names are given for referral.

The consequences of noncooperation should be discussed. If the patient does not wear the appliance and make steady progress, then he or she is placed in a "hold" classification. No periodic payments are to be made, and treatment for the malocclusion is suspended until the patient indicates a desire to resume treatment. Recall examinations, prophylaxis, fluoride treatments, and routine restorative care is continued.

End the treatment planning discussion with a positive comment. For example: "Mrs. Smith, two traits are very important for success: confidence and self-esteem. Your child's smile could well determine success in life. A new appearance could give a feeling of well-being and confidence."

References

1. Andrews, L. F. The six keys to normal occlusion. Am. J. Orthod. 62:296–309, 1972.
2. Legan, H. L., Hill, S. C., and Sinn, D.P. Surgical-orthodontic treatment of dentofacial deformities. Dent. Clin. North Am. 25:131–156, 1981.
3. Burstone, C. J. Lip posture and its significance in treatment planning. Am. J. Orthod. 53:262–284, 1967.
4. Eirew, H. L. An orthodontic challenge. Br. Dent. J. 140:96–99, 1976.
5. Solberg, W. K., and Clark, G. T. Temporomandibular Joint Problems. Chicago: Quintessence Publ. Co., 1980, pp. 147–148.
6. McNamara, J. A., Jr. Functional determinants of craniofacial size and shape. Eur. J. Orthod. 2:131–159, 1980.
7. Grave, K. C., McKinnon, J. D., and Smart, L. M. Reality in orthodontics and a treatment approach for certain malocclusions. Eur. J. Orthod. 3:41–47, 1981.
8. Callender, R. S., and Barbour, A. Effective communication with clients: financial arrangements. J. Clin. Orthod. 15:497–500, 1981.
9. Dewel, B. F. Fixed versus removable orthodontic appliances. Am. J. Orthod. 60:518–519, 1971.
10. Graber, T. Orthodontics, Principles and Practice. 3rd ed. Philadelphia: W. B. Saunders Co., 1972.
11. Dickson, G. C. Symposium on functional therapy. Trans. Br. Soc. Orthod. 1964, pp. 93–96.
12. Björk, A. Principles of the Andresen method of orthodontic treatment. Am. J. Orthod. 37:437–458, 1951.
13. Moyers, R. E. Symposium on functional therapy. Trans. Br. Soc. Orthod. 1964, pp. 107–112.
14. Ahlgren, J., and Laurin, C. Late results of activator treatment: a cephalometric study. Br. J. Orthod. 3:181–187, 1976.

Part 3　　　　　　　　　　　　　　　　　　　　　　　Treatment

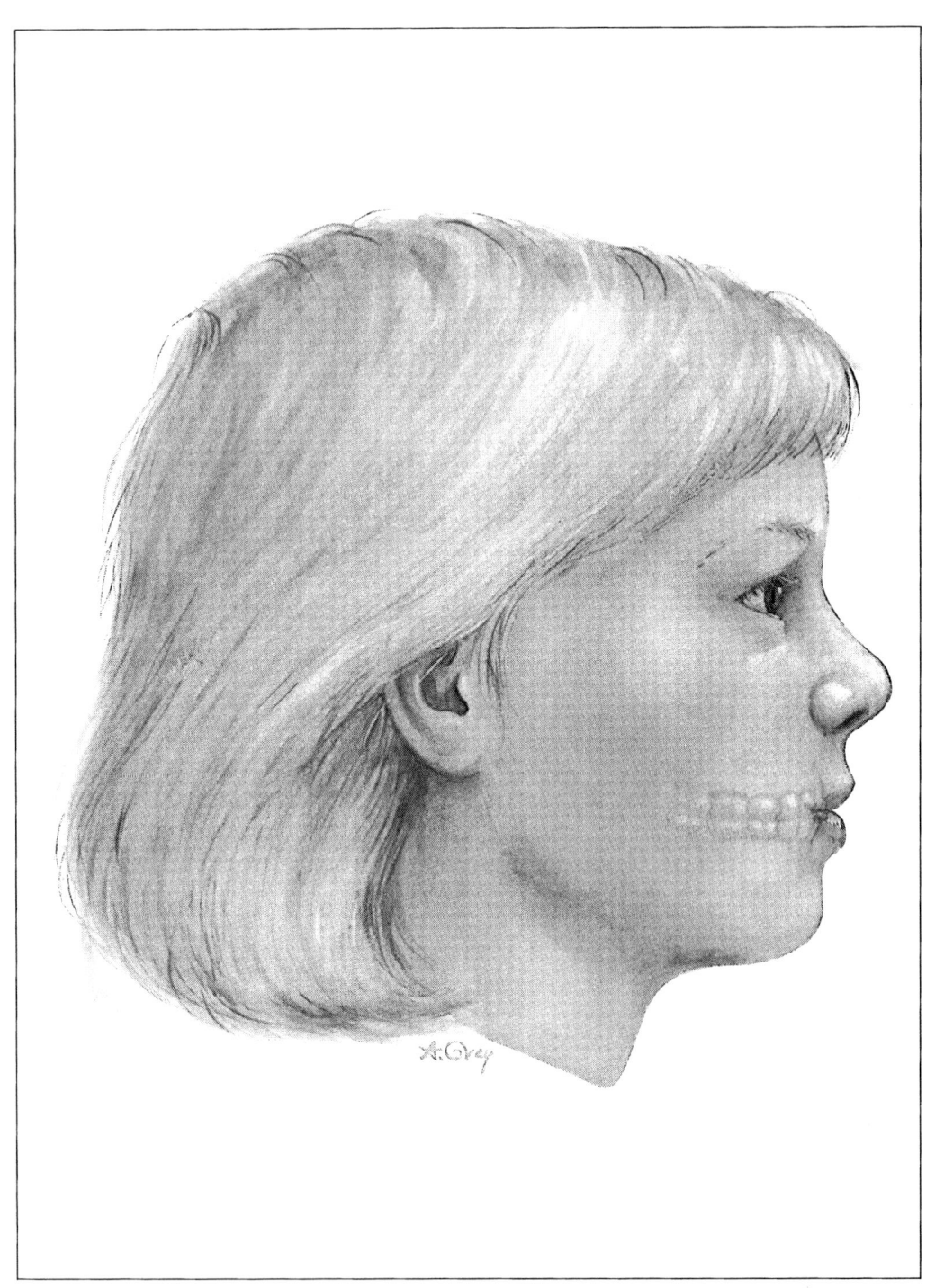

Craniofacial features representing a well-balanced facial structure with Class I malocclusion.

Chapter 7

Class I Malocclusion

Angle Class I (molar and canine) malocclusion may be treated with maxillofacial orthopedic or fixed appliance technique, or a combination of both. Excess dental spacing, occlusal leveling, and severe dental rotation are more easily corrected with a multi-banded-bonded technique. Some clinicians may have more experience with a particular type of orthopedic appliance and hence feel more comfortable using it when indicated. The specific case histories in this section primarily utilize the sagittal, bionator, and orthopedic corrector types of maxillofacial orthopedic appliances. It must be kept in mind that other types of orthopedic appliances could have achieved the same end results. Emphasis has been placed on the sagittal, bionator, and orthopedic corrector appliance variations because of their consistently effective results.

The effectiveness of the bionator and orthopedic corrector appliances is partially due to patient acceptance. When these appliances are utilized with second molar replacement (Chapter 11), the treatment time is reduced; some spontaneous correction occurs as the posterior teeth drift distally to a wider section of the arch.

Record gathering (excluding excessive radiographs) and treatment for malocclusion should ideally begin during the mixed dentition stage of occlusal development. Maxillofacial orthopedic treatment in the early mixed dentition can alter the vector of growth and development of the dentoalveolar process and osseous sutures. The appliances also help to provide a more biologically acceptable balance of the facial musculature.[1] Thilander[2] has summarized four reasons for initiating therapy early:

1. Early occlusal correction of individual teeth may aid spontaneous correction of teeth that erupt later.
2. If functional disturbances are corrected before the pubertal growth increase, further dentoalveolar or skeletal deviations may be prevented.
3. Early correction of Class II and III malocclusion may help establish a normal developmental skeletal pattern and reduce the risk of trauma to protruding incisors.
4. Early treatment will reduce or eliminate treatment during the teenage years when the patient may be more sensitive about treatment or predisposed to a higher incidence of caries and gingivitis.

Stöckli[3] suggests four additional factors that specifically favor early treatment:

1. The relatively flat occlusal surfaces of the primary dentition may facilitate sagittal correction of the maxillary and mandibular dentitions without the more marked cuspal interferences of the permanent premolars.
2. Tooth guidance during eruption is physiologically less harsh on root and periodontal tissues than bodily moving a

fully erupted tooth. Connective tissue seems to be more adaptable in the early stages of growth. If the skeletal structure is altered and guided early, any untoward influences of the lips, cheeks, and tongue can be modified. This enhances neuromuscular adaptation.
3. By waiting for treatment until an increase in growth rate at puberty, the chance to preserve leeway space may be lost. *Complicated mechanotherapy is no substitute for space maintenance and planned guidance of dental eruption.*
4. Ages 8 to 11 generally exhibit three important personality characteristics that lead to success in treatment: the patient is responsive to parental authority, sleeps for 10 to 11 hours per night, and has a more positive attitude toward wearing a functional appliance than might a teenager. Without good patient cooperation, treatment with maxillofacial orthopedic appliances is not successful.

Dental arch crowding

Dental arch crowding is a frequent problem in the mixed and permanent dentitions. It may be the result of premature extraction of primary teeth, interproximal carious lesions, a dental-skeletal discrepancy, oral habits, muscular imbalance, or an abnormal eruption pattern.

Several types of appliances have been developed to prevent or correct malocclusion with dental crowding in the developing child (e.g., the palatal expander and the space regainer). The sagittal appliance increases arch space by anteroposterior and lateral arch expansion.

Indications for the sagittal appliance

1. Class I crowding
2. Class II, Division 1 (as a first appliance)
3. Class II, Division 2 (as a first appliance)
4. early treatment of pseudo-Class III

Contraindications for the sagittal appliance

1. medically compromised patients (e.g., retardation, seizures)
2. poor oral hygiene, multiple caries, periodontal problems
3. poor patient cooperation
4. maxillary or mandibular skeletal and/or dental hyperplasia

Mode of action

Schwarz[4] believed that his appliance operates on the "pressure and tension" concept. He believed that teeth move only within the PDL (periodontal ligament). However, his concept did not take into consideration that the PDL is a continuous hydrostatic system which could transmit variable amounts of pressure to the alveolar bone surface by vessel or matrix distention or compression.[5,6] Baumrind[7] found that bone deflection could be produced routinely by forces lower than those required to produce consequential changes in the PDL width. He also stated that when orthodontic appliances are placed, forces delivered to the tooth are transmitted to all the tissues in the region of force application. In accordance with universally operating physical laws, each of the three structures in the area of force (i.e., tooth, PDL, and bone) are deformed. The amount of deformation produced in a material by a given force is a function of the elastic properties of that material. Bone is a dynamic tissue constantly engaged in active biological processes involving turnover and renewal of both cellular and inorganic components. These renewal processes also proceed, perhaps at an accelerated rate, during the period when the bone is held in a deformed position by appliance therapy. Reorganization proceeds not only at the surface of the alveolus but also on the surface of every trabecula within the corpus of the bone. The force of stress delivered to the tooth is dissipated by the development of stress lines in the deflected bone. This force becomes a stimulus for altered biological activity of cells lying perpendicular to the stress lines. The altered activity of these cells modifies the shape and internal organization of the bone to accommodate the exogenous forces upon it.[7]

The stimulus for bone deformation and destruction is electrical in nature.[6] The appliance is believed to act as a transducer, transforming mechanical energy into electrical forces (piezo) to the cell. The bioelectrical potentials generated by the connective tissues during appliance insertion produce electrical energy through physical transduction. Muscles, vessels, tendons, periosteum, teeth, and cartilage can produce "streaming" potentials that will directly affect bone behavior.[6] For this reason, it is advised that patients eat with the appliance in the mouth (Chapter 2).

Treatment objectives

Treatment in Class I individuals should maximize dental esthetics without harming facial esthetics or changing the healthy condyle-disc-fossa relationship in the temporomandibular joint (see Figs. 4-23 and 4-24 in Chapter 4).

Achievement of treatment goals

Treatment should cause as little iatrogenic trauma as possible. Root resorption, gingivitis, periodontal pockets, and decalcified white lesions on previously healthy teeth are sequelae to be avoided. Sadowsky and BeGole[8] have studied the incidence of periodontal disease 12 years after treatment. Very little difference could be found in the incidence or severity of periodontal disease between a group treated 12 years previously with fixed appliances and a group of patients showing Class I and II malocclusions but not treated. The authors did find some evidence to suggest that patients who had undergone premolar extraction had a greater prevalence of mild to moderate periodontal disease in the posterior regions of the mouth as compared with patients treated without extraction.

Minimizing treatment time so there will be as little biomechanical intervention as possible will result in healthy periodontal and osseous tissues. In a controlled study with a fixed technique, periodontal pocket depth has shown no major change as long as oral hygiene procedures are adequate.[9]

Description and design of the sagittal appliance

The sagittal appliance is a removable appliance made from anterior and posterior acrylic biteplanes connected with precision screws (Fig. 7-1).

The anterior biteplane may extend slightly forward of the maxillary incisors so that it will contact the mandibular incisors when the teeth are in occlusion. This will produce flaring of the maxillary anterior teeth. If flaring is not desired, the acrylic should not be in contact with the palatal surface of the anterior teeth. The acrylic of the posterior biteplane may cover part of the occlusal surfaces of the posterior teeth.

The labial bow, when indicated, is made from 0.40 wire. The purpose of the labial bow is to control labial movement of the anterior teeth and to prevent overflaring of the teeth. The clasps are made from heavy wire and are placed on the posterior segment (e.g., Adams, ball, C-clasps). Canine retractor wires are often used to move "blocked-out" canines distally and lingually when necessary.

Class I Malocclusion

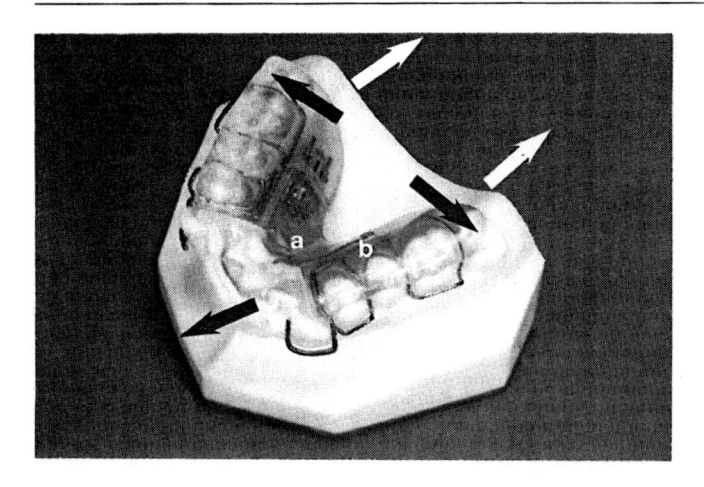

Fig. 7-1 A two-way sagittal appliance. (Courtesy of Dyna-Flex Orthodontic Laboratory, St. Louis, Mo.)

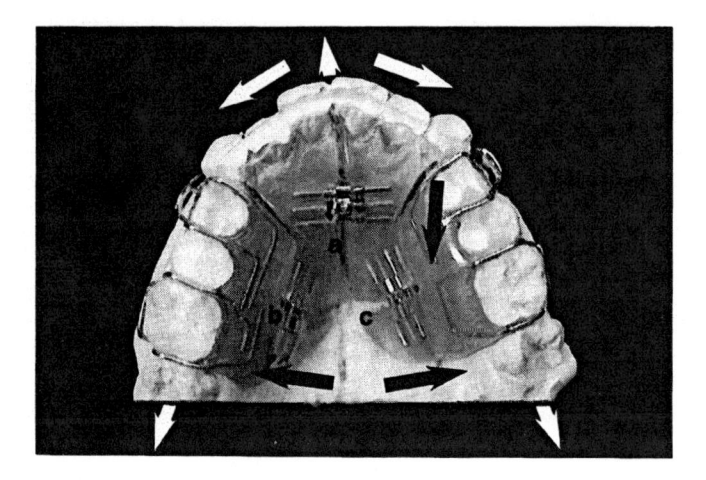

Fig. 7-2 A three-way sagittal appliance as it is returned from the orthodontic laboratory. Additional midline screw will enable the clinician to achieve some midline expansion.

The precision screws are incorporated into the acrylic. The number of screws used depends on the type of appliance desired. The two-way sagittal appliance has two precision screws that connect the anterior with the posterior acrylic parts. The screws are located on the posterior segment and run parallel to the midpalatal suture (Fig. 7-1).

The three-way sagittal has an additional screw that runs perpendicular to the midpalatal suture and is situated in the anterior biteplane (Fig. 7-2).

The two-way sagittal appliance is used when anteroposterior arch expansion is needed; the three-way sagittal appliance provides not only anteroposterior but also some lateral expansion. Both appliances create room for blocked-out canines or premolars and also provide additional space for the eruption of slightly crowded anterior teeth. The space is created by forward movement and anterior advancement of the premaxilla and some distalization of the posterior segment. Whenever the canine is displaced anteriorly because of crowding, the addition of a C-clasp on the appliance helps the distalization of the ectopically erupted canine into the created space (Fig. 7-3). However, the presence of the clasp

158

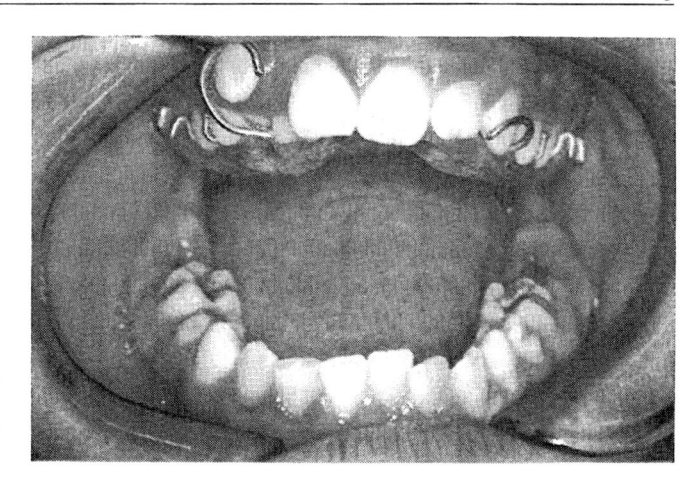

Fig. 7-3 When necessary, clasps are added to the posterior biteplane to facilitate the distal movement of the ectopically erupting canine.

will create some resistance to the distalization of the buccal segment. With the insertion of a two-way sagittal appliance there is more anterior than posterior expansion. The ratio is dependent on the stage of eruption and the presence of second molars. The presence of fully erupted second molars will produce more movement and flaring of the anterior segment.

Whenever a two-way sagittal appliance is considered for the creation of space for blocked-out canines, the clinician should evaluate whether anterior movement is more desirable than distalization of the posterior segment (Figs. 7-4 and 7-5).

When tooth removal is necessary for the correction of the malocclusion, second molar extraction (Chapter 11) may provide the necessary space by distalization of the posterior segments with the use of the sagittal appliance. This is helpful in the treatment of skeletal Class I; Class II, Division 1; and Class II, Division 2 types of malocclusion. Second molar extraction is usually preferable to premolar extractions.[10-15] Removal of second molars reduces the duration of treatment, increases the stability of the treated occlusion, and provides the patient with a better smile and facial profile.[15] In patients with third molars present extraction of second molars not only eliminates the need for premolar extraction, but it also facilitates the eruption of third molars by providing the necessary space (see Chapter 11).

Clinical observation shows that some bite opening is observed in patients treated with a sagittal appliance (Figs. 7-7a to f). Such bite opening is attributed to the distobuccal movement of the posterior segment.

Bite registration

The following steps are required:

1. The patient practices biting in centric occlusion (maximum intercuspation).
2. A pink base plate of wax is softened in hot water (139°F), folded once, trimmed, and placed on the posterior teeth. The patient is asked to close slowly to the correct position (Figs. 7-6a and b).
3. The wax is carefully removed and cooled in water.
4. With straight scissors, the wax is removed beyond the indentations of the maxillary buccal cusps.
5. The bite registration is inserted once more to check for distortion.

Proper maxillary and mandibular alginate

Class I Malocclusion

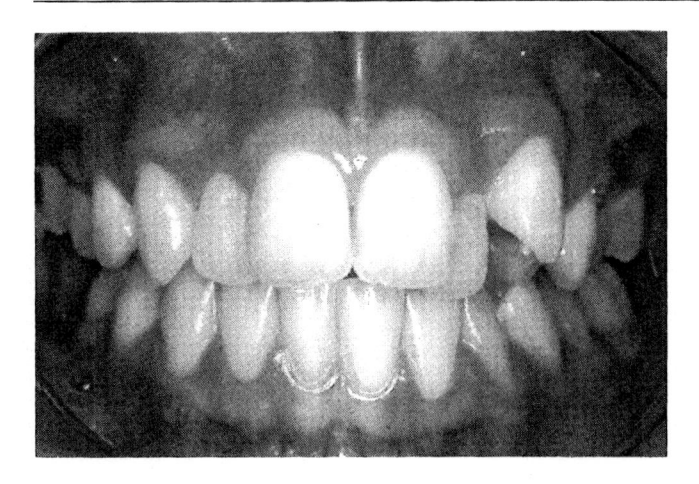

Fig. 7-4a Patient with bimaxillary crowding, resulting in ectopically erupting laterals and a "blocked-out" left canine.

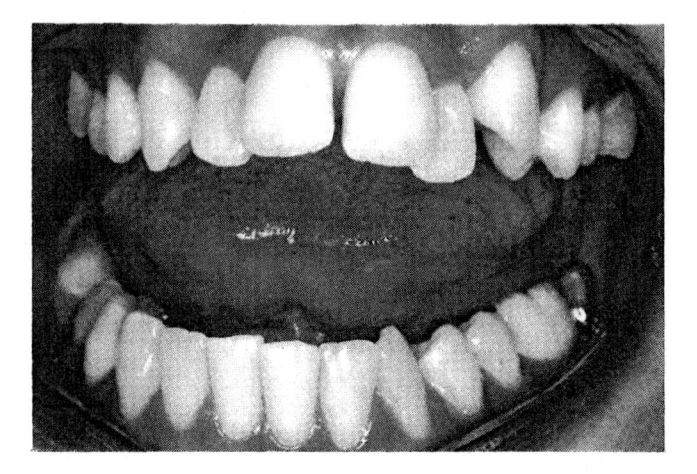

Fig. 7-4b Three months after insertion of a three-way sagittal appliance. Interdental spacing shows that the patient has been wearing the appliance.

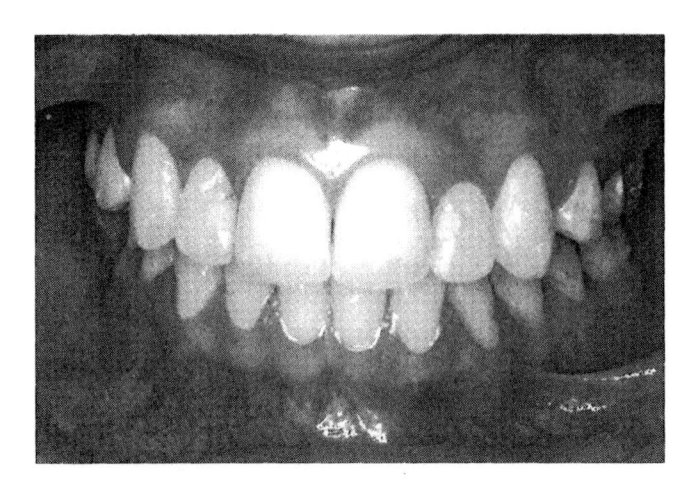

Fig. 7-4c The patient nine months after sagittal appliance treatment. (Reprinted with permission from Chan et al.[1])

Dental Arch Crowding

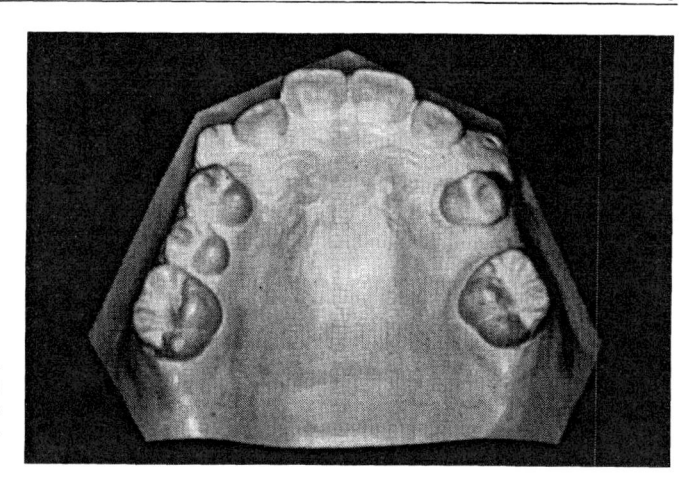

Fig. 7-5a Three-way sagittal inserted on patient with crowding and "blocked-out" maxillary canines and second right premolar.

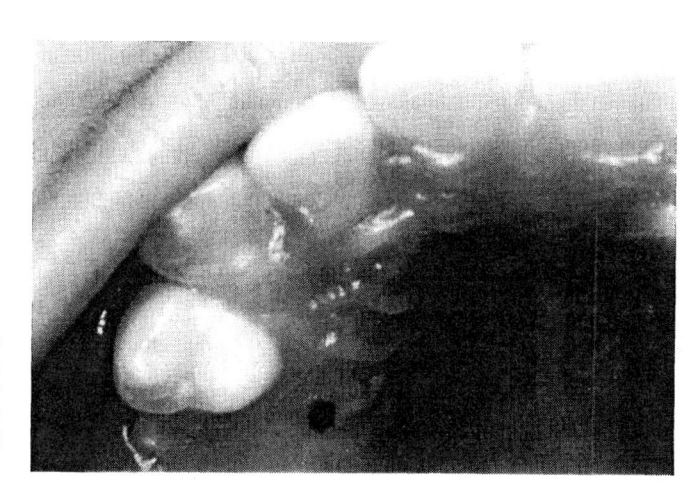

Fig. 7-5b After nine months of treatment, the proper space has been created for the eruption of the permanent teeth. (Reprinted with permission from Chan et al.[1])

impressions are taken. They are poured in orthodontic stone and sent to the laboratory for the fabrication of the appliance.

Instructions to the patient

The cooperation of the patient is very important for successful treatment. Proper wearing, activating, and care of the appliance is necessary. The patient should be instructed to use both hands for insertion and removal, using the molar Adams clasps to avoid distortion. The patient is informed that there will be difficulty in speaking and eating during the first two or three days.

The appliance is worn all the time, *including while eating and sleeping*. It should be removed and cleaned after meals and immediately reinserted.

Although rare, soreness may occur after initial placement. A soft diet is recommended for three or four days until the tissues adjust to the appliance.

The patient, along with the parent, is instructed to properly activate the appliance twice a week (e.g., Wednesdays and Sundays). Progress is checked using a diary that is given to the patient. The patient

Class I Malocclusion

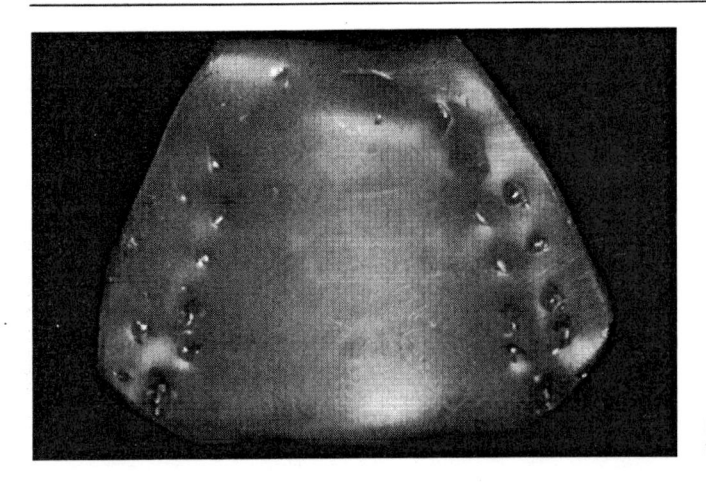

Figs. 7-6a and b Bite registration for the sagittal appliance.

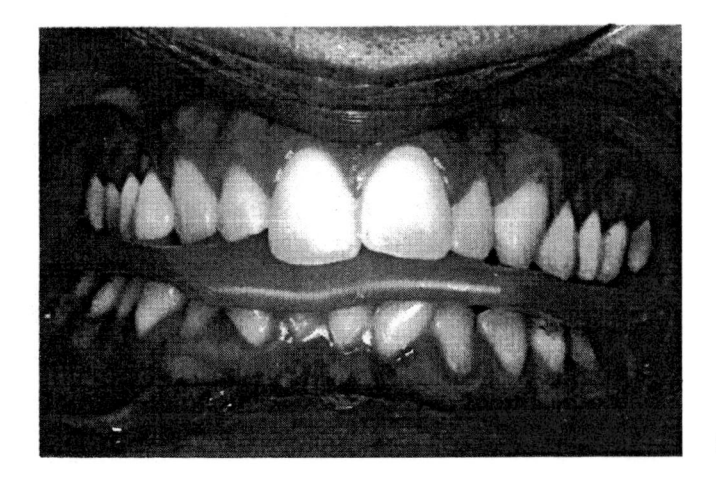

Fig. 7-6b

should bring the diary to every appointment (Chapter 12).

The frequency of follow-up appointments depends on patient cooperation and ability to follow instructions, and on treatment progress. The patient is seen during the first week after the insertion and advised to call immediately if any discomfort should occur. Progress appointments are scheduled monthly.

An atlas-style format is used to best illustrate patient selection, treatment timing, and results of treatment. Adult treatment has not been specifically documented, but several applications for older patient treatment have been suggested in Chapter 10.

Treatment of Class I malocclusion with dental crowding

J.B., age 13 (Figs. 7-7a to f)

J.B. presented with a Class I crowded malocclusion and a flat upper lip. There was crossbite of the maxillary lateral incisors, some mandibular anterior crowding, and insufficient space for the eruption of the maxillary permanent canines. A 1 mm midline discrepancy was also present. Third molar tooth development was faintly visible on the panoramic radiograph.

His medical history was essentially negative except for a mild sinusitis. Space analysis revealed a 5 mm arch discrepancy with minor transverse crowding (Schwarz analysis −1 mm in the premolar area). The maxillary canines were crowded and delayed in erupting. The maxillary lateral incisors were in lingual crossbite. A review of the methods available to correct the crowding suggested three possibilities:

1. expansion
   a. lateral
   b. sagittal
   c. dental tipping
2. tooth removal
   a. extraction of entire tooth
   b. stripping a portion of mesial and distal enamel
3. bone apposition and growth

Since the facial skeletal components were esthetic and well-balanced with the exception of a short upper lip, premolar extraction was eliminated.

The five important, common goals of correction of malocclusion would not have been met by premolar extraction for this patient:

1. Excellent facial esthetics. Proper fullness to the midface area and proper vertical dimension aid in a pleasing frontal and profile view of the face.
2. Protection of the temporomandibular joint. Treatment should not jeopardize the health or function of the TMJ.
3. Attractive smile. A full, attractive smile will encourage the patient's self-esteem.
4. Functional occlusion. The teeth should occlude so that proper masticatory and excursive movements are made without pain or premature occlusal contacts.
5. Stability. The posttreatment dental and skeletal results should be maintained without retentive appliances and with minimal relapse.

A sagittal appliance with no occlusal coverage was used to create space for the maxillary canines and for the final correction of the slightly rotated teeth. The three-way sagittal appliance allows for transverse expansion while creating space for the canines. This appliance is quite effective during the mixed dentition phase of development. If occlusal coverage is not required, it is not utilized. Patient cooperation is improved with a less bulky appliance.

Treatment plan for J.B.	Treatment time
A. orthopedic records	
B. maxillary sagittal appliance	12 months
C. labiolingual or straight-wire appliance for finishing treatment of the malocclusion	6 months

Case discussion

This patient had a negative TMJ history with good facial esthetics. The treatment was planned to ensure a continuation of temporomandibular joint health and improved facial and dental esthetics. Figures 7-7a to c show pretreatment, and Figs. 7-7d to f show posttreatment.

Treatment objectives

The treatment objectives were met by a removal of the source of the malocclusion (dental arch crowding). The treatment objective included a desire for long-term stability of the results without relapse and without prolonged retention. The labiolingual appliance, spring retainer, or preformed positioner are excellent for final finishing and retention of a malocclusion that includes minor rotations of the teeth. Occasionally, slight stripping of the mesial and distal enamel may be necessary for final correction of incisor rotations.[16-20] Slight

Class I Malocclusion

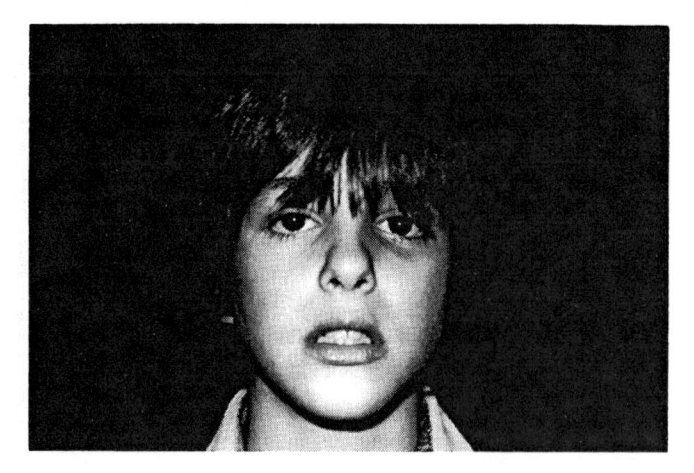

Fig. 7-7a J. B. Full face pretreatment.

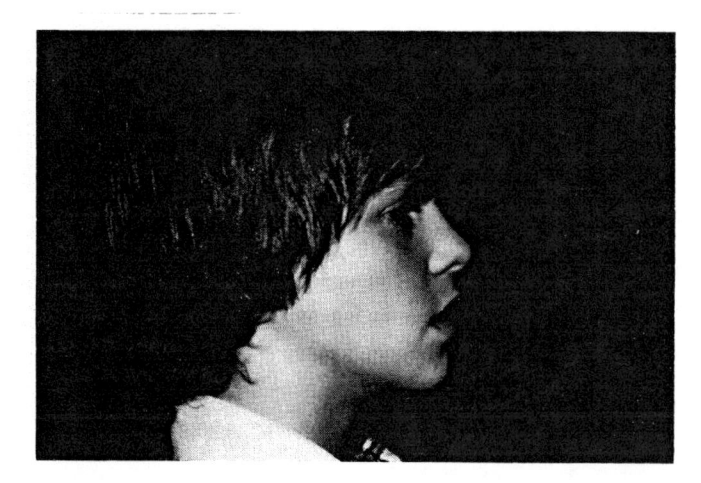

Fig. 7-7b J. B. Pretreatment facial profile.

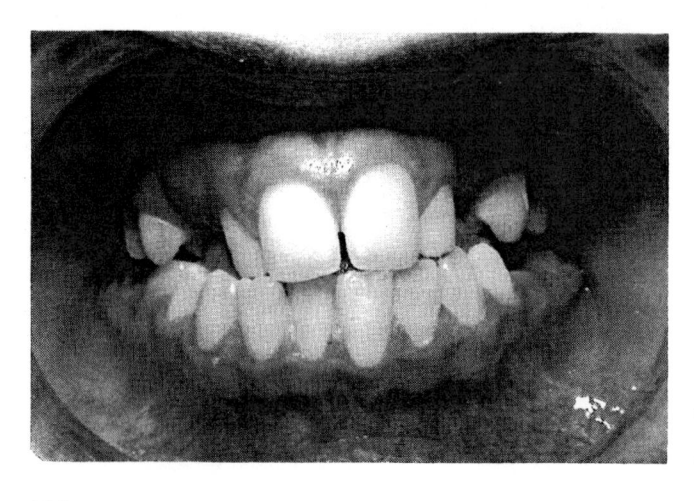

Fig. 7-7c Labial view of patient J. B. showing crowded-out maxillary canines, anterior crossbite, and mandibular crowding.

Dental Arch Crowding

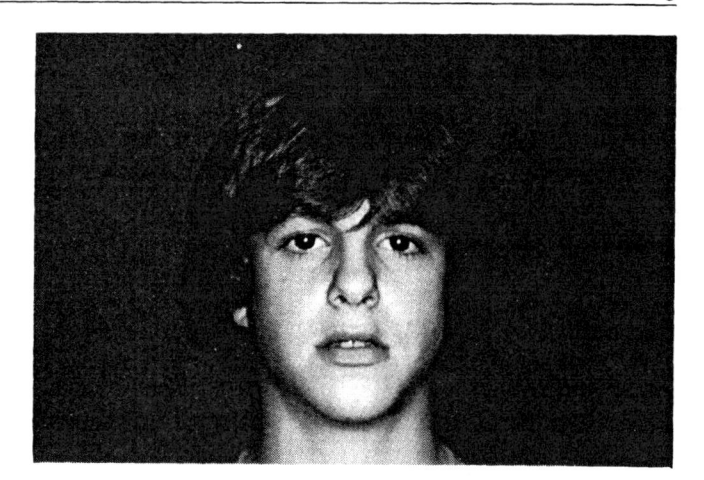

Fig. 7-7d J. B. Full face posttreatment.

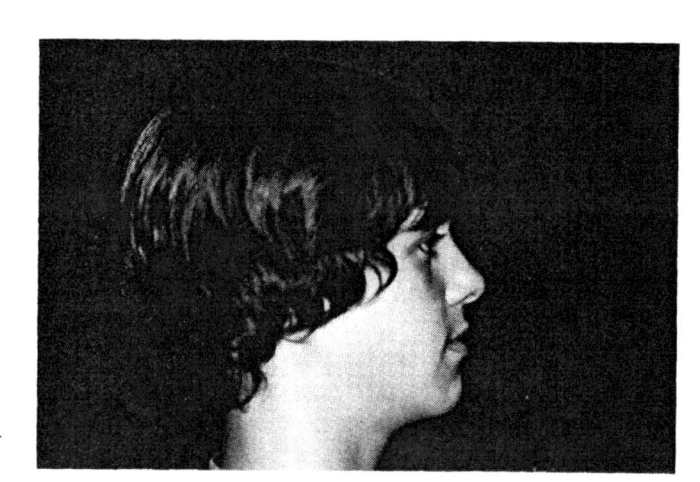

Fig. 7-7e J. B. Posttreatment facial profile.

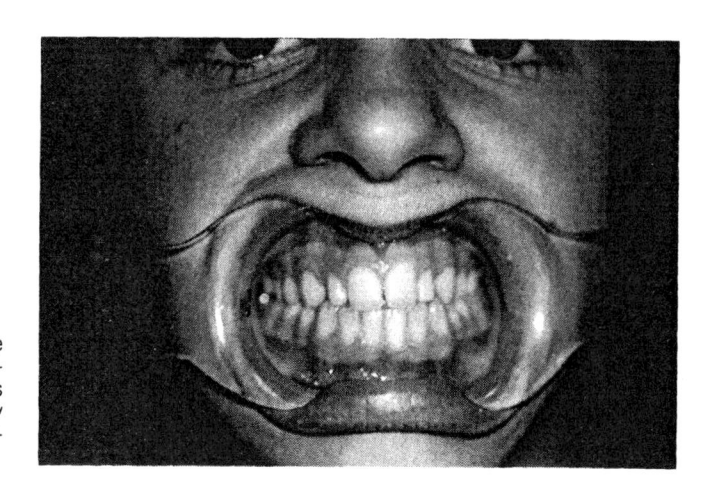

Fig. 7-7f Labial view. Space has been created for the maxillary canines. The final rotations were corrected with maxillary and mandibular labiolingual appliances.

Class I Malocclusion

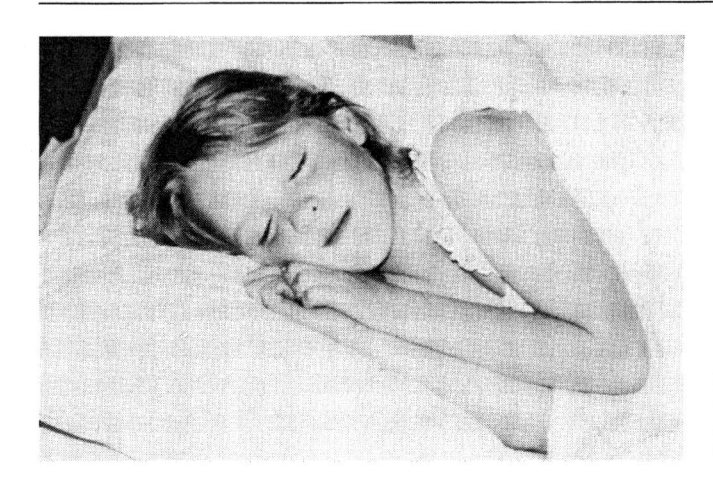

Fig. 7-8a Sleeping on a closed fist may affect the proper growth of the maxilla and cause dental crossbite.

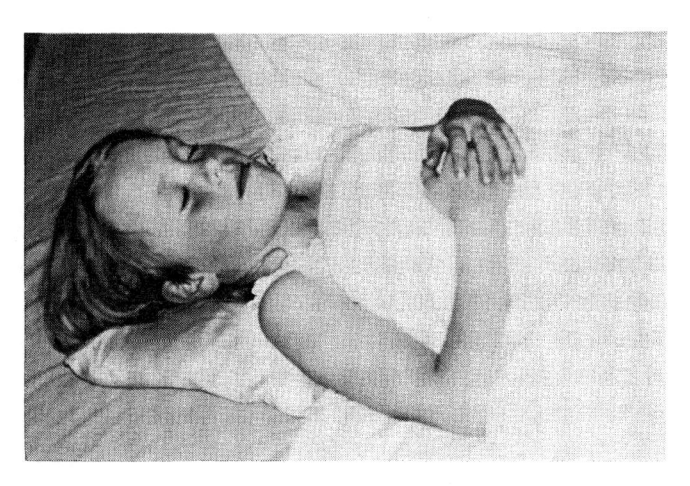

Fig. 7-8b Sleeping on the back with a small pillow under the neck is the best position for growth and orthopedic development.

overcorrection allows for some biological drift (relapse). The fixed straight-wire appliance is effective for achieving final occlusal leveling, root tip, and torque.

Treatment of Class I malocclusion with posterior crossbite

S.L., age 11.5

S.L. presented with a Class I crowded malocclusion with anterior and posterior unilateral crossbite and a history of sleeping on one side. The crossbite might have developed from this sleeping position (such as in Fig. 7-8a).[21] The child was advised to sleep on her back (as in Fig. 7-8b). The maxillary canines had insufficient arch length for proper eruption. The medical and other dental history were unremarkable except for advising sealants for the posterior teeth with deep fissures.

The Straight-wire Appliance in Clinical Practice

Treatment timing

Dental and skeletal crossbites are corrected as soon as reasonable cooperation can be elicited from the patient. Cohen[22] suggests early treatment to take advantage of skeletal growth. Treatment during a rapid growth phase of skeletal development can shorten the treatment time and diminish the chances of untoward iatrogenic sequelae (e.g., tipping the teeth). Houston[23] also recommends timing the correction of skeletal discrepancies with favorable growth patterns (see Chapter 2).

Treatment plan for S.L.	Treatment time
A. orthopedic records	
B. maxillary and mandibular second molar replacement	
C. maxillary sagittal appliance	6 months
D. bionator appliance to correct the vertical and sagittal discrepancy	12 months
E. labiolingual appliance or straight-wire appliance for final correction of the malocclusion	6 months

Since most of the dental crowding occurred in the maxillary arch, the maxillary second molars were removed in order to allow eruption of the maxillary third molars. Mandibular second molars were also removed to allow the mandibular third molars to erupt.

A sagittal appliance was used to correct the sagittal skeletal discrepancy. Maxillary slow dysfunction (via the maxillary expansion appliance) corrected the posterior crossbite without the danger of buccal root surface resorption that is possible with rapid maxillary expansion.[24]

The bionator and sagittal appliances have proven most effective for the dentoalveolar correction of developmental malformation in the prepubertal growth period of the transitional dentition.[25] After the dental crowding was corrected for S.L., the dentoalveolar response to bionator treatment was rapid (eight months) and easily tolerated. The labiolingual appliance was used to correct the final dental rotation.

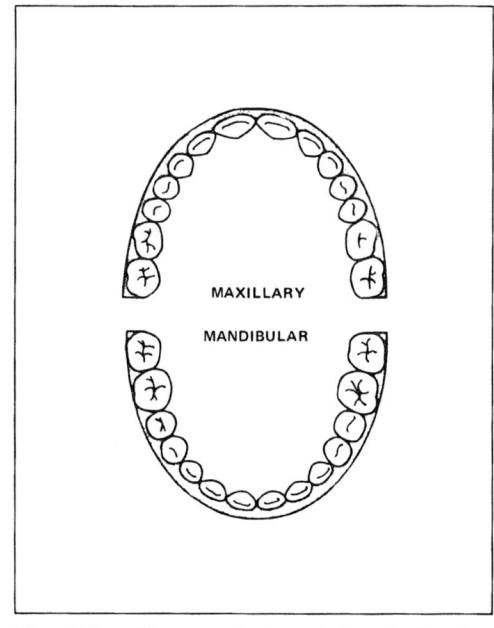

Fig. 7-9a The required variation in bracket thickness. The bracket must fill the space between the tooth and the outer edge of the shaded area to eliminate first-order arch wire bends. (Figs. 7-9 to 7-14 courtesy of The A-Company, San Diego, Calif.)

The straight-wire appliance in clinical practice

Proper finishing details are important for long-term stability and esthetics of a treated malocclusion. With the use of maxillofacial orthopedic technique, many rotations and labial/lingual discrepancies can be corrected during treatment. However, root angulation or tip, torque, in/out, moderate-

Class I Malocclusion

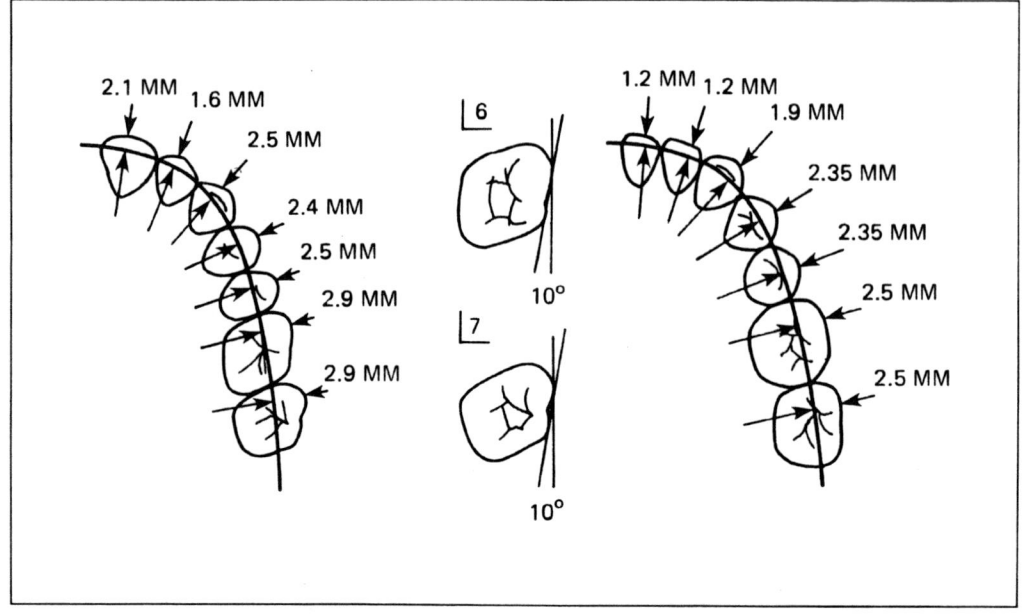

Fig. 7-9b In/out variables are measured from the contact points for the upper teeth *(left)* and the lower teeth *(right)*. A 10° offset for the distal cusps of the upper molars is incorporated into the straight-wire brackets for those teeth.

to-severe rotations, and occlusal plane corrections are best completed with the straight-wire appliance.

The straight-wire bracket

In/out crown relationship

The straight-wire bracket is constructed to help minimize time-consuming wire bending. The thickness of the bracket is constructed to reflect the proper in/out location for utilization of a preformed arch wire (Figs. 7-9a to c).

Crown inclination

Each straight-wire appliance bracket provides the torque required for the proper inclination of each specific tooth type. Having a specific bracket for each tooth type makes it possible to coordinate the bracket bases with the slot. Torque is cast in the base of each straight-wire bracket.

Torque in the base allows the slots of all brackets to line up horizontally without varying the bracket height. The torque in the bracket base allows the center of the slot and the center of the base to be always on the same plane. This makes bracket placement consistent (Fig. 7-10).

Skeletal differences and the success of maxillofacial orthopedic treatment can alter the amount of incisor bracket torque needed for each patient. Incisor brackets are available in prearranged sets for the three most common skeletal variations. Set I (Standard) is recommended for a Class I skeletal tendency. Set II is recommended for Class II skeletal tendencies and Set III is recommended for Class III skeletal tendencies (Fig. 7-11).

The Straight-wire Appliance in Clinical Practice

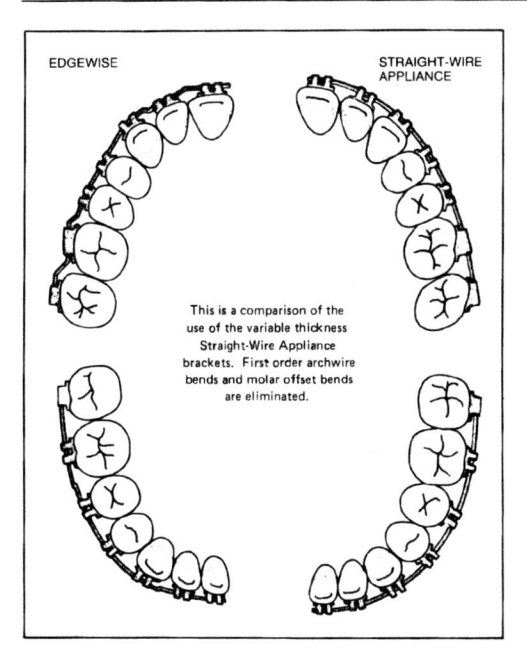

Fig. 7-9c A comparison of the variable-thickness straight-wire appliance brackets and edgewise brackets. First-order arch wire bends and molar offset bends are eliminated when the straight-wire brackets are used.

Fig. 7-10 With two cuspids in correct position, the conventional edgewise bracket requires arch-wire torque for slot engagement. The straight-wire appliance bracket base is pre-torqued, eliminating arch-wire torque.

Crown angulation

The proper root tip (angulation) is built into the slot on the bracket. Each crown in normally occluded teeth has the gingival portion of the long axis distal to the occlusal portion of the long axis.[26,27] The degree of tip varies with each tooth; each bracket is designed to accommodate proper root tip and eliminate tip bends in the arch wire (Fig. 7-12).

Tip bends are eliminated, since slot tip is built into every bracket. Angulating the slot within the bracket instead of angulating the entire bracket allows the bracket base to adapt properly to the long axis of the dental crown. This eliminates bracket rock and band distortion and preserves the specific in/out and torque built into each bracket.

Angulating the slot rather than the bracket also provides for a uniform system of bracket/band placement. The vertical long axis of each bracket is designed to coincide with the vertical long axis of the crown.

Treatment should result in contact points that abut. Each tooth type must be angulated individually to achieve a proper contact-to-contact positioning of all crowns.

With placement of the straight-wire appliance after utilization of the maxillofacial orthopedic appliance, the final minor rotations, torque, and in/out and occlusal leveling movements occur rapidly in a three-dimensional direction. Use of the fixed bonded appliance usually is required for six months or less.

Bracket placement

Bracket positioning is critical for the effec-

169

Class I Malocclusion

CROWN TORQUE:

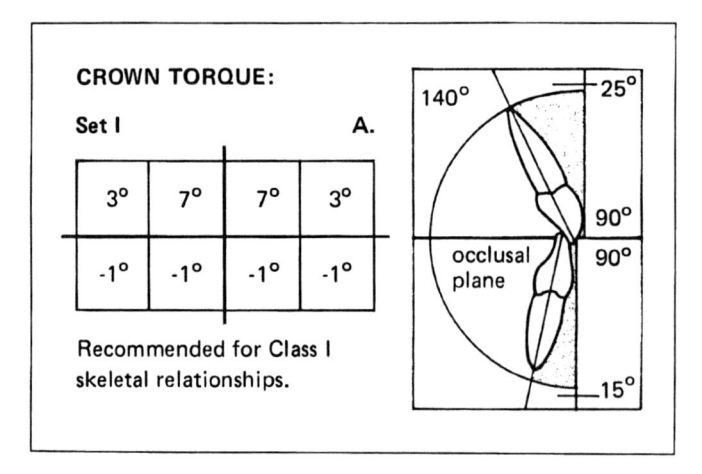

Set I — A.

3°	7°	7°	3°
-1°	-1°	-1°	-1°

Recommended for Class I skeletal relationships.

Set II — B.

-2°	2°	2°	-2°
4°	4°	4°	4°

Recommended for Class II skeletal tendencies.

Set III — C.

8°	12°	12°	8°
-6°	-6°	-6°	-6°

Recommended for Class III skeletal tendency.

Figs. 7-11a to c Different crown torques are built into brackets to maximize esthetics for various skeletal types.

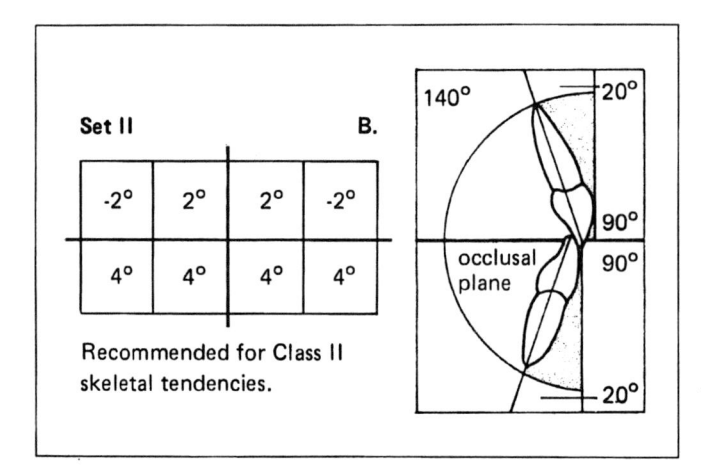

Fig. 7-11b

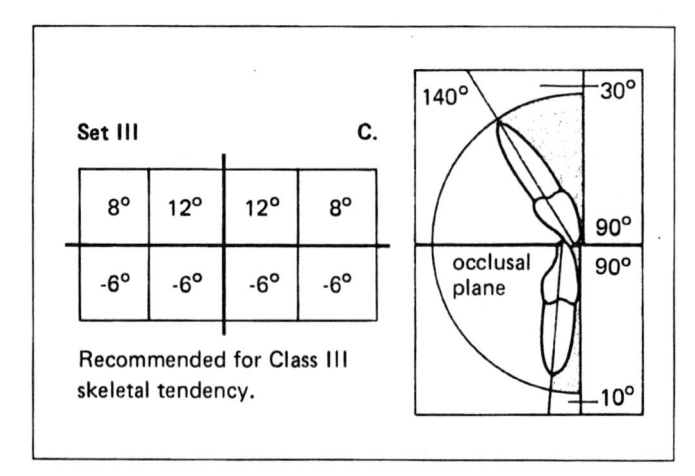

Fig. 7-11c

The Straight-wire Appliance in Clinical Practice

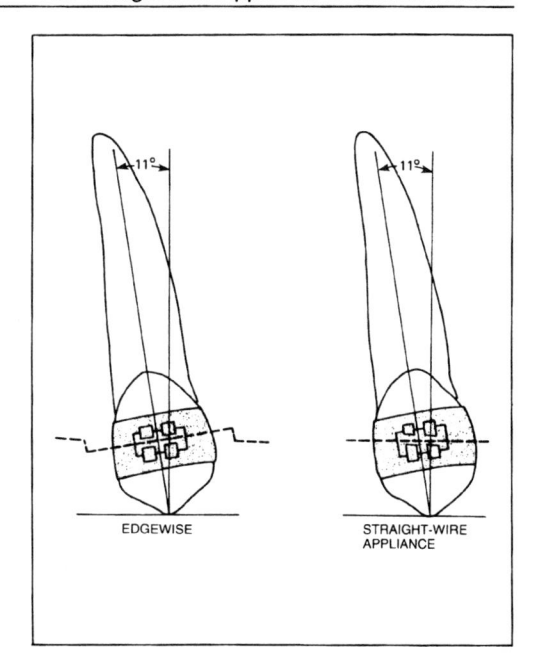

Fig. 7-12a An **edgewise bracket** placed on the long axis of the clinical crown requires wire bending to achieve the desired tip. A **straight-wire bracket** placed on the long axis of the clinical crown requires no wire bending because the desired tip is built into the bracket.

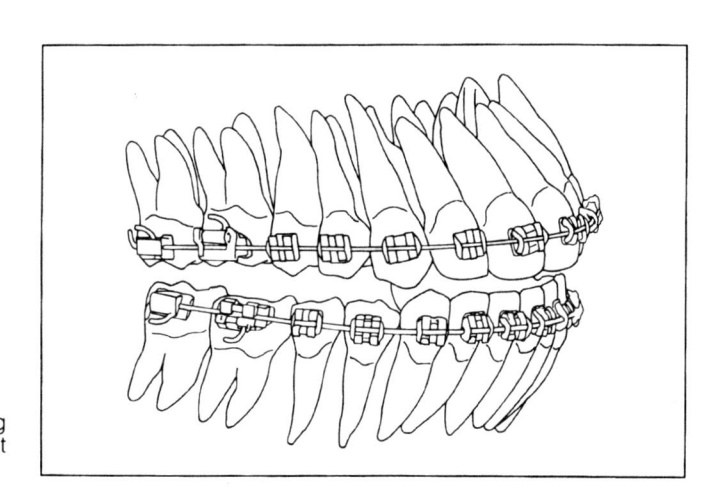

Fig. 7-12b Artist's drawing showing consistent bracket placement.

tive utilization of the straight-wire appliance. If bracket positioning is accomplished carefully, first, second, and third order bends in the wires are not necessary for most patients. Reverse and compensating curves are required for the rectangular arch wire, but most wire bending is reserved for arch form. Minimal arch form wire bending is accomplished by the selection of a broad cuspid preformed arch wire. This broad intercanine form will best accommodate the full skeletal arch development obtained with the maxillofacial orthopedic appliances and a non-premolar extraction technique.

Wire bending is occasionally necessary

171

Class I Malocclusion

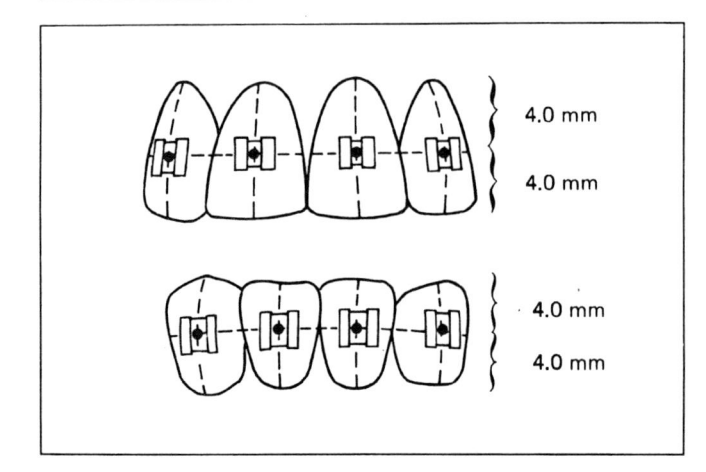

Fig. 7-13 The middle of the clinical crown on the lateral incisor is the LA point. The Anderson gauge is used to measure in millimeters the distance from the incisal edge to the LA point. All four anterior brackets are placed at this height.

to accommodate individual arch variation. The mechanics built into the individual straight-wire bracket help minimize most arch wire bends. Before bending the wire, bracket placement should be checked. Bracket repositioning will usually eliminate the need to bend the arch wire (Fig. 7-12).

The lateral incisor is used as the guide for bracket placement. The midpoint of the long axis of the clinical crown (not anatomical crown) or LACC is located at the mid-developmental vertical ridge and is the most prominent portion in the central area of the labial or buccal surface. The long axis of molar crowns can be identified by the dominant vertical groove on the buccal surface. The Anderson gauge is used to measure from the incisal edge of the lateral incisor to the midpoint of the clinical crown (LA point). Bracket placement for all four incisors will be at the same height. The tie wings on the bracket are placed parallel to the LACC with the midpoint of the slot directly over the LA point (Fig. 7-13).

The center of the bracket is centered directly over the LA point to avoid extruding or intruding the tooth and to avoid altering the correct tooth torque.

The canine bracket is placed 0.5 mm more gingivally in order to obtain the correct occlusal height and proper disclusion of the posterior teeth. Each successive posterior tooth will have a bracket height of 0.5 mm less than the tooth anterior to it. Proper bracket height ensures a correct marginal ridge height, correct crown torque, and proper intercuspation (Fig. 7-14).

Bonding technique

The brackets are directly or indirectly bonded to the buccal surface of each tooth. There is some evidence that the indirect bonding technique may save chair time and result in more accurate bracket placement with a stronger bond than with direct placement. This is especially true when utilizing a lingual bonded technique.[28] The contours of the lingual surfaces of the anterior teeth can be quite irregular. Precontouring the lingual surface and adapting the bracket to the model will enhance the strength and placement accuracy of the bracket when utilizing a lingual orthodontic technique for final finishing of the malocclusion.

Arch wire placement

Selection of the arch wire depends on the

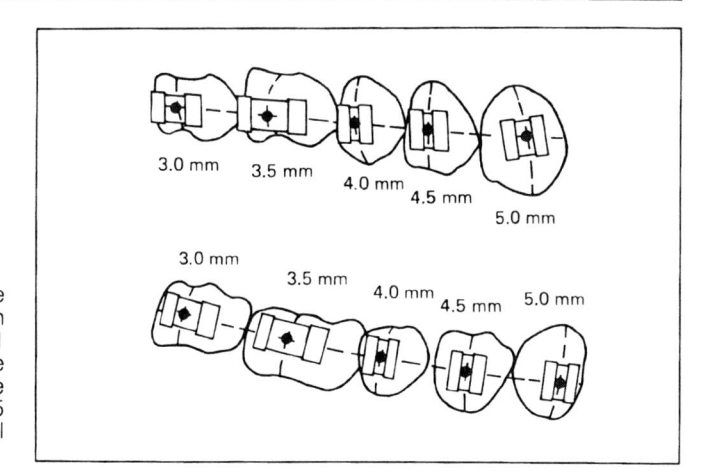

Fig. 7-14 The distance from the incisal edge to the LA point on the canine is increased by 0.5–1 mm for proper positioning. The LA point for each successive posterior tooth is reduced 0.5 mm to achieve ideal marginal ridge height and occlusion.

degree of malocclusion, clinical preference, and the specific problem. Selecting arch wire flexibility by finger pressure can be misleading; some arch wires appear more flexible than deformation tests indicate.[29] The appropriate arch wire will minimize adjustments for the clinician. Thurow[30] has defined "working range" as the distance a wire can potentially move a tooth by a single adjustment. The highly flexible arch wires eliminate most interbracket loops and allow all the brackets to be tied to the arch wire. Office visits are reduced and oral hygiene is enhanced for the patient. If required, flexible multistrand, nickel titanium (Nitinol Activ-arch*), or beta titanium wire (broad cuspid-arch form) is used for correction of rotations, leveling, and in/out alignment. These movements should be completed *before* going to the next sized round wire.

The 0.018 or second arch wire is utilized only after the 0.016 or 0.0175 arch wire is lying passively in the brackets. The 0.018 Tru Arch Form† or 0.018 Nitinol (broad cuspid arch form) is suggested. The 0.020 arch wire is utilized as a third wire unless it lies passively in the brackets. The 0.021 × 0.025 rectangular arch wire is utilized for final root torque. The rectangular wire will also prevent the molars from tipping or rolling toward the lingual.

Final finishing with the straight-wire appliance can maximize stability and esthetic results of maxillofacial orthopedic techniques. The appliance is easily placed by the dental assistant and is required only for a minimal period of time, if placed after the utilization of maxillofacial orthopedic appliances.

Summary

Class I crowded malocclusions are readily treated with maxillofacial orthopedic techniques. Excess interdental spacing, discrepancies in the levels of occlusion, torque, and dental rotation may require a combination of orthopedic and fixed appliance technique for final completion. Tooth structure removal is usually limited to interdental lower incisor stripping (Chapter 12) or the careful evaluation and removal of the second permanent molars (Chapter 11).

*Unitek Corporation, Monrovia, Calif.

†The A-Company, San Diego, Calif.

References

1. Chan, W. B., Tsamtsouris, A., and Saadia, A. M. The sagittal appliance. J. Pedod. 7:18–35, 1982.
2. Thilander, B. Treatment in the mixed dentition with special regard to the indications for orthodontic treatment. Trans. Eur. Orthod. Soc. 215–228, 1975.
3. Stöckli, P. W. Treatment timing. Trans. Eur. Orthod. Soc. 61–65, 1975.
4. Schwarz, A. M. Tissue changes incidental to orthodontic tooth movement. Int. J. Orthod. 18:331–352, 1932.
5. Enlow, D. H. Handbook of Facial Growth. 2nd ed. Philadelphia: W. B. Saunders Co., 1982.
6. Bassett, C. A. L. Biophysical principles affecting bone structure. pp. 1–76. In The Biochemistry and Physiology of Bone: Development and Growth. New York: Academic Press, 1971.
7. Baumrind, S. A consideration of the propriety of the "pressure-tension" hypothesis. Am. J. Orthod. 55:12–22, 1969.
8. Sadowsky, C., and BeGole, E. A. Long-term effects of orthodontic treatment on periodontal health. Am. J. Orthod. 80:156–172, 1981.
9. Eliason, L. A., et al. The effects of orthodontic treatment on periodontal tissues in patients with reduced periodontal support. Eur. J. Orthod. 4:1–9, 1982.
10. Wilson, H. E. Extraction of second permanent molars in orthodontic treatment. The Orthodontist 3:1–7, 1971.
11. Graber, T. M. The role of upper second molar extractions in orthodontics. Am. J. Orthod. 41:354–361, 1955.
12. Graber, T. M. Maxillary second molar extractions in Class II malocclusions. Am. J. Orthod. 56:331–353, 1969.
13. DeAngelis, V. Selection of teeth for extractions as an adjunct to orthodontic treatment. J. Am. Dent. Assoc. 87:610–615, 1973.
14. Wilson, H. E. Long-term observation on the extraction of second permanent molars. Trans. Eur. Orthod. Soc. 215–222, 1974.
15. Lehman, R. A consideration of the advantages of second molar extraction in orthodontics. Eur. Orthod. Soc. 1:119–124, 1979.
16. Betteridge, M. A. The effects of interdental stripping on the labial segments evaluated one year out of retention. Br. J. Orthod. 8:193–197, 1981.
17. Riedel, R. Retention and relapse. J. Clin. Orthod. 10:454–471, 1976.
18. Gardner, S., and Chaconas, S. Posttreatment and postretention changes following orthodontic therapy. Angle Orthod. 46:151–161, 1976.
19. Lombardi, A. Mandibular incisor crowding in completed cases. Am. J. Orthod. 61:374–383, 1972.
20. Boese, L. R. Fiberotomy and reproximation without lower retention nine years in retrospect: part II. Angle Orthod. 50:169–178, 1980.
21. Huggins, H. A. Why Raise Ugly Kids. Westport, Conn.: Arlington House Publishers, 1981.
22. Cohen, A. M. The timing of orthodontic treatment in relation to growth. Br. J. Orthod. 7:69–74, 1980.
23. Houston, W. J. B. The current status of facial growth prediction: a review. Br. J. Orthod. 6:11–17, 1979.
24. Odenrick, L., Lilja, E., and Lindbäck, K-F. Root surface resorption in two cases of rapid maxillary expansion. Br. J. Orthod. 9:37–40, 1982.
25. Janson, I. Skeletale and dentoalveoläre Änderungen durch die Bionatorbehandlung in der vorpubertären und pubertären wachstumszeit. Fortschr. Kieferorthop. 39:62–76, 1978.
26. Holdaway, R. A. Bracket angulation as applied to the edgewise appliance. Angle Orthod. 22:227–236, 1952.
27. Andrews, L. F. The six keys to normal occlusion. Am. J. Orthod. 61:297–309, 1972.
28. Scholz, R. P., and Swartz, M. L. Lingual orthodontics: a status report: Part 3 Indirect bonding—laboratory and clinical procedures. J. Clin. Orthod. 16:812–820, 1982.
29. Barrowes, K. J. Archwire flexibility and deformation. J. Clin. Orthod. 16:803–811, 1982.
30. Thurow, R. C. Edgewise Orthodontics. St. Louis: The C. V. Mosby Co., 1982, p. 18.

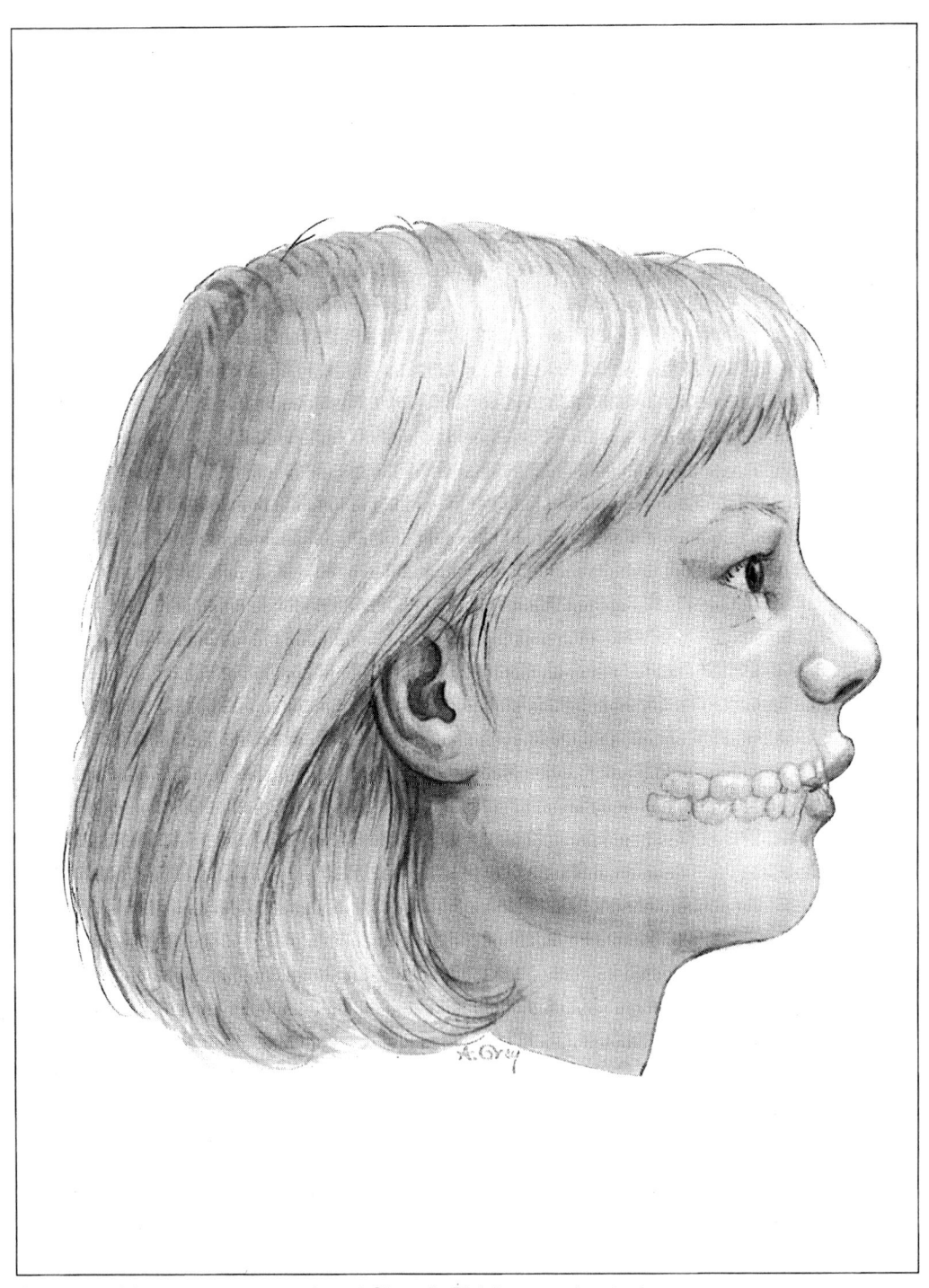

Craniofacial features representative of Class II, Division 1 malocclusion.

Chapter 8

Class II Malocclusion

Class II malocclusion can present a significant challenge to the clinician. Abnormal tooth position and abnormal bone and muscular relationships may exist in all structural components of the stomatognathic system in all three planes of space: horizontal, vertical, and sagittal. The ideal treatment plan should correct skeletal and muscular as well as dental relationships.

Class II, Division 1 malocclusion

Traditionally, the correction of a Class II, Division 1 malocclusion has been accomplished in the United States with the use of extraoral maxillary anchorage (headgear): the maxillary discrepancy has been considered the primary etiological factor of this malocclusion. The headgear produces a mechanical posterior force component to the maxillary teeth and maxilla. The theory was to arrest the normal forward growth of the maxilla, while the unrestricted mandible could grow anteriorly. These changes would achieve a normal sagittal relationship and a Class I molar position. However, the mechanical limitations of these conventional techniques do not allow for biological three-dimensional changes. Orthopedic appliances encourage growth changes while fixed appliances induce tooth movement mechanically.

Growth changes produced by orthopedic appliances affect the dentition, the alveolus, the facial musculature, the craniomandibular articulation, the tongue position, and the function of the perioral and suprahyoid muscles.

Class II, Division 2 malocclusion

Class II, Division 2 malocclusion presents a combination of anteroposterior and vertical skeletal discrepancies. This malocclusion can be established in the mixed dentition stage and is frequently characterized by insufficient mandibular growth. A deep overbite may be responsible for restricting the development of the forward growth of the mandible. The mandible achieves an upward and backward displacement resulting in a shortened lower face height and abnormal facial muscular activity.

The short lower face allows the hyperactive mentalis muscle to pull the lower lip upward, and a force is exerted on the maxillary central incisors. This force is responsible for the lingual version of the central incisors. The lateral incisors are in labial version under the influence of the orbicular oris muscle.

Class II correction

Maxillofacial orthopedic appliances correct Class II malocclusion by a combination of the following:

1. Effect on nonskeletal tissues. Abnormal muscle function is interrupted and harmonious muscular development is encouraged.
2. Proper positioning of the mandible. This allows for a more favorable pattern of horizontal and vertical growth of the dentofacial complex.
3. Restraint of maxillary growth. As the mandible attempts to return to its original posterior position, the muscles contract, creating an intermaxillary force. The retractive muscular pull is transmitted to the maxilla via the appliance.
4. Elimination of mentalis muscle interference. In Class II, Division 1 dentoalveolar malocclusion, the mentalis muscle can exacerbate the overjet by wedging the lower lip between the maxillary and mandibular incisors. This force results in the proclining of the maxillary incisors and retroclining of the mandibular incisors. Mandibular repositioning by the orthopedic appliance eliminates the interference of this muscle.

Early treatment

Treatment of Class II malocclusion is easier and more rapid if accomplished in the mixed dentition. For the most effective resolution of Class II malocclusion, Björk[1] advocates very early treatment, even as early as the primary dentition. The results are improved mastication, respiration, stability, and esthetics. Class II, Division 1 malocclusion is the most common and most easily recognized type of dentoalveolar malformation. Parents of children aged 3 or 4 with finger habits frequently ask the clinician whether the open bite, flaired incisors, or dental crowding might signal later orthodontic problems. If the permanent incisors erupt with significant overjet (5 mm or more) or exhibit labial flairing, then the increased chance for fracture of these teeth is reason enough to consider early analysis and some form of early treatment. Treatment with orthopedic appliances will discourage digit sucking habits in most Class II patients and resolve the adverse growth pattern early.

Class II, Division 2 malocclusion is treated in the late mixed dentition phase of dentoalveolar development unless symptoms (headache, neckache, backache) are a factor in the medical history. Early treatment is suggested if symptoms appear related to the malocclusion [2,3] (Chapter 10).

Patient motivation and treatment timing

With careful regard for the work of Thilander[4] and Stöckli[5] (as reviewed in Chapter 7), treatment time is guided by patient cooperation. Weiss and Eiser[6] have indicated that preadolescent patients wear removable appliances better than do older patients. However, early treatment does not guarantee cooperation. The preadolescent years—particularly ages 11, 12, and 13—are puzzling, frustrating, and rebellious. The child is between development stages: not exactly a child, but not yet an adolescent. The body is changing and preparing for puberty. These physical changes often raise anxieties that manifest themselves in obnoxious behavior. The clinician must realize that such behavior is normal and temporary. Preadolescent antics may delay, but should not disrupt entirely, a well-planned course of treatment. *Cooperation is much more dependent on patient motivation than on age* (see Chapter 6).

Deep-bite malocclusion

Treatment goals need careful consideration for patients with deep-bite malocclusion. Several investigators[7-9] have commented on the relationship of deep overbite and temporomandibular joint symptoms. Protection and improvement of the condylar-disc-fossa relationship is discussed in Chapter 10. Emphasis is placed on the concept of protection of the temporomandibular joint; virtually all treatment for malocclusion can affect this joint.

Premolar extraction

It has been suggested that maxillary premolar extraction followed by retrusion of the maxillary anterior teeth would be adequate and beneficial treatment for some patients with maxillary skeletal and dental protrusion. This has proven incorrect. None of the treatment goals was met fully by premolar extraction. By retruding the maxillary anterior segment, the mandibular skeletal component is often deflected distally as the anterior teeth come into contact. Instability and pathology within the temporomandibular joint is a possible long-term result. Janzen[10] urges careful consideration for facial esthetics by an improvement of the maxillary incisor position. However, reduction of the ANB difference via a posterior migration of point A and premolar extraction may have an adverse effect on the temporomandibular joint.

Wilson[11] has suggested that anterior bite closing and arch contraction will result when teeth mesial to the first molars are extracted. Extraction of teeth distal to the first molars was regarded as having no significant effect on the level of occlusion. If extractions are planned to alleviate dental crowding, care must be taken not to damage the condyle-disc-fossa relationship in the temporomandibular joint. Moffett[12] has discussed the importance of maintaining a dynamic equilibrium between form and function in the healthy temporomandibular joint. Suddenly deepening the bite by extracting premolars could upset the smooth function of the condylar head and articular disc with the articular surface of the temporal portion of the zygomatic bone.

Maximizing an esthetic profile

The finest facial esthetic results depend on facial harmony and symmetry or balance. *Facial harmony* as defined by Peck and Peck[13] should consider *the orderly and pleasing arrangement of the facial structures from the profile view*. The profile landmarks are identified in Fig. 8-1.

The facial profile line is an effective method of clinically evaluating lower lip position.[14] A line tangent to the soft-tissue pogonion and to the most anterior point of the upper lip will give the facial profile line. According to Merrifield,[15] the lower lip should be tangent or slightly behind the profile line (Fig. 8-2). Many patients desire a somewhat more forward position of the chin. With pogonion anteriorly positioned, the lower face tends to have a more "filled-out" appearance.

Utilization of maxillofacial orthopedic appliances with a non-premolar extraction technique ensures facial fullness. Lower facial height is maximized; the lower lip is brought out to the facial profile line. *Facial proportion, or the comparative relation of the facial structures from the profile view*,[13] is effectively achieved with orthopedic appliances. An increase in lower facial height results in esthetically pleasing chin fullness.

Facial orientation considers the relationship of the facial profile elements to the cranium. Since premolar teeth are generally not removed when using orthopedic appliances, deleterious side effects are not a

Class II Malocclusion

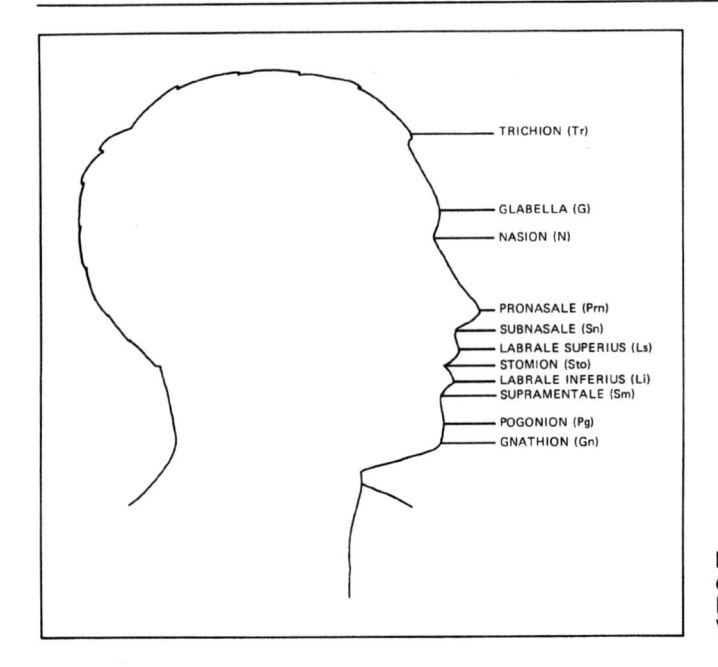

Fig. 8-1 Landmarks on the facial profile. (From Peck and Peck[13] with permission of The C. V. Mosby Co., St. Louis, Mo.)

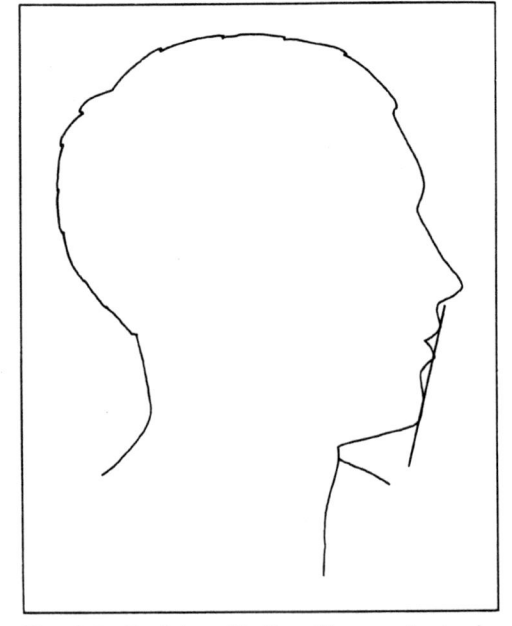

- TRICHION (Tr)
- GLABELLA (G)
- NASION (N)
- PRONASALE (Prn)
- SUBNASALE (Sn)
- LABRALE SUPERIUS (Ls)
- STOMION (Sto)
- LABRALE INFERIUS (Li)
- SUPRAMENTALE (Sm)
- POGONION (Pg)
- GNATHION (Gn)

Fig. 8-2 Facial profile line. Many patients desire the more "filled-out" facial profile that is routinely achieved with maxillofacial orthopedic techniques.

factor for facial orientation and condylar position.

Developmental response to maxillofacial orthopedic therapy

Meach[16] has studied the bony profile changes in Class II, Division 1 patients treated with extraoral force and orthopedic appliances. This study found a significant increase in the facial angle and a high percentage of forward mandibular positioning with orthopedic appliance forces as compared with extraoral forces. Figures 8-3a and b represent diagrammatically the force vectors of extraoral and orthopedic appliances.

Meach contends that the growth process of the Class II, Division 1 patient is "normalized" with orthopedic appliance therapy. Functional and esthetic improvement are brought about "through alteration of the

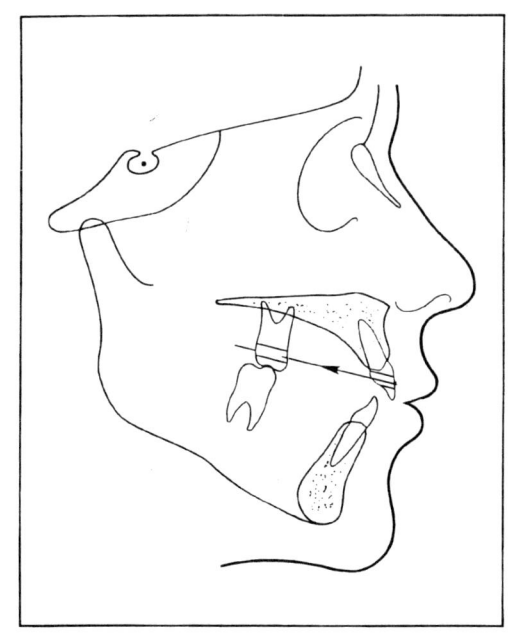

Fig. 8-3a A diagrammatic representation of the force vector with the use of extraoral force. (Modified from Meach[16] with permission of The C. V. Mosby Co., St. Louis, Mo.)

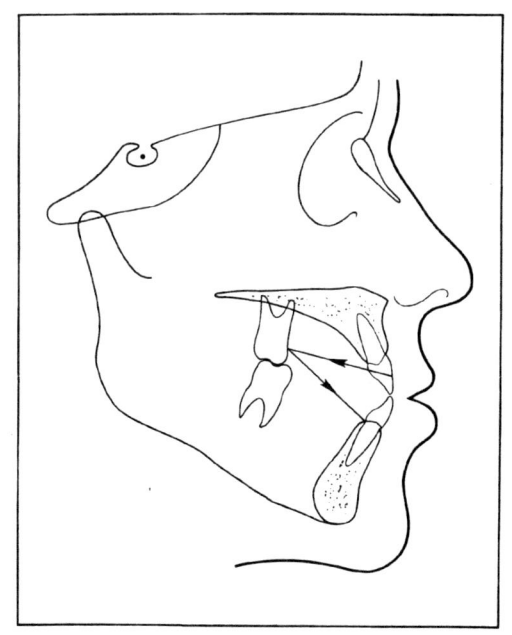

Fig. 8-3b Maxillofacial orthopedic technique distributes the force vectors to the maxillary and mandibular arches.

horizontal and vertical components of growth of the dentofacial complex, especially the mandibular condyle."[16] These findings are in agreement with those of Korkhause in 1954,[17] that the growth pattern of the alveolar process and condyle is altered during orthopedic therapy, and in 1960,[18] that the mandible can be repositioned forward into a correct occlusion with an orthopedic appliance. The correction results from the growth stimulation imparted to the muscles and temporomandibular joint.

Baume, in 1961,[19] reported that condylar cartilage was highly responsive to mechanical stimulation and highly adaptive to environmental influences. Moss[20] contended that condylar cartilage growth occurs because of the change in mandibular position. Alteration in the mandibular "functional matrix" can alter the rate and direction of mandibular growth. Harris[21] reported on an analysis of annual growth increments of the mandible in an elementary school group. The velocity of mandibular growth was strongly stimulated in patients treated with orthopedic appliances as compared with the untreated group.

Holtz[22] considered muscle tension to be the primary "power source" of maxillofacial orthopedic therapy. In his work the construction bite was taken with the mandible repositioned forward and opened for Class II patients. The muscle tension exerted an intermaxillary force on the maxilla. As the mandibular musculature attempted to retract the mandible to the former position, the force was transmitted through the orthopedic appliance to the maxilla. This force has a distalizing effect on the maxillary teeth via the interproximal acrylic and a mesializing force on the mandibular teeth.

In the Meach study,[16] the osseous profile was improved with maxillofacial orthopedic therapy. Pogonion was favorably influenced with orthopedic appliances and negatively influenced in a group treated with headgear extraoral force. The orthopedic improvement was attributed to alteration of the growth (amount and direction) of the mandibular condyle. Success of maxillofacial orthopedic correction is partially dependent on the growth potential of the mandible.

Ricketts[23] has commented that the real problem for many Class II patients is mandibular position. When there is a pathological discrepancy in the maxillary-mandibular relationship, the fault most often lies in the mandible.[24,25]

Insertion of an orthopedic appliance may alter the capsular matrix of the oral cavity. The bionator, by repositioning the mandible downward and forward, increases the volume of space that is occupied by the tongue and teeth. The teeth are encouraged to erupt into a wider, less crowded arch. The dental component is encouraged to develop to the limits of a new functional, capsular matrix.

Developing a treatment philosophy

There are many types of fixed and removable orthodontic and orthopedic appliances. Most appliances and techniques, if properly used, will correct most types of malocclusion.[26] The important goal of treatment planning is to match realistic treatment objectives with the real needs of the patient. The best results are accomplished by keeping an open mind and having the ability to utilize several techniques. Often the least complicated treatment method is the most efficient.[27]

A combined approach

Utilization of maxillofacial orthopedic, fixed, and removable appliances gives the greatest amount of flexibility for achieving treatment objectives. Pfeiffer and Grobety[28] have discussed the advantages of correcting skeletal and muscular imbalances before final tooth movement. It is stressed that tooth movement alone does not discourage the "perverting forces" of basal osseous tissue disharmony or muscular dysfunction.

Maxillofacial orthopedic appliances are designed to redirect and stimulate growth of the skeletal elements of the craniofacial structure. In addition, these appliances help to alter, improve, and balance any deleterious habits or patterns in the craniofacial neuromusculature (e.g., digit sucking, lip biting, cheek chewing).

Types of removable appliances

There are several types of removable orthodontic and orthopedic appliances. Each is designed for a particular type of malocclusion or occlusal discrepancy. Some are effective for a broad range of problems; others are more specific in purpose. A partial listing of various types includes the Andresen-Häupl activator, Bimler adaptor, bionator, Crozat, duoblock, Fränkel functional regulator, Harvold activator, Hawley retainer, oral screen, orthopedic corrector, Planas, propulsor, sagittal appliance, Schwarz expansion appliance, Stockfisch kinetor, and univator.

Advantages of orthopedic appliances

Korkhause[18] and others[24-30] have discussed the advantages and disadvantages of orthopedic appliances. The appliances are primarily used in combination with a non-premolar extraction technique.

1. Appliances are kind to the tissues. There is *less* chance of iatrogenic damage to the patient: root resorption, tipped teeth, periodontal pockets, decalcified areas on the teeth, and TMJ disorder. Since the appliances are removable, flossing, brushing, and rinsing with a fluoride rinse are all easily accomplished. When it is necessary, the surgical procedure for second molar removal is usually less stressful for the patient than third molar extraction.
2. The final result gives an excellent functional occlusion with a full complement of 28 teeth. Since premolar teeth are not extracted, there is no constricted tongue space or loss of vertical dimension. For patients with posterior crowding, the first molar will upright after second molar removal. The result is a spontaneous increase in vertical dimension as the premolar teeth are able to erupt to full potential. Third molars are allowed to erupt into the second molar position.
3. Three-dimensional movement of the skeletal component (vertical, horizontal, and sagittal) can be accomplished simultaneously. This shortens the treatment time and reduces expensive chair time for the clinician. Utilization of the orthopedic corrector can reduce the number of appliances and further reduce treatment time.
4. Some emergencies do not have to be seen immediately. Since the appliances are removable, the patient does not have to endure discomfort until the problem is corrected.
5. Excellent esthetic results. Facial esthetics are enhanced because the patient has a full broad smile without loss of vertical dimension. The patients and parents are pleased with the final esthetic results and encourage others to seek similar treatment.

Disadvantages of orthopedic appliances

1. Orthopedic appliances cannot solve all problems of malocclusion. Excess dental spacing, occlusal height discrepancies, dental rotation, and root tip and torque are more easily corrected with a multibonded straight-wire technique. Severe skeletal Class III malocclusion in adolescent or adult patients would probably require surgical correction.
2. Since the appliances are easily removed, special-needs children may have difficulty with cooperation. An adolescent between the ages of 15 and 18 may not be motivated enough to wear an appliance that can hinder enunciation. The appliances can be lost through carelessness.

Procedure for the construction bite

A proper construction bite is required to achieve the optimum results with bionator treatment. The patient should practice bringing the mandible forward with the anterior teeth in a protruded position. The degree of the forward movement of the mandible and the position of the teeth depend on the amount of overjet to be corrected and the age of the patient. For example, with Class I deep bite or Class II, Division 2 patients, the lower anterior teeth should occlude to an end-to-end relationship. When a severe skeletal overjet discrepancy exists, the mandible is brought anteriorly to the point that does not cause discomfort for the patient.

The need for a second construction bite and a new appliance at a later time may be avoided with the use of the orthopedic corrector. The construction of the orthopedic corrector is similar to that of the bionator except for the addition of two screws (one on each side) in the premolar region. These screws allow further sagittal repositioning of the mandible during treatment. Activation of the screws (two turns once a week) prouces gradual advancement of the mandible. This gradual repositioning will minimize patient discomfort (Figs. 8-4a to c).

The construction bite is taken with the wax softened to approximately 140° F and folded and placed over the posterior teeth. The thickness of the wax depends on the amount of space between the occlusal surfaces of the posterior teeth after end-to-end positioning of the anterior teeth (approximately 4 to 6 mm).

Opening the bite too much may make the patient uncomfortable. After the wax construction bite is chilled and trimmed, it is placed back in the mouth to check for occlusal or midline discrepancies. Two additional construction bites in the same position will help avoid errors and give the laboratory technician some flexibility during construction of the appliance.

Changes observed with bionator use

Maxilla

1. slight posterior expansion (accomplished by the activation of the coffin spring)
2. vertical alveolar bone growth (contributes to the correction of a deep bite)
3. downward rotation of the premaxilla (contributes to the correction of an open bite)
4. improved muscular balance and tone

Mandible

1. slight expansion of the anterior segment (accomplished by the once-a-week activation of the lingual midline screw)
2. repositioning of the mandible

3. improved muscular balance and tone
4. vertical alveolar bone growth

Check for proper appliance construction

After initial insertion of the appliance, the following should be checked to ensure patient comfort:

1. The appliance is held against the maxillary arch with the wires in the desired position.
2. The acrylic and the coffin spring wire should not impinge on the soft tissues.
3. With the patient closing into the appliance, the distal extension of the acrylic should not extend beyond the middle portion of the last molar and should not impinge on the floor of the mouth.
4. Stability is evaluated with the appliance seated in the mandibular arch. There should be no rocking or lateral tipping of the appliance.
5. There should be no patient discomfort with the appliance inserted.

Instructions to patients

Patient cooperation is important for successful bionator treatment (Chapter 13). A close rapport between the clinician and the patient is especially helpful at the beginning of treatment. Better appliance acceptance is noted when the patient is prepared for the difficulties in swallowing and speaking that will be encountered during the first few days. The clinical assistant should have the patient practice talking and swallowing with the teeth closed into the appliance.

The patient should be encouraged to always wear the appliance except during meals. If the child reports an inability to sleep because "the appliance keeps falling out," then cooperation is doubtful; this may

Changes Observed With Bionater Use

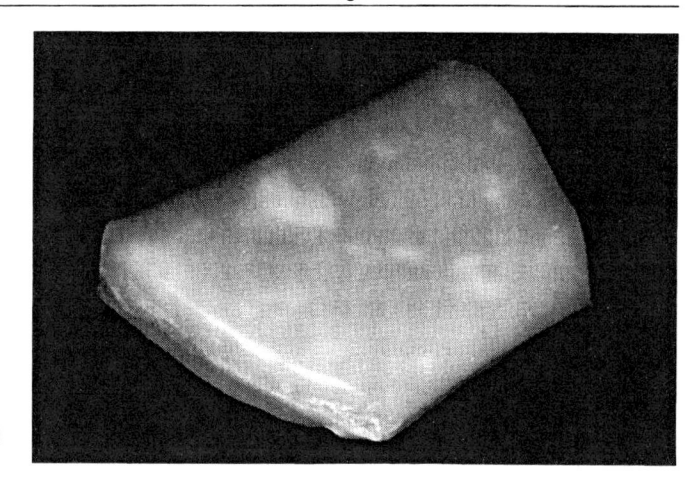

Figs. 8-4a to c Construction bite for the Class II bionator.

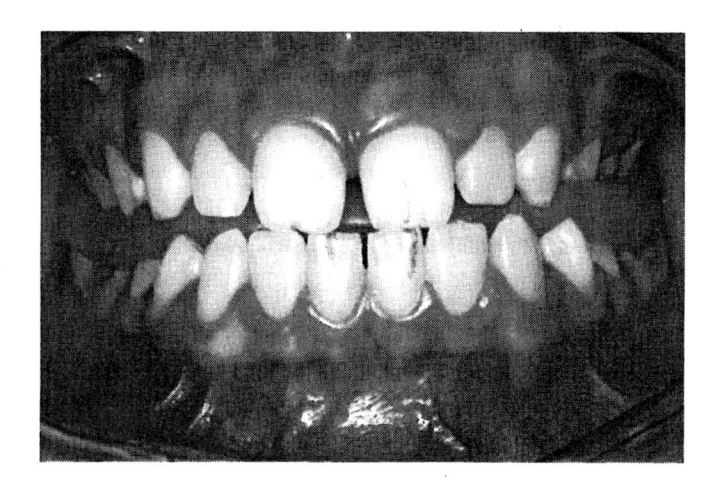

Fig. 8-4b

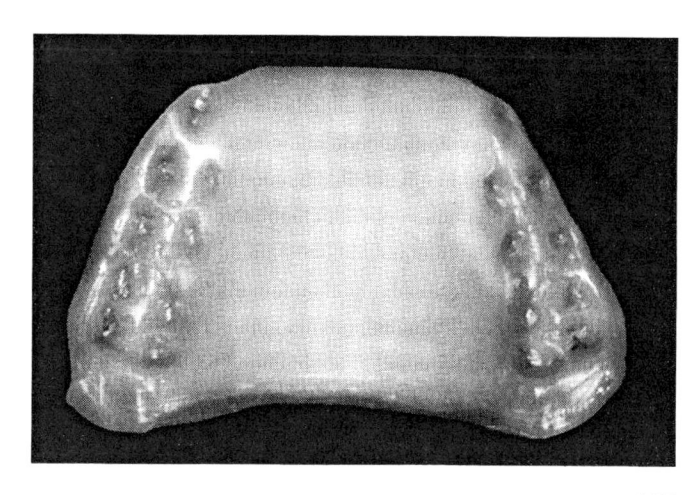

Fig. 8-4c

Class II Malocclusion

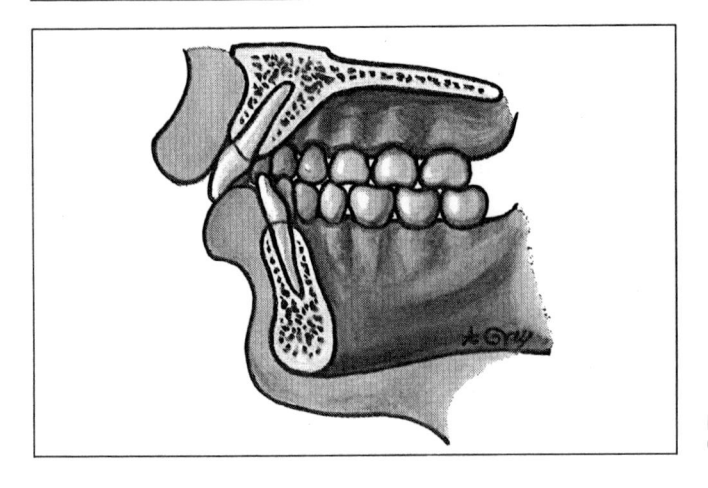

Fig. 8-5 Cross section of a Class II malocclusion.

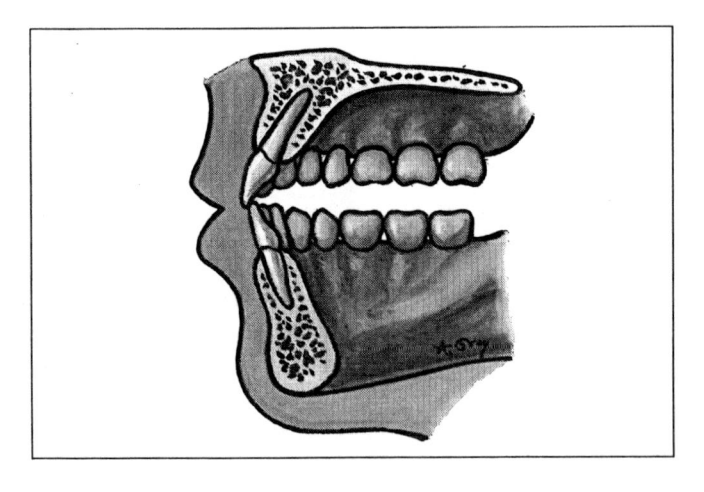

Fig. 8-6 Cross section of a forwardly repositioned mandible. Notice the improved facial esthetics, Class I occlusal position, and the posterior interocclusal space.

indicate that the patient is not wearing the appliance during the day.

If there is a mandibular midline screw, activation is usually once a week.

Verbal reinforcement (praise) at the periodic adjustment appointments helps achieve good patient cooperation and successful results.

After the anticipated results are accomplished, the bionator may be worn at night only for two to six months before being discarded. Relapse is usually minimal, if the appliance has been worn properly (Chapter 3).

The best form of motivation is the individual patient diary or orthodontic progress report (Fig. 12-3). Repeated praise gives the patient confidence that minor speech problems can be overcome.

Method of appliance action

The bionator appliance is especially effective for patients with mandibular retrognathism and shortened lower facial height (Fig. 8-5). An immediate improvement in facial esthetics is noted when the patient repositions the mandible forward (Fig. 8-6).

Generalized Treatment Plan

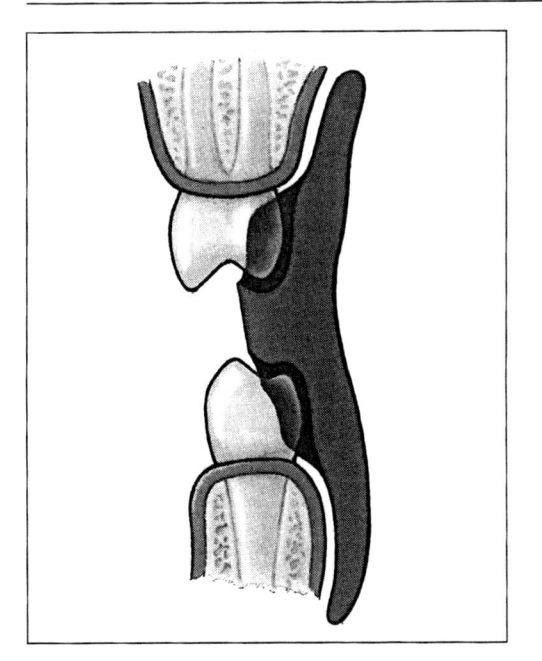

Fig. 8-7 The interproximal acrylic is generally present between the premolars and molars.

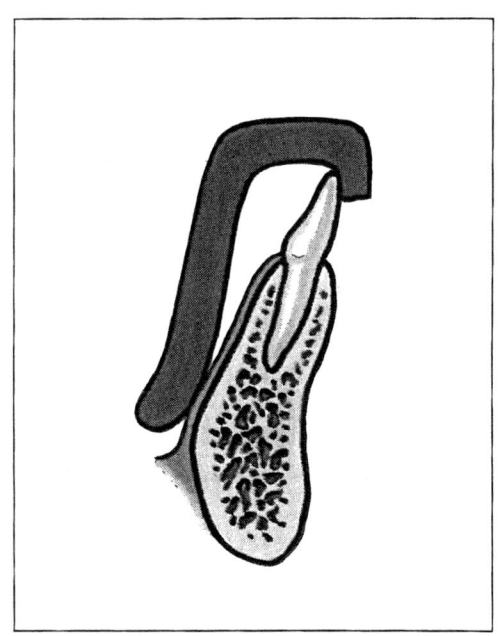

Fig. 8-8 The acrylic in the anterior lingual portion should be free from the tooth and alveolar bone contact in order not to produce overflaring of the anterior teeth. The only contact exists on the lowest portion of the acrylic. This serves as a propioceptive mechanism. The acrylic coverage prevents overeruption of these teeth.

The bionator resists the distal pull of the musculature toward the rest position. This is accomplished by the interproximal acrylic wedged between the teeth (Fig. 8-7) and by the lingual acrylic in the area of the mandibular anterior incisors (Fig. 8-8). The acrylic in the bionator acts as a transducer, changing mechanical energy into electrical stimuli, which activate the growth response (Chapter 2).

Interocclusal acrylic is utilized for patients with anterior open bite (Figs. 8-9 and 8-10). The interocclusal acrylic appears to produce an autorotation of the mandibular arch and a downward rotation of the premaxilla.

For patients with a deep bite, alveolar growth is encouraged when no interocclusal acrylic is present (Figs. 8-11a and b).

To aid interarch leveling, occlusal acrylic can be placed on the maxillary and mandibular teeth to encourage alveolar development (Figs. 8-12a and b).

Minor dental corrections can be accomplished by selective removal of the interproximal acrylic. On appliance insertion, the interproximal acrylic should completely fill the interproximal spaces (Fig. 8-13). During treatment, the interproximal acrylic is removed to encourage final dental positioning (Figs. 8-14a and b).

Generalized treatment plan

Each patient and malocclusion requires an individualized treatment plan based on the

Class II Malocclusion

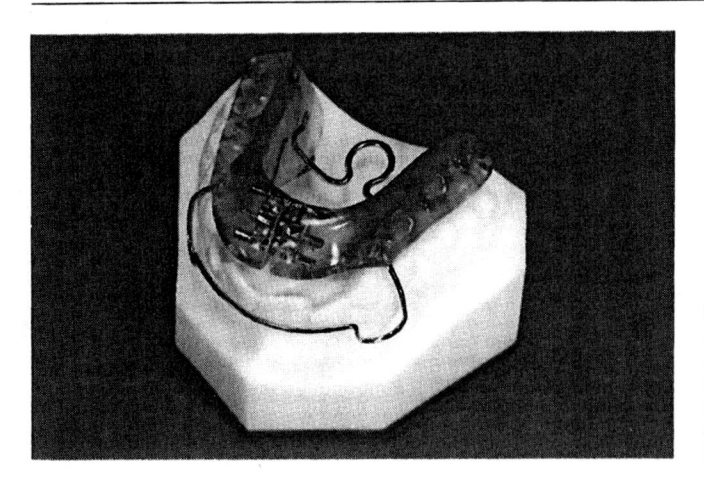

Fig. 8-9 Bionator for treatment of an open bite: interocclusal acrylic with no lingual wire and no coverage of the mandibular anterior teeth. (Courtesy of Dyna-Flex Orthodontic Laboratory, St. Louis, Mo.)

history and documented examination. It is helpful, however, to have an overall plan of treatment sequence. A written sequential treatment plan will shorten treatment time and avoid communication errors with the patient. The following order is suggested for correcting many types of malocclusion:

1. correction of anterior or posterior crossbite
2. elimination of crowding in the dental arches and achievement of a stable maxillomandibular skeletal and neuromuscular relationship, and correction of vertical discrepancy
3. correction of rotated and excessively spaced dental components, leveling of the occlusal plane, and final correction of in/out, root tip, and root torque

A standard treatment sequence with a set time allotted for each phase will help shorten the treatment time and keep the patient positively motivated. Treatment plan modification and individualization is expected. Maxillary crowding is usually treated before maxillomandibular skeletal harmony is attained. An atlas-style presentation of examples of Class II malocclusion will demonstrate individualized treatment plans and goals.

K.M., age 10.6 (Figs. 8-15a to h)

K.M. presented with a Class II, Division 1 malocclusion. Overjet was 7 mm and overbite was 6 mm (deep). She had a history of prolonged thumb sucking and was still occasionally observed sleeping with her thumb in her mouth. The patient was self-conscious about her appearance and wanted treatment for her malocclusion but was skeptical about wearing an appliance. A treatment plan was formulated to minimize appliance intrusion and interrupt the thumb habit.

Treatment plan for K.M.	*Treatment time*
A. orthopedic records	
B. orthopedic corrector	12 months
C. rest	6 months
D. bionator, night only	6 months
E. removal of third molars at age 15 to 20	

Treatment time was 20 visits over 24 months.

Mandibular growth

Some investigators have found a change in

Mandibular Growth

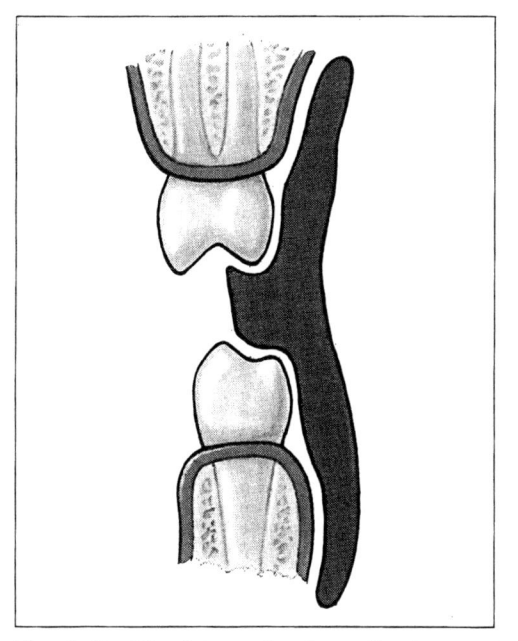

Fig. 8-10 The interocclusal acrylic does not encourage posterior alveolar bone growth.

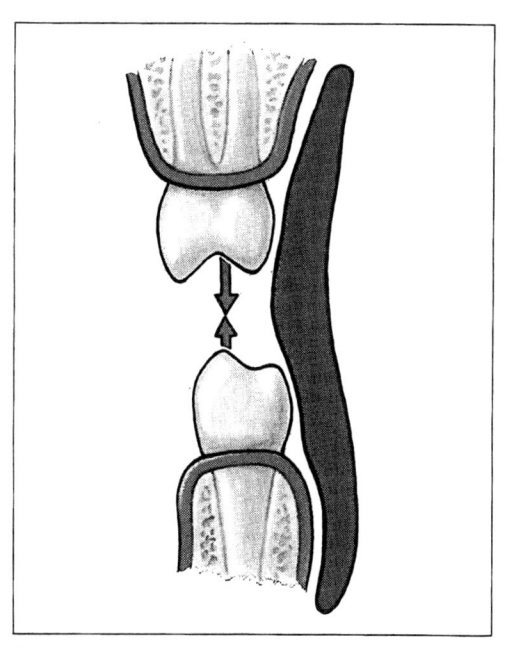

Fig. 8-11a In order to stimulate posterior alveolar bone development, interocclusal acrylic coverage is not utilized for patients with short lower alveolar facial height.

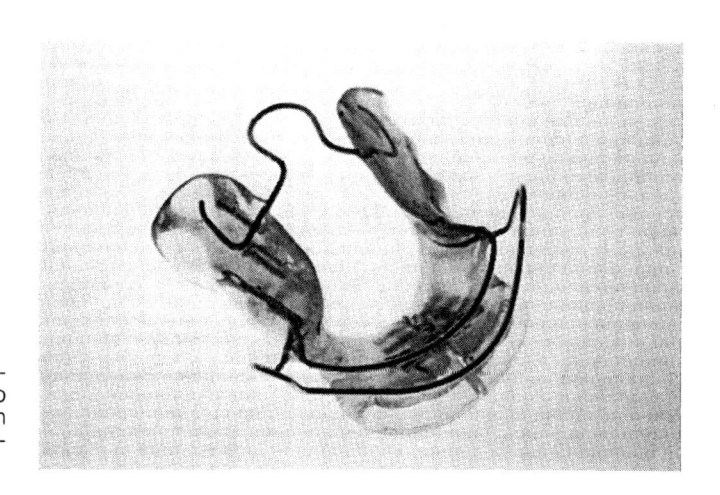

Fig. 8-11b Bionator for treatment of a deep bite. There is no interocclusal acrylic. There is an acrylic cap over mandibular anterior teeth, and a lingual wire.

skeletal development that is greater than normal when mandibular growth is stimulated with an orthopedic appliance.[31,32] Other researchers feel that although growth per se is not stimulated, the direction of mandibular growth is altered. Jakobsson[33] reported a small increase in the gonial angle and an increase in lower face height. Later studies by Ahlgren and Laurin,[34] and Pancherz[35] did not, however, confirm any

189

Class II Malocclusion

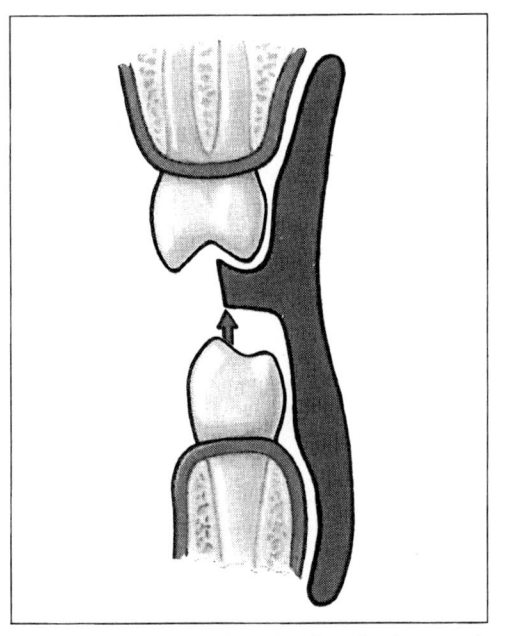

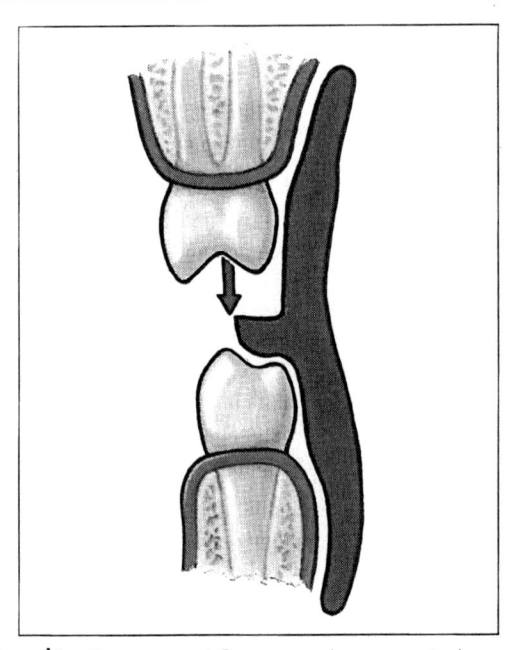

Figs. 8-12a and b By adjusting the interocclusal acrylic, the curve of Spee may be corrected.

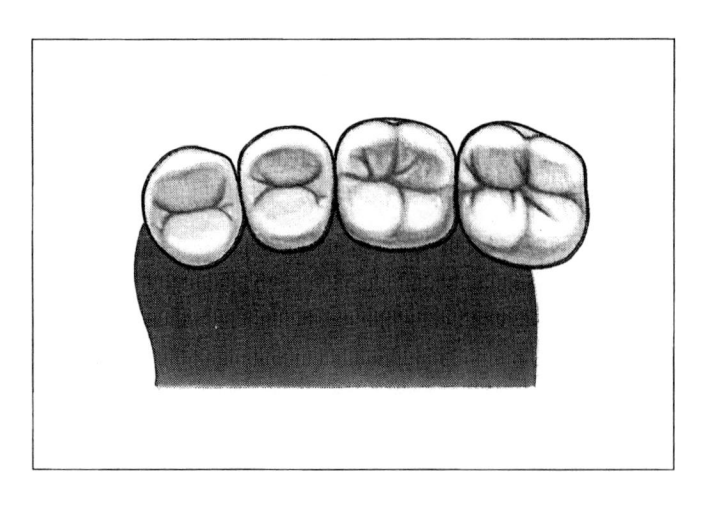

Fig. 8-13 The interproximal acrylic should not be blunted. It should fill the interproximal spaces.

permanent opening rotation of the mandible with orthopedic therapy.

Maxillary growth is also affected in maxillofacial orthopedic appliance therapy. The force of the activated musculature transmitted through the appliance (Fig. 8-3b) to the maxillary dentition has an inhibitory effect on forward maxillary growth. Mills[36] has shown that the most retruded part of the skeletal maxilla (cephalometric point A) is really an alveolar, not a basal, landmark. The maxillary distalizing force of the appli-

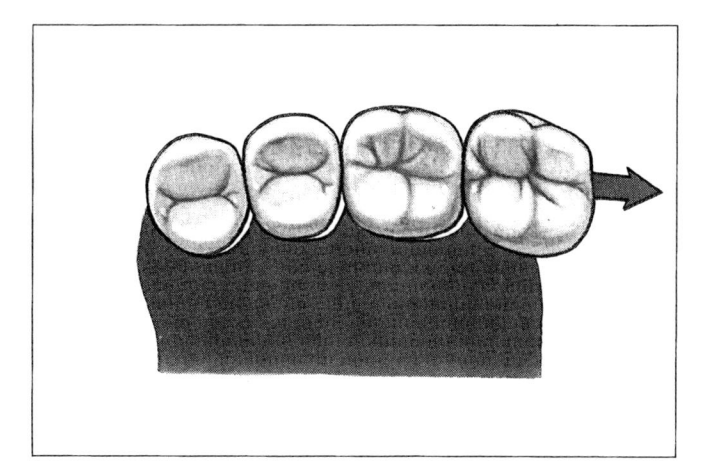

Figs. 8-14a and b Selective removal of interproximal acrylic can direct final tooth movement. If an end-to-end molar relationship exists toward the end of treatment, Class I correction can be achieved by grinding the distal interproximal maxillary acrylic and the mesial interproximal mandibular acrylic.

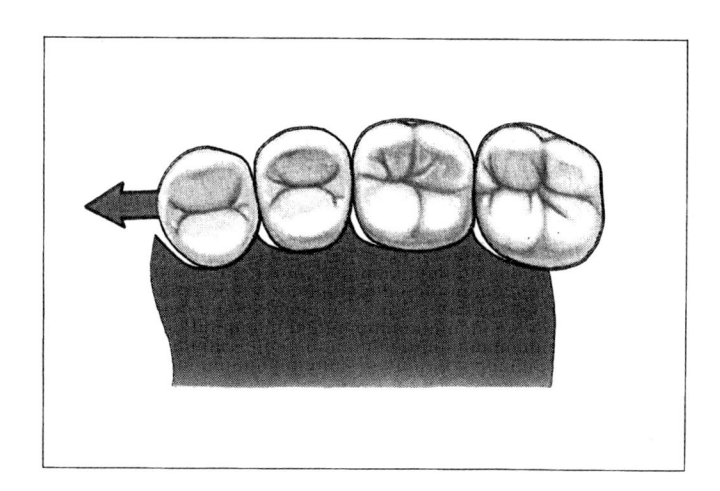

Fig. 8-14b

ance will also serve to induce osseous remodeling in the maxillary skeletal tissues.

Most investigators agree that dentoalveolar changes account for the additional occlusal results achieved with maxillofacial orthopedic appliances. Woodside,[37] and Reey and Eastwood[38] have demonstrated overbite reduction via posterior dentoalveolar growth and eruption. Calvert[39] has shown that the amount of mandibular growth stimulation with the Andresen appliance is small. Changes in the skeletal profile and dental occlusion result from a combination of mandibular growth, maxillary skeletal remodeling, and dentoalveolar changes that include some slight tipping of anterior teeth and eruption of posterior teeth.

Craniofacial response to maxillofacial orthopedic appliance therapy

Although Jakobsson[33] and others[31,32,39] do not agree that condylar growth and a forward position of pogonion can be attained

Class II Malocclusion

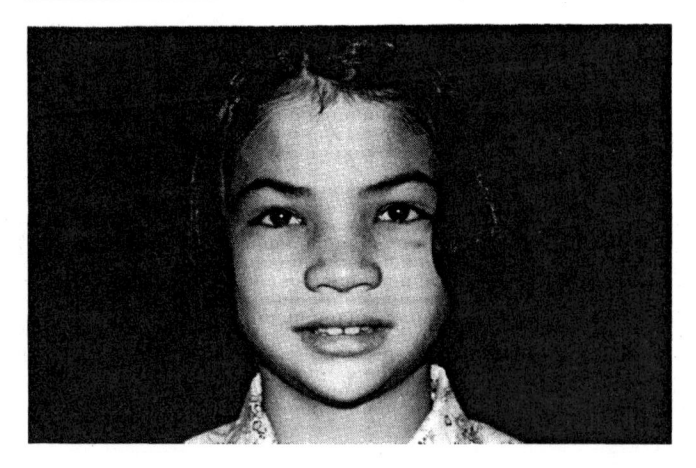

Fig. 8-15a K. M. Full face, pretreatment.

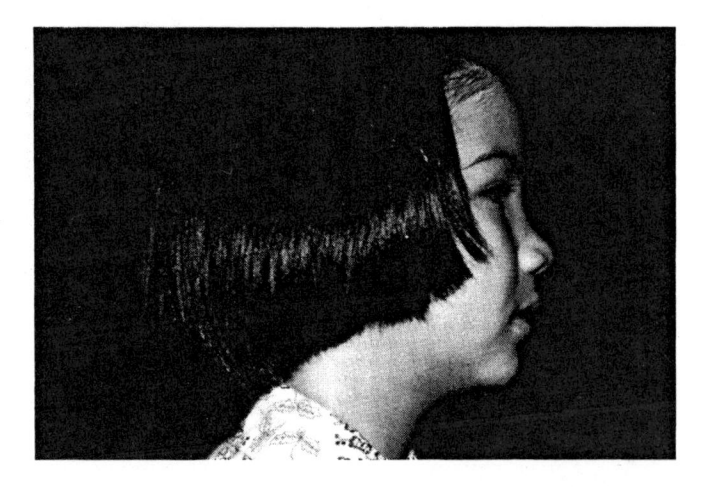

Fig. 8-15b Pretreatment facial profile.

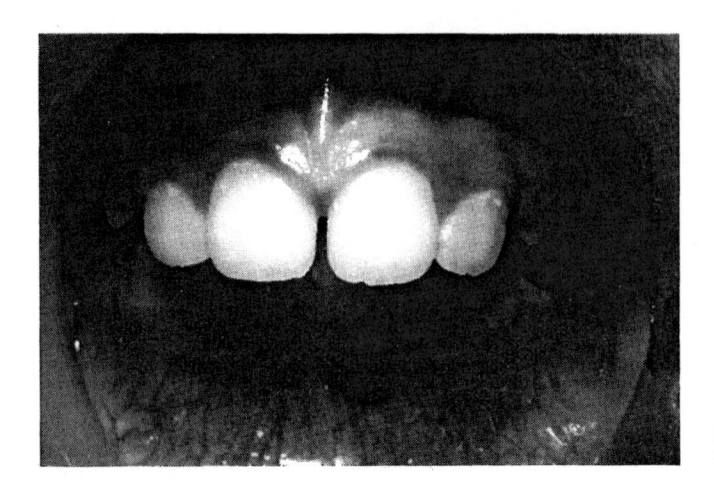

Fig. 8-15c Pretreatment labial view.

192

Craniofacial Response to Maxillofacial Orthopedic Appliance Therapy

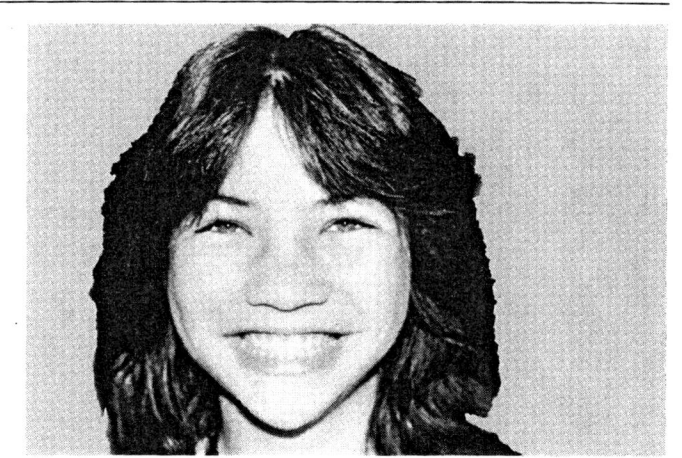

Fig. 8-15d K. M. Full face, post-treatment.

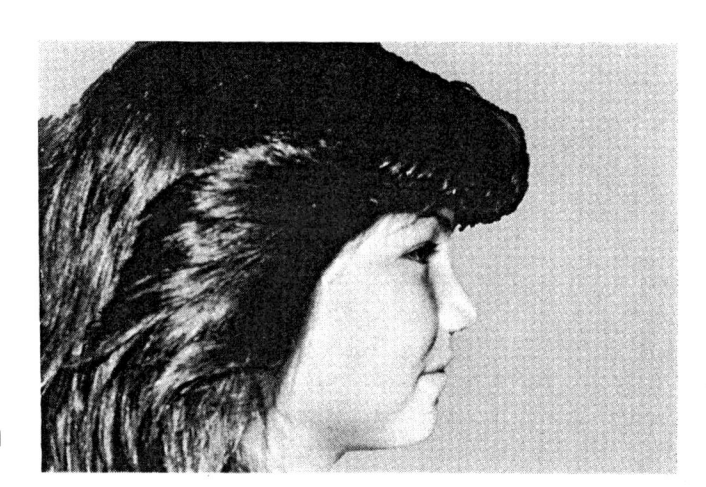

Fig. 8-15e Posttreatment facial profile.

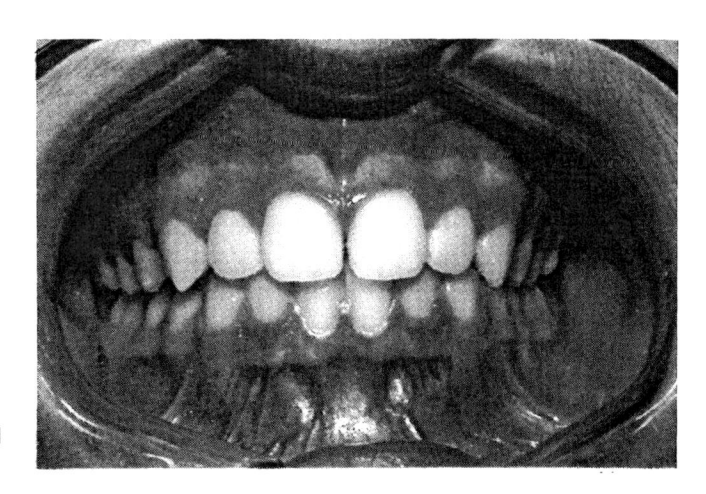

Fig. 8-15f Posttreatment labial view.

193

Class II Malocclusion

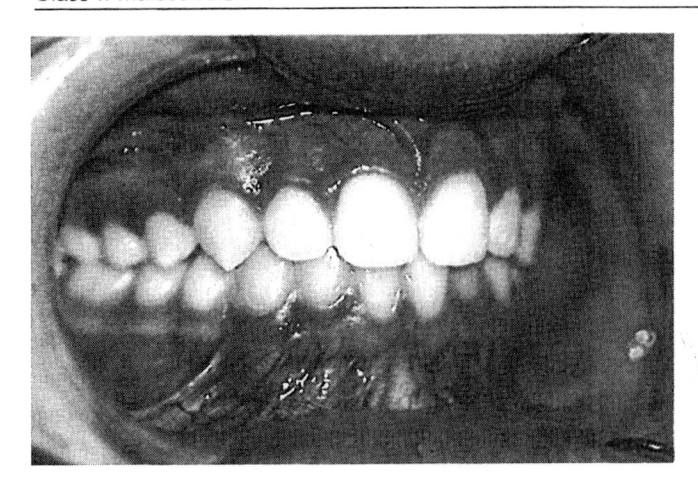

Fig. 8-15g Posttreatment right buccal view.

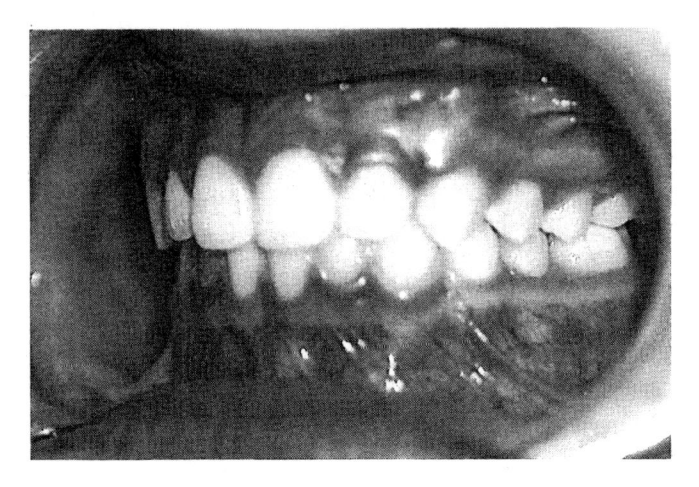

Fig. 8-15h Posttreatment left buccal view.

with maxillofacial orthopedic technique, other investigators[40-47] have shown positive growth results.

In a comparative study of the Fränkel and activator appliance and extraoral traction, Righellis[48] found the Fränkel appliance to have the following effect for 16 patients in the mixed dentition:

1. no significant horizontal effect on maxillary growth
2. mandibular length was significantly increased
3. variable effects on lower face height
4. some increase in molar eruption, especially in the mandible

Gianelly et al.,[49] in a statistical evaluation of condylar position and mandibular length changes in 10 patients after one year of Fränkel appliance therapy, found large variations in mandibular growth. The results of Fränkel appliance therapy were not significantly different from the means of patients treated with an edgewise appliance. The authors doubt that mandibular repositioning appliances can stimulate condylar growth in humans under clinical conditions.

Studies by Woodside et al.[50] suggest that chronic or continuous alteration in mandibular position within the neuromuscular environment can produce extensive condylar remodeling and size changes in the mandible.

Mandibular growth, as reviewed in Chapter 2, occurs from apposition on the distal border of the ramus and resorption on the mesial border. Moss and Salentijn[40] have theorized that as the oral capsule grows downward and forward, it carries the mandible. Growth is induced along the distal border of the ramus. Enlow[41] has shown that condylar growth occurs as a compensatory response to fill the space left by the mandible as it is carried forward by the facial musculature.

Craniofacial response to maxillofacial orthopedic therapy (Chapter 3) is well-documented by scientific study.[42-46] As the appliance is placed, the neuromusculature gives the condyle and all the osseous facial tissues feedback indicating forward mandibular growth. The condylar cartilage responds by proliferating and stimulating the production of osseous tissue.

Stöckli and Willert,[42] in 1971, studied the growth response of the temporomandibular joint in growing Macacus Iris monkeys after placing splints that caused mandibular protrusion. The study found that mechanical stimuli could produce adaptive changes in the temporomandibular joint of the monkeys, and that the new condylar position demonstrated a high resistance against relapse after the splints were removed.

Petrovic et al.,[43] in 1975, studied mandibular hyperpropulsion in rats. These investigators found that mandibular growth rate increased with forward positioning of the rat mandible. Mandibular growth response was found to be closely linked with the level of circulating somatotrophic growth hormone.

McNamara et al.[44] in 1975, McNamara[45] in 1979, and McNamara[46] in 1980 have studied forward mandibular repositioning in growing Macaca Mulatta monkeys. Electromyographical changes were noted in the superior head of the lateral pterygoid muscle. The frequency and amplitude of muscle activity increased until four to eight weeks before slowly returning to normal after 12 weeks. These changes in muscle activity paralleled histologic proliferation of the chondroblastic layer of the condylar growth cartilage (Fig. 2-14). Skeletal changes that were similar in pattern and time to the electromyographical changes of the superior head of the lateral pterygoid muscle were also observed in the mandibles of the monkeys.

The increased muscle activity of the superior head of the lateral pterygoid muscle, the histologic change in the condylar cartilage, and increased mandibular growth were all found to occur simultaneously after insertion of a mandibular repositioning appliance. When young adult patients were studied,[51] it was shown that mandibular length did not increase significantly with functional regulator treatment. However, increases in vertical dimension were noted. Bass has summarized the clinical application of an appliance system that utilizes a neurogenic feedback mechanism for growing children:[47]

1. Forward mandibular repositioning in response to an appliance will cause continuous contraction of the lateral pterygoid muscle.
2. Appliance activation is increased at six- to eight-week intervals to limit muscular adaptation and continuously stimulate condylar growth.
3. A rapidly growing patient ensures an effective level of somatotrophic circulating hormone in order to significantly influence condylar growth cartilage.

Class II Malocclusion

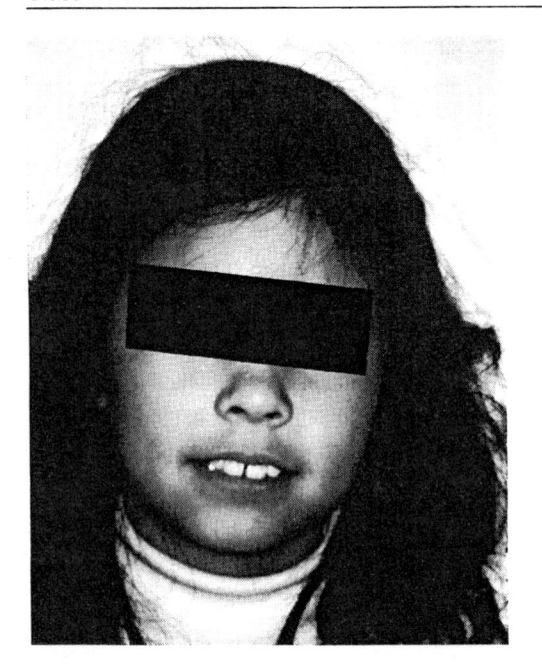

Figs. 8-16a to c T. G. Pretreatment photographs.

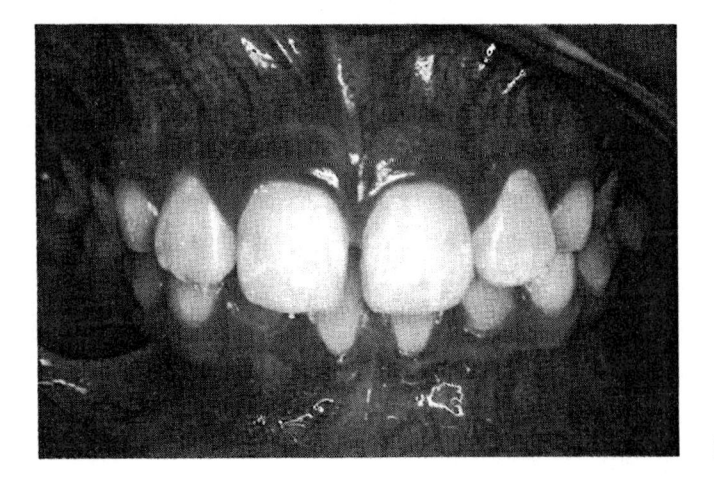

Fig. 8-16b

T.G., age 9.5 (Figs. 8-16a to i)

T.G. presented with a Class II, Division 1 malocclusion. Overjet was 6.5 mm and overbite was 5 mm. The parent was concerned about the excessive overjet and the facial appearance (Figs. 8-16a to c).

Cephalometrically, this patient presented with a Class II skeletal mandibular retrusion and protruded maxillary incisors (Fig. 8-16d).

Treatment plan for T.G.	Treatment time
A. orthopedic records	
B. bionator	18 months
C. bionator, night only	6 months

196

Craniofacial Response to Maxillofacial Orthopedic Appliance Therapy

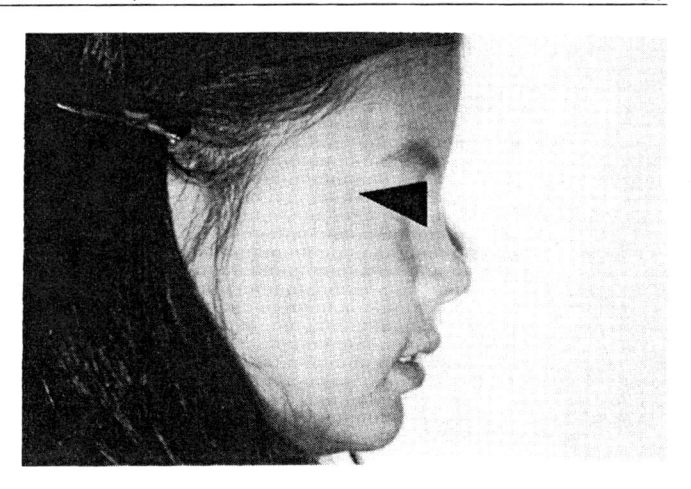

Fig. 8-16c

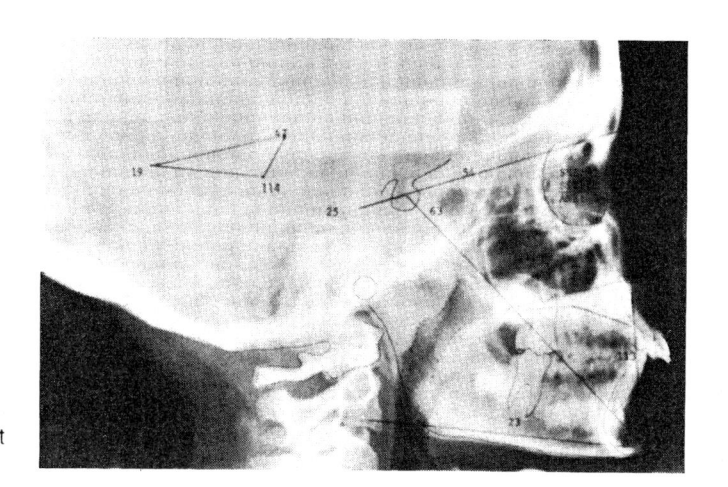

Fig. 8-16d Before treatment cephalogram.

Ongoing treatment photographs reveal an improvement in facial esthetics and occlusion (Figs. 8-16e to g). The post-bionator treatment cephalogram demonstrates an improved skeletal pattern with a normal interincisal angle (Fig. 8-16h). Superimposition of the pre- and post-bionator treatment radiographs on the S-N plane show a downward and forward growth of the mandible and some downward displacement of the maxilla (Fig. 8-16i). The labial wire has helped with the correction of the maxillary protrusion.

The skeletal component of this malocclusion was corrected early because Class II malocclusion tends to get worse over time. Future treatment may include additional correction of the dental component with the straight-wire appliance (Chapter 7).

Summary

The patients presented, animal studies,

Class II Malocclusion

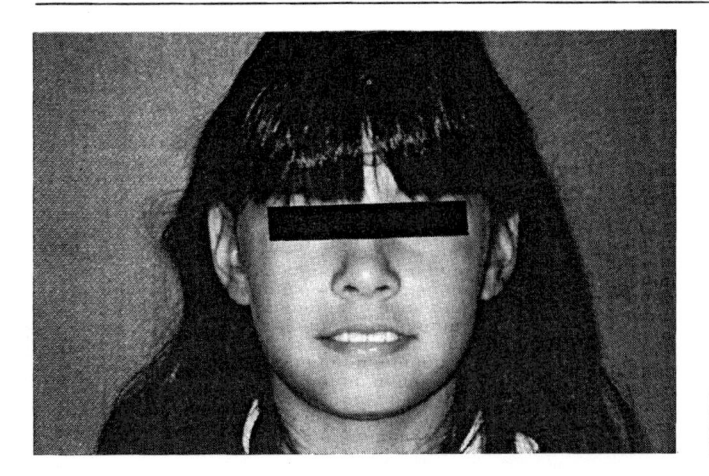

Figs. 816e to g T. G. Post-bionator treatment photographs in the mixed dentition.

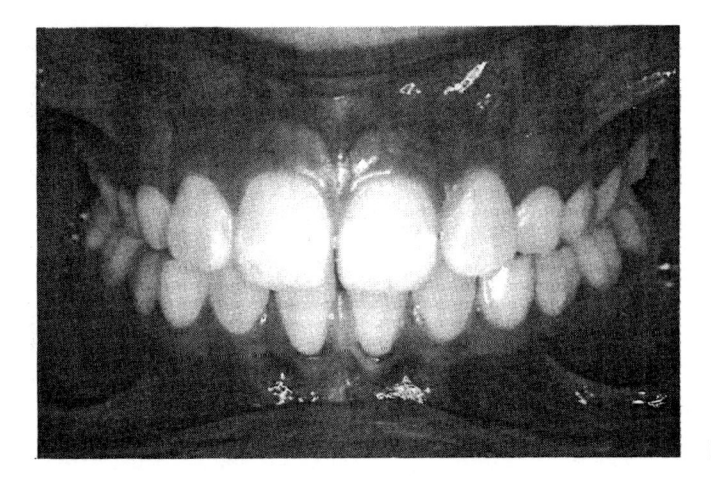

Fig. 8-16f

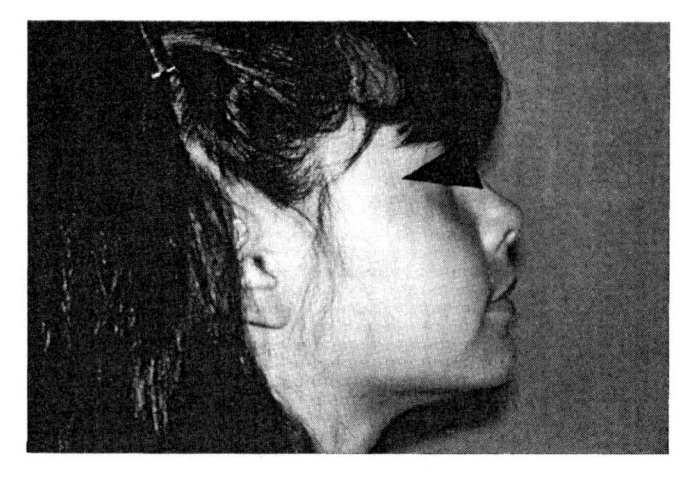

Fig. 8-16g

198

Summary

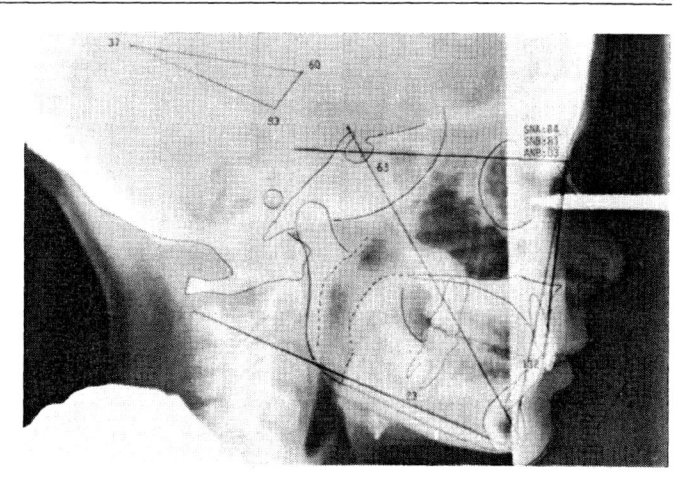

Fig. 8-16h Post-bionator treatment cephalogram.

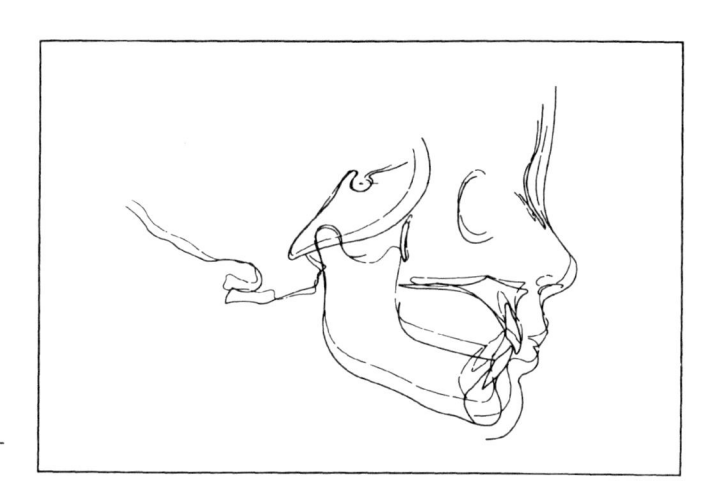

Fig. 8-16i Cephalometric superimposition.

and the bulk of scientific evidence indicate positive histological, skeletal, dental, and esthetic results from the use of maxillofacial orthopedic techniques. Final dental correction and occlusal refinement may require a fixed technique during the last few months of treatment. A fixed appliance that includes the indirect technique of bracket bonding can save the clinician significant chair time.[52] The maxillofacial orthopedic treatment for Class II discrepancy should be initiated as soon as the clinician feels effective results will be obtained. Management of the developing craniofacial complex with orthopedic appliances will shorten treatment time. Since prediction of rapid growth is difficult,[53,54] treatment of anteroposterior skeletal discrepancies is initiated when patient cooperation is evident (see Chapter 6).

References

1. Björk, A. Andresen method of orthodontic treatment. Am. J. Orthod. 37:437–458, 1951.
2. Ahlin, J. H., and Ramos-Gómez, F. J. Treatment of temporomandibular joint related headaches in the pedodontic patient: a preliminary report. J. Pedod. 6:164–175, 1982.
3. Stack, B., and Funt, L. Temporomandibular joint dysfunctions in children. J. Pedod. 1:240–247, 1977.
4. Thilander, B. Treatment in the mixed dentition with special regard to the indications for orthodontic treatment. Trans. Eur. Orthod. Soc. 215–228, 1975.
5. Stöckli, P. W. Treatment timing. Trans. Eur. Orthod. Soc. 61–65, 1975.
6. Weiss, J., and Eiser, H. M. Psychological timing of orthodontic treatment. Am. J. Orthod. 72:198–204, 1977.
7. Williamson, E. H. Temporomandibular dysfunction in pretreatment adolescent patients. Am. J. Orthod. 72:429–433, 1977.
8. Rickets, R. M. Laiminography in the diagnosis of temporomandibular joint disorders. J. Am. Dent. Assoc. 46:620–648, 1953.
9. Prentiss, H. J. Preliminary report upon the temporomandibular articulation in the human. Dent. Cosmos 60:505–512, 1918.
10. Janzen, E. K. A balanced smile—a most important treatment objective. Am. J. Orthod. 72:359–372, 1977.
11. Wilson, W. L. The development of a treatment plan in the light of one's concept of treatment objectives. Am. J. Orthod. 45:561–573, 1959.
12. Moffett, B. The morphogenesis of the temporomandibular joint. Am. J. Orthod. 52:401–415, 1966.
13. Peck, H., and Peck, S. A concept of facial esthetics. Angle Orthod. 40:284–318, 1970.
14. Holdaway, R. H. Changes in relationship of points A and B during orthodontic treatment. Am. J. Orthod. 42:176–193, 1956.
15. Merrifield, L. L. The profile line as an aid in critically evaluating facial esthetics. Am. J. Orthod. 52:804–822, 1966.
16. Meach, C. L. A cephalometric comparison of bony profile changes in Class II, Division 1 patients treated with extraoral force and functional jaw orthopedics. Am. J. Orthod. 52:353–370, 1966.
17. Korkhause, G. Die Kieferorthopädische Bissverlagerung. In G. Korkhause (ed.) Zahn-, Mund-, und Kieferheilkunde in Vorträgen. Munich: Carl Hanser, 1954.
18. Korkhause, G. Present orthodontic thought in Germany. Am. J. Orthod. 46:270–287, 1960.
19. Baume, L. Principles of cephalofacial development revealed by experimental biology. Am. J. Orthod. 47:881–901, 1961.
20. Moss, M. L. Functional analysis of human mandibular growth. J. Pros. Dent. 10:1149–1159, 1960.
21. Harris, J. D. A cephalometric analysis of mandibular growth. Am. J. Orthod. 48:161–174, 1962.
22. Holtz, R. P. Application and appliance manipulation of functional forces. Am. J. Orthod. 58:459–477, 1970.
23. Ricketts, R. M. A foundation for cephalometric communication. Am. J. Orthod. 46:330–357, 1960.
24. Harvold, E. P. Some biologic aspects of orthodontic treatment in the transitional stage. Am. J. Orthod. 49:1–27, 1958.
25. McNamara, J. A., Jr. Components of Class II malocclusion in children 8–10 years of age. Angle Orthod. 51:177–202, 1981.
26. Grave, K. C., McKinnon, J. D., and Smart, L. M. Reality in orthodontics and a treatment approach for certain malocclusions. Eur. J. Orthod. 3:41–47, 1981.
27. Rose, J. S. Choice of appliance in relation to demand for orthodontic treatment. Eur. J. Orthod. 4:55–64, 1982.
28. Pfeiffer, J. P., and Grobety, D. A philosophy of combined orthopedic-orthodontic treatment. Am. J. Orthod. 81:185–201, 1982.
29. Fränkel, R. The treatment of Class II, Division 1 malocclusion with functional correctors. Am. J. Orthod. 55:265–275, 1969.
30. Harvold, E. P., and Vargervik, K. Morphogenetic response to activator treatment. Am. J. Orthod. 60:478–490, 1971.
31. Trayfoot, J., and Richardson, A. Angle Class II, Division 1 malocclusions treated by the Andresen method. Br. Dent. J. 124:516–519, 1968.
32. Parkhouse, R. C. A cephalometric appraisal of cases of Angle's Class II, Division 1 malocclusion treated by the Andresen appliance. Dent. Practit. 19:425–433, 1969.
33. Jakobsson, S. O. Cephalometric evaluation of treatment effect on Class II, Division 1 malocclusion. Am. J. Orthod. 53:446–457, 1967.
34. Ahlgren, J., and Laurin, C. Late results of activator treatment: a cephalometric study. Br. J. Orthod. 3:181–187, 1976.
35. Pancherz, H. Long-term effects of activator (Andresen appliance) treatment. Odontologisk Rev. 25:suppl. 35, 1976.
36. Mills, J. R. E. The effect of orthodontic treatment on the skeletal pattern. Br. J. Orthod. 5:133–143, 1978.
37. Woodside, D. G. The activator. pp. 557–591. In J. A. Salzmann (ed.) Orthodontics in Daily Practice. Philadelphia: Lippincott, 1974.
38. Reey, R. W., and Eastwood, A. The passive activator: case selection, treatment response and corrective mechanics. Am. J. Orthod. 73:378–409, 1978.
39. Calvert, F. J. An assessment of Andresen therapy on Class II Division I malocclusion. Br. J. Orthod. 9:149–153, 1982.
40. Moss, M. L., and Salentijn, L. The capsular matrix. Am. J. Orthod. 56:474–490, 1969.
41. Enlow, D. M. Handbook of Facial Growth. Philadelphia: W. B. Saunders Co., 1975, pp. 196–205.
42. Stöckli, P. W., and Willert, H. G. Tissue reactions in the temporo-mandibular joint resulting from an-

References

terior displacement of the mandible in the monkey. Am. J. Orthod. 60:142–155, 1971.
43. Petrovic, A. G., Stutzmann, J. T., and Oudet, C. L. Control processes in the postnatal growth of the condylar cartilage of the mandible. pp. 101–153. In Determinants of Mandibular Form and Growth. Monogr. no. 4, Craniofacial Growth Series. Ann Arbor: Center for Human Growth and Development, Univ. of Michigan, 1975.
44. McNamara, J. A., Jr., Connelly, T. G., and McBride, M. C. Histological studies of temporomandibular joint adaptations. pp. 209–277. In Determinants of Mandibular Form and Growth. Monogr. no. 4, Craniofacial Growth Series. Ann Arbor: Center for Human Growth and Development, Univ. of Michigan, 1975.
45. McNamara, J. A., Jr. Quantitative analysis of temporomandibular joint adaptations to protrusive function. Am. J. Orthod. 76:593–611, 1979.
46. McNamara, J. A., Jr. Functional determinants of craniofacial size and shape. Eur. J. Orthod. 2:131–159, 1980.
47. Bass, N. M. Dento-facial orthopaedics in the correction of Class II malocclusion. Br. J. Orthod. 9:3–31, 1982.
48. Righellis, E. G. Treatment effects of Fränkel, activator and extraoral traction appliances. Angle Orthod. 53:107–121, 1983.
49. Gianelly, A. A., et al. Mandibular growth, condyle position and Fränkel appliance therapy. Angle Orthod. 53:131–142, 1983.
50. Woodside, D. G., et al. Primate experiments in malocclusion and bone induction. Am. J. Orthod. 83:460–468, 1983.
51. McNamara, James A., Jr. Dentofacial adaptations in adult patients following functional regulator therapy. Am. J. Orthod. 85:57–71, 1984.
52. Aguirre, M. J., King, G. J., and Waldron, J. M. Assessment of bracket placement and bond strength when comparing direct bonding to indirect bonding techniques. Am. J. Orthod. 82:269–275, 1982.
53. Bishara, S. E., et al. Longitudinal changes in standing height and mandibular parameters between 8 and 17 years of age. Am. J. Orthod. 80:115–135, 1981.
54. Jamison, J. E., et al. Longitudinal changes in the maxilla and maxillary-mandibular relationship between 8 and 17 years of age. Am. J. Orthod. 82:217–230, 1982.

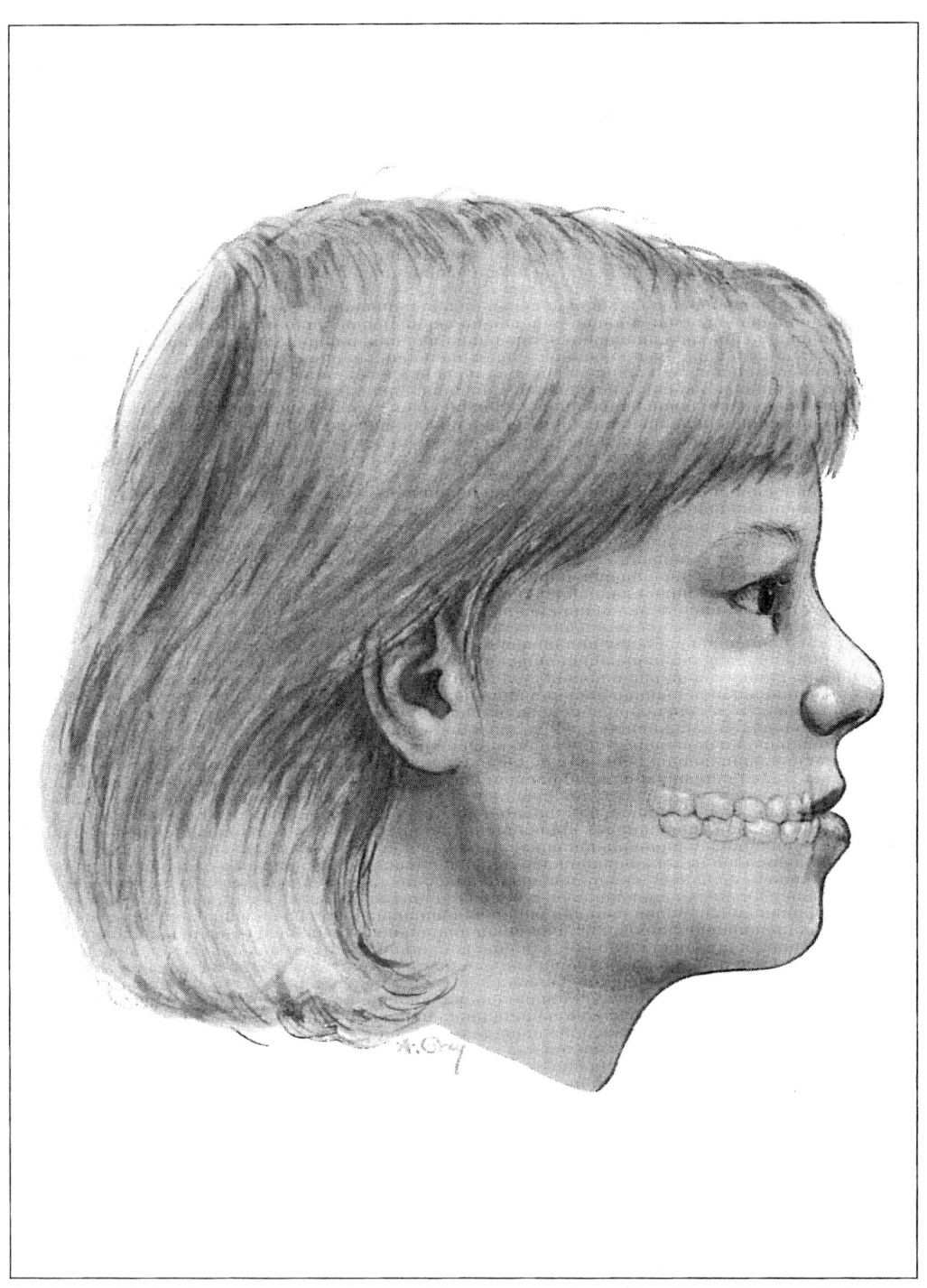

Craniomandibular features representing mandibular prognathism with a Class III malocclusion.

Chapter 9

Class III Malocclusion

Class III malocclusion is the dental result of mandibular hypertrophy, a deficient maxillary component, or a combination of both. The dental result is anterior crossbite with mandibular overjet. From the profile, the mandibular skeletal condition is prognathic or the maxillary skeletal condition is retrognathic. The most common Class III facial pattern occurs when the maxilla is within or less than the normal cephalometric range of standards and the mandible exceeds the cephalometric range of normal. Jacobson et al.[1] have suggested that approximately 25% of Class III patients show a relative maxillary deficiency.

When the maxillary primary incisors are lost early (e.g., 18 to 36 months), there can be a resulting lack of premaxillary alveolar development. The lack of anterior maxillary growth can cause the maxillary anterior teeth to erupt in a pseudo-Class III malocclusion. The permanent maxillary incisors tend to erupt crowded and in crossbite. The resulting malocclusion requires lengthy treatment because there is insufficient maxillary osseous tissue for the mesial-distal width of the maxillary central and lateral incisors (Fig. 9-1). Maxillary dental crowding and a pseudo-Class III malocclusion can also occur if the maxilla is more fully developed (Fig. 9-2).

Orthopedic treatment for Class III malocclusion represents the use of reciprocal biological and mechanical forces. Maxillary skeletal growth is encouraged and mandibular skeletal growth is restricted. Success of treatment depends upon the age at which treatment is initiated, severity of the Class III condition, and patient cooperation.

Without sufficient maxillary alveolar osseous tissue, the teeth cannot be uncrowded and moved to a corrected incisal relationship out of crossbite. This type of malocclusion requires early diagnosis and possible maxillary advancement with sagittal appliance therapy. Every possible preventive measure should be undertaken to prevent the maxillary primary incisors from becoming carious, abscessed, and extracted. A home-applied fluoride gel in a preformed tray may prolong the retention of carious primary incisors.[2]

Class III types of malocclusion

1. skeletal
   a. mandibular prognathism
   b. maxillary retrognathism
2. neuromuscular
   a. mesial functional mandibular displacement
   b. mandibular rotation
3. dentoalveolar
   a. maxillary collapse
   b. excess mandibular dental arch length

Class III Malocclusion

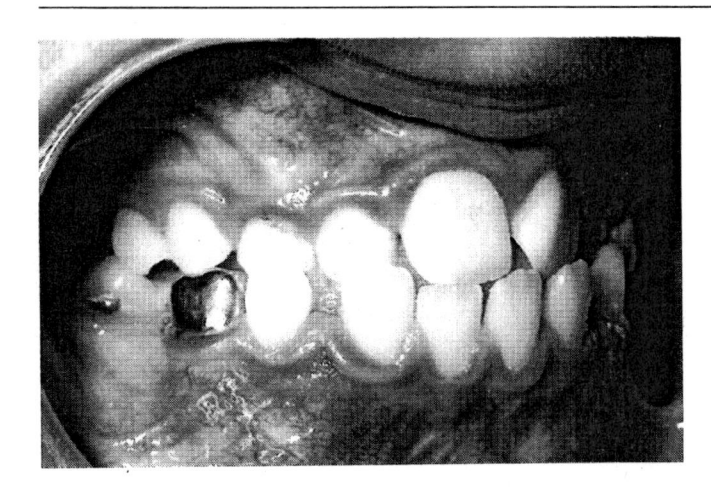

Fig. 9-1 This 9-year-old patient had her four infected maxillary primary incisors extracted at age 3.5 years. The crossbite and crowding may be due to poor maxillary development.

    c. small maxillary dental arch length
4. any combination of the above

Surgical consultation

Treatment of severe Class III skeletal malformations require the combined efforts of dental and surgical consultation. Orthopedic treatment of Class III malocclusion in adult patients (or in children past the pubertal growth period) is more time-consuming than in younger children,[3] and the patient should have the benefit of surgical consultation. Since 5% or less of the Caucasian population develop skeletal mandibular prognathism,[4-6] the research has not been as intensive in the U.S.A. as it has for other types of malocclusion. In Japan, however, almost 50% of treated malocclusions are Class III.

Early treatment

Several authors have suggested early treatment for malocclusion. Barich[7] suggested early treatment of all types of malocclusion in order to bring natural forces into function as early as possible. Sturman[8] equated early treatment with improved chances for success. Hahn[9] thought treatment in the primary dentition would improve conditions for a second period of treatment. King[10] suggested early treatment of malocclusion in proportion to the severity of the problem. Tweed[11] has maintained that early correction of malocclusion is desirable, but cautions that analysis and treatment "in the mixed dentition are more complicated than in the permanent dentition because, in young children, greater growth changes occur in the dento-facial complex." Early treatment for Class III malocclusion in the late primary and early mixed dentition has proven more successful than treatment delayed until puberty. Bernstein[12] suggests early treatment to eliminate sucking or atypical swallowing habits and to restore a "normal functional balance in the oro-facial region."

There are some clinicians that prefer to wait for Class III treatment until eruption of all of the permanent dentition. Delaying maxillofacial orthopedic treatment for these patients may have far-reaching physical and psychological ramifications: a delay in treatment may impose a more lengthy or surgically based treatment plan, or, because of the facial deformity, place undue

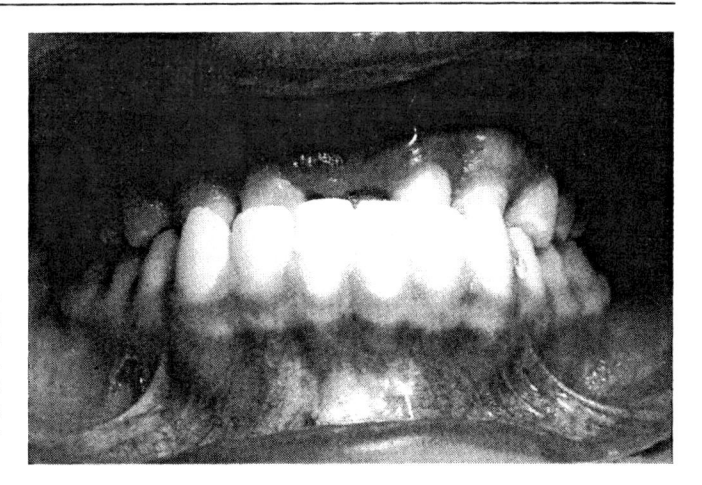

Fig. 9-2 Note the lack of anterior maxillary development in this 14-year-old male. The maxillary central incisors were traumatically exfoliated in an automobile accident at age 9 years. Before the teeth were lost, maxillary development was normal.

hardship on a child during the early teenage years.

Salzmann,[13] in 1966, advocated treatment of Class III patients "as soon as the abnormality is diagnosed." Although patient cooperation may make early treatment difficult, he utilized a chin cup to alter the growth vector of the mandible.

Bell, Profitt, and White,[14] in 1980, have discussed the complexity of treating Class III patients. They suggest that the excessive mandibular development may only be part of the problem, and that a deficient maxillary component may contribute significantly to the malocclusion.

In 1980, Nanda[15] utilized a modified protraction headgear for correction of a maxillary deficiency in a clinical study of 20 patients. The chin cup was also used during a 24 to 36 month posttreatment period. Typical clinical and cephalometric changes included lingual tipping of the mandibular incisors, remodeling at point B, downward mandibular rotation, and flaring of the maxillary incisors.

It is evident that early treatment of Class III malocclusion would be of significant benefit to the patient. Treatment planning is accomplished early (between ages 4 and 7); actual treatment is begun as soon as the maxillary permanent central and lateral incisors and maxillary first permanent molars have erupted, and patient cooperation is assured. It is important to inform the parent and child that the treatment is apt to be lengthy, and that surgical intervention is a possibility.

Campbell,[16] in 1983, reported the effective use of a reverse-pull face crib on 14 patients with Class III malocclusion. He suggests early treatment in order to achieve four definitive goals:

1. provide a more favorable environment for normal growth
2. achieve as much relative maxillary advancement as possible
3. improve occlusal relationships
4. improve facial esthetics for more normal psychosocial development

Campbell found the reverse-pull face crib effective for early interceptive treatment of Class III malocclusion and observed the following phenomena after reverse-pull mechanics:

1. relative maxillary advancement
2. mandibular rotation
3. labial tipping of the maxillary incisors
4. lingual tipping of the mandibular incisors

Class III Malocclusion

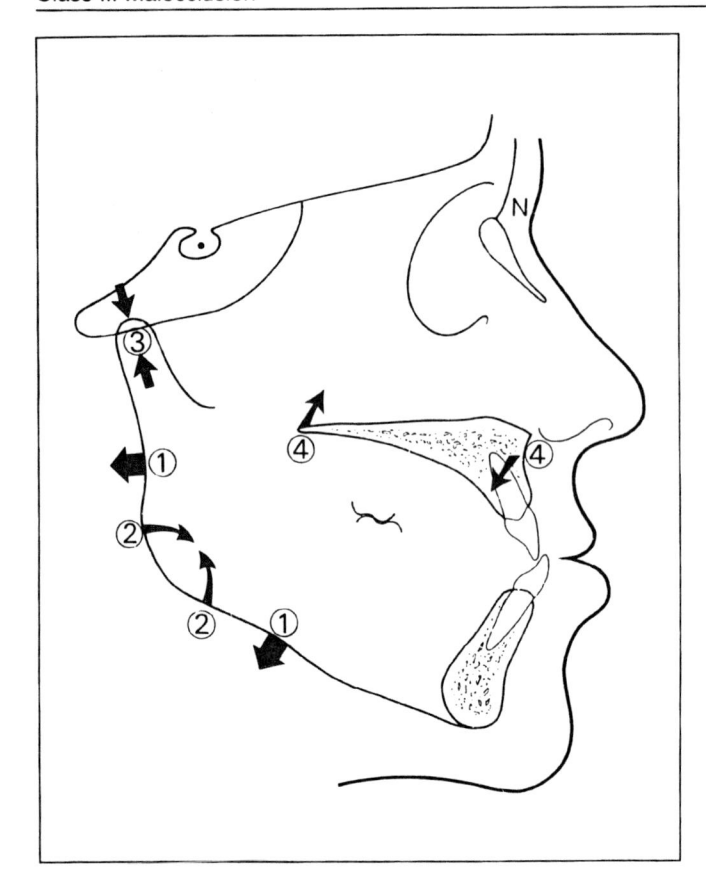

Fig. 9-3 Major contributions to correction of the Class III skeletal malocclusion. *(1)* The mandible was rotated posteriorly, placing the ramus in a more vertical orientation to the cranial base. *(2)* The gonial angle was decreased, reestablishing the mandibular plane by overcoming changes introduced by posterior mandibular rotation. *(3)* Vertical condylar growth was restricted. *(4)* The maxilla was rotated slightly in a clockwise direction.

5. mesial movement of the maxillary molars
6. changes in ANB differences toward a more positive value

Chin-cup therapy

The use of the chin cup to slow mandibular growth for Class III malocclusion has met with some success. Lavergne and Gasson[17] studied the effect of night-only chin-cup force (800 g/side) on patients with Class III malocclusion. The patients with a tendency for posterior rotation of the mandible had effective treatment results with crossbite elimination in six to 12 months. Other studies[18-20] have shown that mandibular rotation is a growth mechanism that allows adjustment of the mandibular length to the maxillary length. This adjustment mechanism functions in a narrow range of mandibular and maxillary growth increments. A malocclusion results when growth exceeds the limits of the adjustment mechanism. The Class III malocclusion develops with an increase in the gonial angle and a posterior growth direction of the condylar cartilage.

Experimental studies with animals[21-24] have indicated that temporomandibular joint growth can be altered by a distalizing force placed against the mandible. The studies with chin-cup application to human patients have shown varying degrees of success.[17,25-32] The failures seem to occur when light chin-cup forces are used with older patients. The more successful results were noted when strong orthopedic forces of 600 to 800 g were used with younger patients (5 to 10 years of age).

Graber[32] has studied chin-cup therapy for mandibular prognathism in patients 5 to 8 years of age. The results encouraged early orthopedic forces (450 to 900 g/side) in order to change the craniofacial growth pattern and correct Class III malocclusion. The following results noted in the Graber study are reprinted here with the permission of Dr. Graber and The C. V. Mosby Co.:[32]

1. retardation of vertical ramus growth
2. retardation of vertical development in the posterior aspect of the mandibular body
3. retardation of vertical development in the posterior maxilla
4. closure of the gonial angle
5. distal rotation of the mandibular complex
6. decreased anteroposterior anterior cranial base growth
7. redirection of the predominantly horizontal mandibular growth pattern to a more vertical direction
8. reduction of the maxillomandibular malrelationship toward normative values
9. production of an Angle Class I dental relationship following the establishment of normal maxillomandibular relations
10. lack of detectable localized effect on the symphyseal region or incisor position as a direct result of chin cup placement and pressure
11. development of soft-tissue profile changes in harmony with underlying skeletal changes

Diagrammatic representation of the craniofacial changes that add to Class III resolution are shown in Fig. 9-3.[32]

In this study, most of the craniofacial changes from the chin cup were in the mandible and posterior face. The good results obtained indicate that orthopedic chin-cup forces are successful in young patients with skeletal mandibular prognathism.

Sassouni[33] has shown that orthopedic force systems can be helpful in correcting several types of malocclusion. Chin-cup therapy with cervical anchorage is recommended for downward rotation of the mandible, which reduces the protrusion of the chin. Occipital anchorage, with the force directed through the condyles, may alter mandibular growth. Cleall[34] has also shown good results with chin-cup therapy when used over a period of three years.

Consideration for the health of the temporomandibular joint is of vital importance in deciding on the amount of force to use in chin-cup therapy. Stress has been observed in the posterior portion of the glenoid fossa and the contacting posterior part of the condylar head when a high-pull chin cup is utilized.[35]

Teuscher[36] suggests that functional deviations in the sagittal plane be eliminated at the earliest opportunity. Additional Class III growth correction may be compensated within the dentofacial complex (multilocal compensation). Since compensating procedures are limited,[37] particularly in postpubertal patients, the necessity for surgical correction is a consideration for young adults.

Reduced anterior lower facial height

Class III malocclusion associated with a deep bite, reduced facial height, and other mild skeletal discrepancies responds favorably to maxillofacial orthopedic intervention. Correction is accomplished by the downward and backward rotation of the

Class III Malocclusion

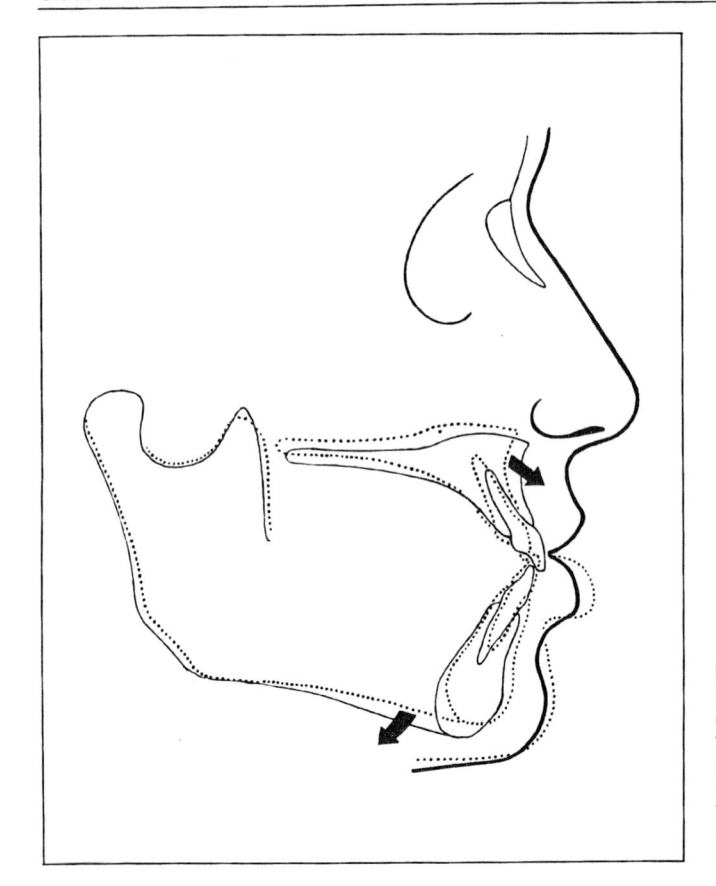

Fig. 9-4 Class III malocclusions in patients with a short lower face (broken line) are successfully treated with maxillofacial orthopedic appliances. These appliances rotate the mandible downward and backward while increasing the forward maxillary displacement.

mandible, accompanied by a change in the postural position of the tongue (Fig. 9-4). Mandibular repositioning increases the lower face height, and will improve the skeletal relationship. Maxillofacial orthopedic treatment is contraindicated in children with a normal to long lower facial height. Vertical skeletal changes can be controlled in patients treated with the activator, Fränkel, and bionator appliances by covering the occlusal surfaces of the posterior teeth with acrylic. However, mandibular forward growth cannot be controlled with acrylic coverage, and a Class III malocclusion may be exacerbated using this technique.

Role of the tongue

In Class III malocclusion, the tongue is generally placed in a lower and more protruding position in the oral cavity. Little tongue stimulation is applied to the premaxillary area. The balance between the tongue and the perioral musculature is lost, and tension in the orbicularis oris muscle can restrict midfacial growth.

One of the treatment objectives of Class III malocclusion with maxillofacial orthopedic appliances is the upward and backward repositioning of the tongue. This can be accomplished with the bionator appliance by positioning the coffin spring anteriorly instead of posteriorly, as with the Class

II bionator. The tongue is stimulated to withdraw posteriorly as it contacts the loop during swallowing.[38]

Consideration for open bite

The lack of a vertical overbite makes correction of Class III malocclusion more difficult. Anterior rotation and growth stimulation of the maxillary complex is aided when there is sufficient vertical overbite. Force vectors that enhance maxillary growth will tend to open a vertical overbite but will exacerbate an existing open bite. Posterior occlusal coverage on the sagittal appliance will help minimize anterior bite opening. However, fixed appliance treatment or possible surgical intervention may be necessary when the anterior incisal relationship is open or edge-to-edge.

Haas[39] contends that some downward and forward displacement of the maxilla is possible with rapid palatal expansion. Biederman[40] has discussed the "orthopedic nature" of rapid palatal expansion in the young patient and suggests this treatment "unless the skeletal disharmony is so extreme that only surgical treatment will reconcile the skeletal disharmony."

Langford and Sims[41] have shown that care is necessary with rapid maxillary expansion because of root resorption damage to the anchor teeth when a fixed appliance technique is used. A later study[42] demonstrates repair of most resorptive root defects, although repair remained incomplete one year after rapid maxillary expansion.

The periodontal status of the supporting tissues after palatal expansion has been studied by Greenbaum and Zachrisson.[43] Both slow and rapid fixed palatal expansion therapy had little effect on the periodontal condition when compared with a control group receiving fixed appliance (but no expansion) treatment. Some periodontal breakdown at the central aspect of the first molars was noted in a few patients in the rapid maxillary expansion group.

Open bite: treatment

Class III open bite patients are difficult to treat with sagittal appliances alone. One or more surgical procedures is frequently necessary in conjunction with a period of interarch fixed retention.

Mandibular rotation

Bryant[44] found that Class III patients demonstrated an opening rotation of the mandible before and during occlusal correction. The patients with the best treatment results demonstrated a reversal of the opening rotation and achieved an overall forward rotation after treatment.

A combination of maxillary stimulation and mandibular inhibition has been successful for many patients with Class III malocclusion. Although this chapter reviews several successful treatment modalities, the sagittal appliance has shown excellent esthetic results without the necessity of external anchorage in patients that demonstrate maxillary growth deficiency.

Of all of the studies reviewed, those that have shown an attempt to incorporate the natural intrinsic compensatory growth processes into a logical plan of treatment have been successful. Enlow[45] has discussed the value of utilizing growth stimulation to achieve the desired skeletal results. If the nasal and oral parts of the midface do not balance with the growth of the mandible, then early maxillary growth stimulation may be required.

Case studies of two patients with closed anterior crossbite and Class III malocclusion demonstrate excellent long-term stability after sagittal appliance therapy (courtesy of J. W. Witzig, D.D.S.).

Class III Malocclusion

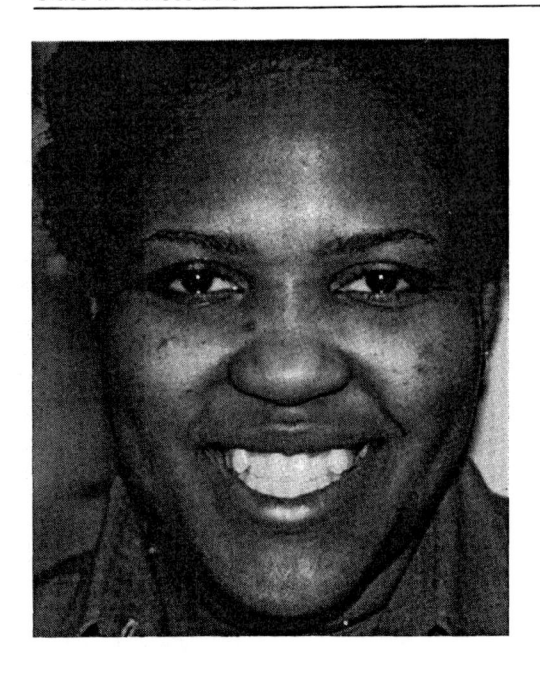

Fig. 9-5a A. L. Full face, pretreatment.

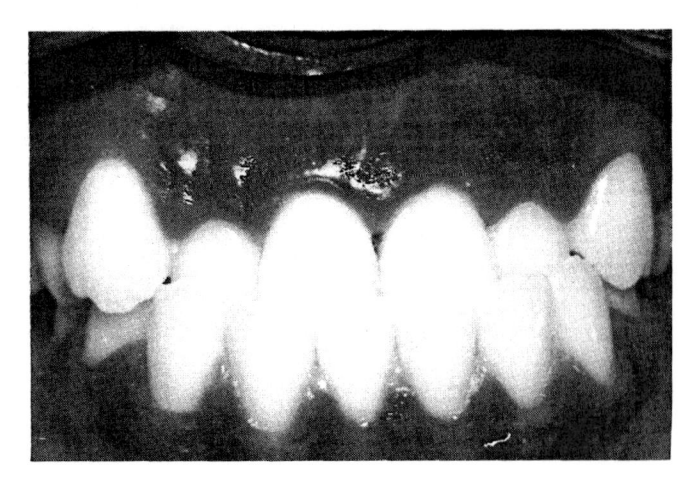

Fig. 9-5b Pretreatment labial view of crossbite.

A.L., age 13 (Figs. 9-5a to d)

A.L. was treated with two maxillary sagittal appliances over a two-year period. No other appliances were required. Posttreatment results show excellent occlusal stability three years after appliances have been removed.

F.S., age 10 (Figs. 9-6a to h)

F.S. required two maxillary sagittal appliances over an 18-month treatment period. Posttreatment results demonstrate excellent occlusal stability and facial esthetics five years after all appliances have been removed.

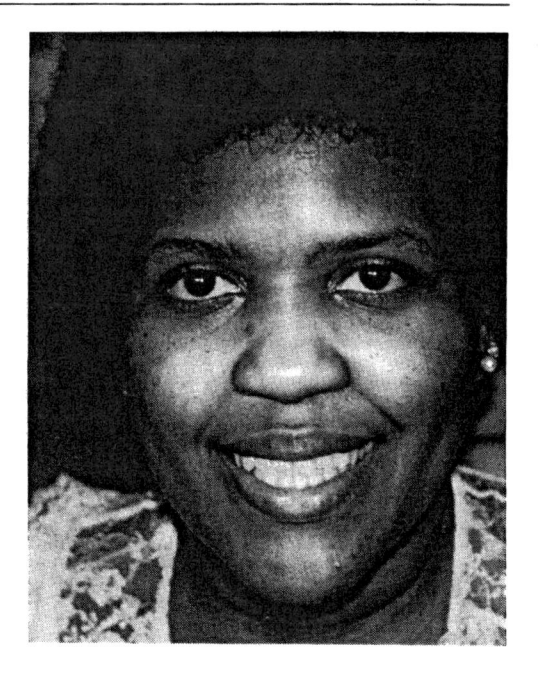

Fig. 9-5c A. L. Full face, posttreatment.

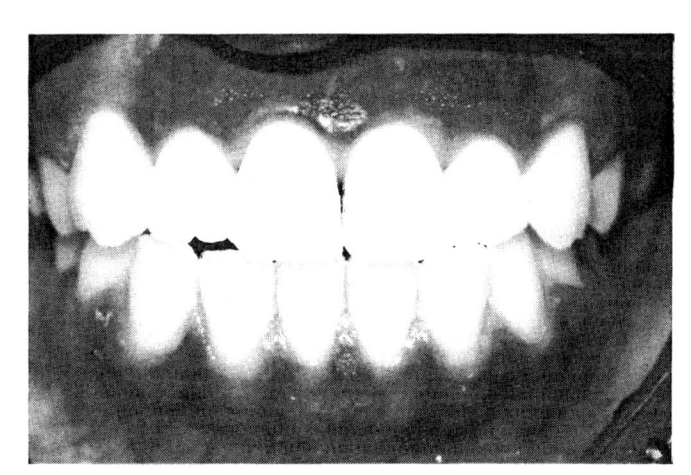

Fig. 9-5d Posttreatment labial view.

Treatment Plan for A.L. and F.S.
- A. orthopedic records
- B. maxillary sagittal appliance
- C. labiolingual appliance or fixed appliance for final dental correction

Class III orthopedic appliances

The Class III activators, Class III Fränkel appliance, and fixed interarch appliances are constructed to utilize reciprocal and multilocal actions.[36] The primary goal is to reposition or displace the mandible in a

Class III Malocclusion

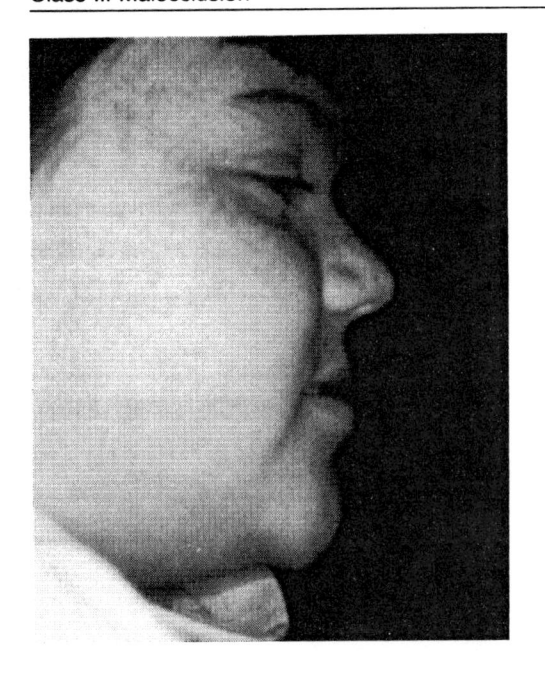

Fig. 9-6a F. S. Pretreatment facial profile.

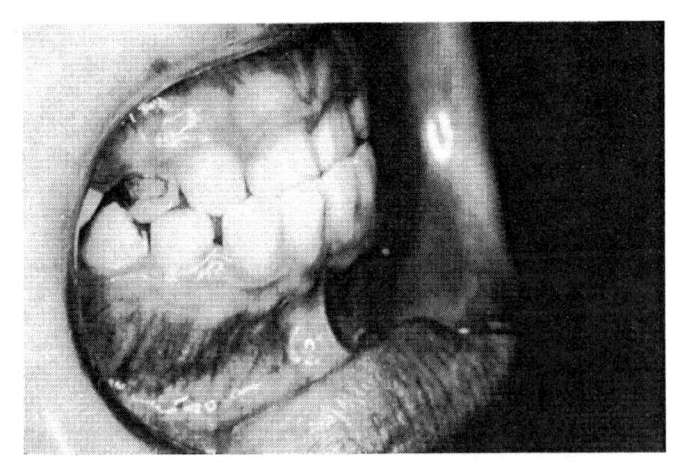

Fig. 9-6b Pretreatment anterior crossbite occlusion.

posterior and downward direction and to compensate for excessive condylar growth at other sites within the craniofacial complex.

Bite registration

Occlusal bite registration depends on the appliance to be used for the downward and backward rotation of the mandible.

In activator treatment, the bite is generally opened 6 to 8 mm, with the mandible in the most retruded position. Because the appliance can be uncomfortable to wear full-time, it is only recommended that it be worn a few hours a day. On the other hand, the bite registration for the bionator or the

Class III Orthopedic Appliances

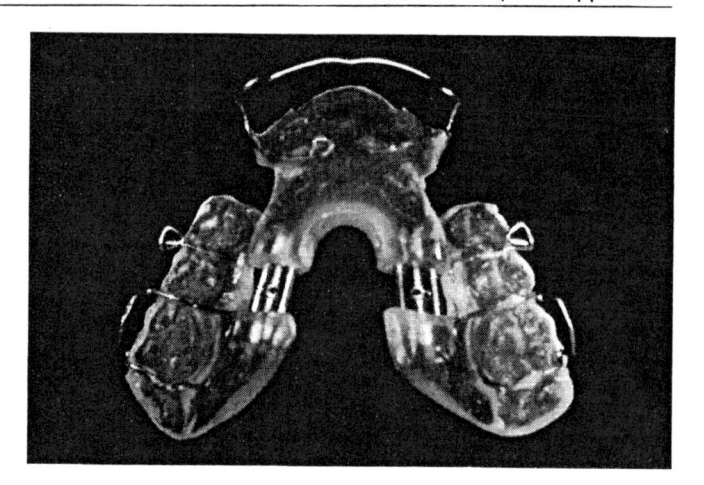

Fig. 9-6c First of two sagittal appliances used during treatment.

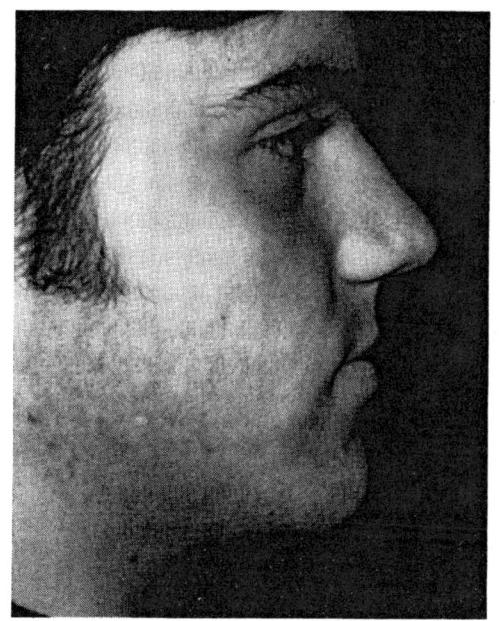

Fig. 9-6d F. S. Facial profile, five years posttreatment.

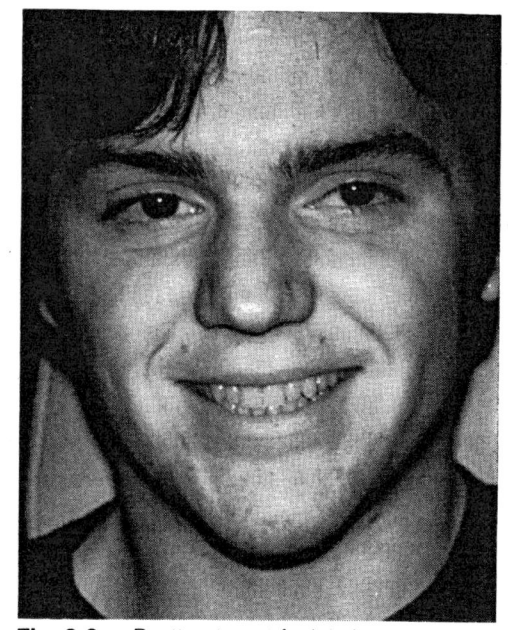

Fig. 9-6e Posttreatment facial view.

Fränkel appliance is only opened 1 to 2 mm with the mandible in the most retruded position. This encourages full-time wear.

The correction generally seen is associated with posterior rotation of the mandible and maxillary advancement. In all appliances, the mandibular anterior teeth are capped with acrylic during the first interception. This will allow the maxillary teeth to erupt downward and forward, creating a Class I molar relationship. The acrylic is initially trimmed at the mesial surface of the first permanent molar, and later in the premolar area (see Fig. 8-12 in Chapter 8).

213

Class III Malocclusion

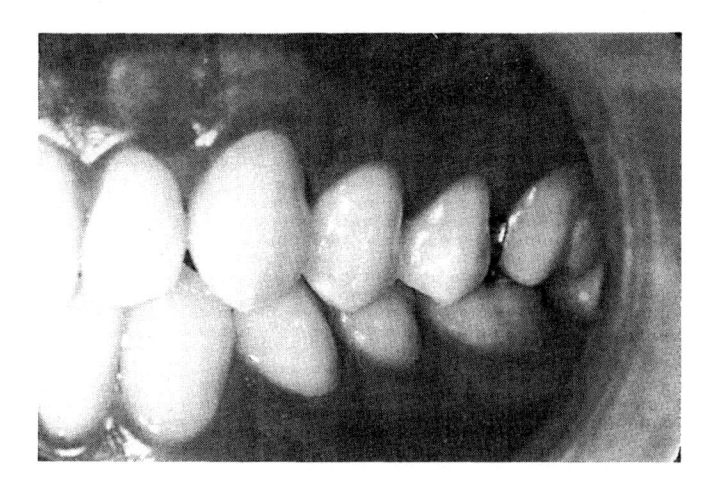

Fig. 9-6f Right buccal segment, posttreatment.

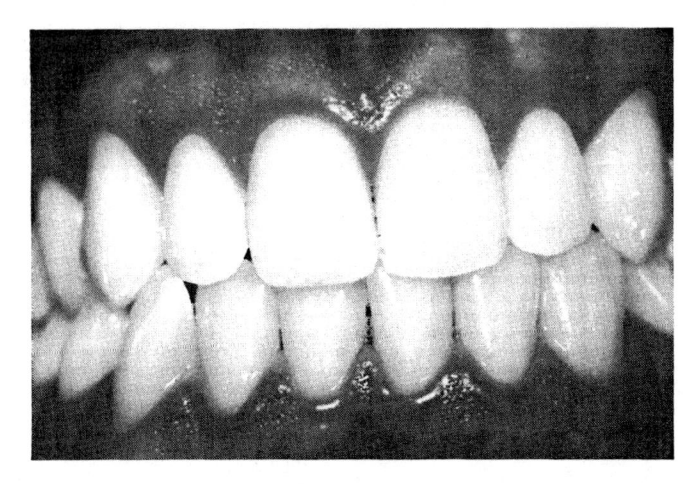

Fig. 9-6g Posttreatment labial view prior to final correction with the straight-wire appliance.

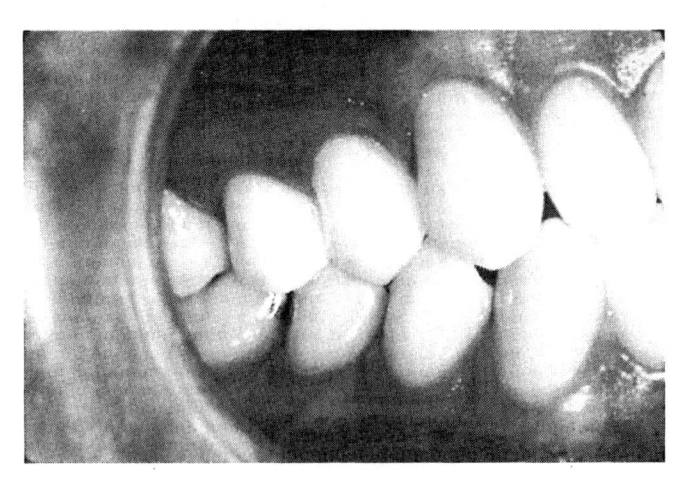

Fig. 9-6h Left buccal segment, posttreatment.

Andresen retractor

Hjulstad[46] has described the use of the Andresen retractor appliance for treating Class III malocclusion. The appliance is designed for treatment of the early and mixed dentition in patients with a dual bite. The best results occur when the patient can reposition the mandible toward an edge-to-edge anterior occlusion. The construction bite is taken with the mandible in the furthest retruded position.

The retractors are made with lingual wings in the lower arch to give the mandibular teeth better guidance during bite closure. The appliance is trimmed so that each tooth in the lateral segments of the maxilla has just one small contact point with the acrylic. The appliance is relieved behind the maxillary anterior teeth, so that all contact with the teeth is at three points: the appliance engages the distolingual cusps of the lower first permanent molars and the labial arch wire makes the third contact point by exerting lingually directed pressure on the lower incisors. Unless there is any small rotation to be corrected the incisors have no contact with the acrylic.

The initial trimming is carried out on the model and the appliance is further trimmed in the mouth. Then, cold-curing acrylic is added behind the maxillary anterior teeth; before it sets, the appliance is placed in the mouth and the patient is instructed to bite the teeth hard together. When the acrylic has set, all contact between the new acrylic and the maxillary incisor teeth is removed, so that all pressure is directed onto the palatal gingiva. Further additions of acrylic are made every six weeks until a good vertical anterior overbite has been attained. The retractor appliance has the advantage of being effective without the necessity of waiting for premolar eruption for a fixed technique.

Summary

The overall long-term goal is to give the patient a chance for orthopedic or orthodontic correction utilizing the best available treatment plan before surgical intervention becomes necessary. Parental history, early childhood diet, allergies, mouth breathing, patient cooperation, and chronologic-skeletal age all require careful consideration when planning treatment.

References

1. Jacobson, A., et al. Mandibular prognathism. Am. J. Orthod. 66:140–171, 1974.
2. Frigoletto, R. Update—simplified treatment of baby-bottle syndrome. J. Dent. Child. 49:374–376, 1982.
3. Shapira, Y., and Zilberman, Y. The orthodontist's role in the correction of facial malformations. Trans. Eur. Orthod. Soc. 1977, pp. 245–251.
4. Mills, L. F. Epidemiologic studies of occlusion. IV. The prevalence of malocclusion in a population of 1,455 school children. J. Dent. Res. 45:332–336, 1966.
5. Horowitz, S. L., Converse, J. M., and Gerstman, L. J. Craniofacial relationships in mandibular prognathism. Arch. Oral Biol. 14:121–131, 1969.
6. Thilander, B., and Myrberg, N. The prevalence of malocclusion in Swedish schoolchildren. Scand. J. Dent. Res. 81:12–20, 1973.
7. Barich, F. T. Treatment in the mixed dentition period. Am. J. Orthod. 38:625–633, 1952.
8. Sturman, H. A. Early treatment. Angle Orthod. 28:94–107, 1958.
9. Hahn, G. W. A panel on treatment in deciduous dentition. Am. J. Orthod. 41:255–261, 1955.
10. King, E. W. Variations in profile change and their significance in timing treatment. Angle Orthod. 30:141–153, 1960.
11. Tweed, C. H. The diagnostic facial triangle in the control of treatment objectives. Am. J. Orthod. 55:651–667, 1969.
12. Bernstein, K. Early oral orthopaedic functional diagnosis and treatment. Trans. Eur. Orthod. Soc. 1973, pp. 151–161.
13. Salzmann, J. A. Practice of Orthodontics. Philadelphia: Lippincott, 1966.
14. Bell, W. H., Profitt, W. R., and White, R. P., Jr. (eds.) Surgical Correction of Dentofacial Deformities. Philadelphia: W. B. Saunders Co., 1980.

15. Nanda, R. Biochemical and clinical considerations of a modified protraction headgear. Am. J. Orthod. 78:125–139, 1980.
16. Campbell, P. M. The dilemma of Class III treatment: early or late? Angle Orthod. 53:175–191, 1983.
17. Lavergne, J., and Gasson, N. Rotational pattern of the mandible—an indication for treatment of Class III malocclusion with chin cap. Trans. Eur. Orthod. Soc. 237–243, 1977.
18. Lavergne, J., and Gasson, N. Operational definitions of mandibular rotation. Angle Orthod. 46:144–150, 1976.
19. Lavergne, J., and Gasson, N. Operational definitions of mandibular morphogenetic and positional rotations. Scand. J. Dent. Res. 85:185–192, 1977.
20. Lavergne, J., and Gasson, N. Direction and intensity of mandibular rotation in the sagittal adjustment during growth of the jaws. Scand. J. Dent. Res. 85:193–199, 1977.
21. Breitner, C. Bone changes resulting from experimental orthodontic treatment. Am. J. Orthod. Oral Surg. 26:521–547, 1940.
22. Janzen, E. K., and Bluher, J. A. The cephalometric, anatomic and histologic changes in *Macaca mulatta* after application of a continuous-acting retraction force on the mandible. Am. J. Orthod. 51:823–855, 1965.
23. Petrovic, A. G., Stutzman, J. J., and Oudet, C. L. Control processes in the postnatal growth of the condylar cartilage of the mandible. pp. 101–154. *In* J. A. McNamara (ed.) Determinants of Mandibular Form and Growth. Monogr. no. 4, Craniofacial Growth Series. Ann Arbor: Center for Human Growth and Development, Univ. of Michigan, 1975.
24. Joho, J. P. The effects of extraoral low-pull traction to the mandibular dentition of *Macaca mulatta*. Am. J. Orthod. 64:555–577, 1973.
25. Graber, T. M., Chung, D. D. B., and Aoba, T. J. Dentofacial orthopedics versus orthodontics. J. Am. Dent. Assoc. 75:1145–1160, 1967.
26. Matsui, Y. Effect of chin cap on the growing mandible. J. Jap. Orthod. Soc. 24:165–181, 1965.
27. Armstrong, C. J. A clinical evaluation of the chin cup. Aust. Dent. J. 6:338–346, 1961.
28. Thilander, B. Treatment of Angle Class III malocclusion with chin cap. Trans. Eur. Orthod. Soc. 384–398, 1963.
29. Thilander, B. Chin cap treatment for Angle Class III malocclusion: a longitudinal study. Trans. Eur. Orthod. Soc. 311–327, 1965.
30. Irie, M., and Nakamura, S. Orthopedic approach to severe skeletal Class III malocclusion. Am. J. Orthod. 67:377–392, 1975.
31. Suzuki, N. A cephalometric observation on the effect of the chin cap. J. Jap. Orthod. Soc. 31:64–74, 1972.
32. Graber, L. W. Chin cup therapy for mandibular prognathism. Am. J. Orthod. 72:23–41, 1977.
33. Sassouni, V. Dentofacial orthopedics: a critical review. Am. J. Orthod. 61:255–269, 1972.
34. Cleall, J. F. Dentofacial orthopedics. Am. J. Orthod. 66:237–250, 1974.
35. De Alba, J. A., et al. Stress distribution under high-pull extraoral chin cup traction. Angle Orthod. 52:69–78, 1982.
36. Teuscher, U. Compensation procedures in Class III treatment. Trans. Eur. Orthod. Soc. 217–227, 1977.
37. Graber, T. M., Chung, D. D. B., and Aoba, J. T. Dentofacial orthopedics versus orthodontics. J. Am. Dent. Assoc. 75:1145–1166, 1967.
38. Balters, W. Eine Einführung in die Bionator-Heilmethod. Ausgewalte Schriften und Vorträge. Heidelberg: Herman, 1973.
39. Haas, A. J. Rapid palatal expansion: a recommended prerequisite to Class III treatment. Trans. Eur. Orthod. Soc. 311–318, 1973.
40. Biederman, W. Rapid correction of Class III malocclusion by midpalatal expansion. Am. J. Orthod. 63:47–55, 1973.
41. Langford, S. R., and Sims, M. R. Root surface resorption, repair, and periodontal attachment following rapid maxillary expansion in man. Am. J. Orthod. 81:108–115, 1982.
42. Langford, S. R. Root resorption extremes resulting from clinical RME. Am. J. Orthod. 81:371–377, 1982.
43. Greenbaum, K. R., and Zachrisson, B.U. The effect of palatal expansion therapy on the periodontal supporting tissues. Am. J. Orthod. 81:12–21, 1982.
44. Bryant, P. M. F. Mandibular rotation and Class III malocclusion. Br. J. Orthod. 8:61–75, 1981.
45. Enlow, D. H. Craniofacial growth. J. Clin. Orthod. 17:669–679, 1983.
46. Hjulstad, B. The almost forgotten chapter of the Norwegian System. Trans. Eur. Ortho. Soc. 229–236, 1977.

Chapter 10

Treatment of Craniomandibular Disorders With Maxillofacial Orthopedic Appliances

A patient suffering from temporomandibular joint disorder is one of the most misunderstood of all dental patients. Frustration can become acute as one medical or dental specialist after another is visited and rejected because no permanent relief for the symptoms can be found. Understanding the patient is helpful in determining a plan for treatment. It is not suggested that all or even most patients suffering from TMJ disease can or should be treated with orthopedic appliances. However, patients with capsular dysfunction have shown long-term improvement with orthopedic appliance therapy.

Patient profile

More than 50% of all patients seen for dental examination present with some signs of temporomandibular joint disorder. Patients as young as 4 years old have had documented TMJ problems. Richards and Brown[1] studied degenerative changes in the temporomandibular joints of Australian aboriginal skeletal remains from the South Australian Museum; no association was found between age and degeneration of the temporomandibular joint. The temporal bone was the most frequent site of pathology, but degenerative changes were observed on the condylar head and on all joint regions of affected skulls. Funt[2] has described headache as a common symptom of TMJ disorder. The pain can be near the anterior or medial segment of the insertion of the temporalis muscle. Muscle pain in other trigger areas is common. Women seem to have more symptoms than men.

It is important to understand the patient as well as the symptoms. As the psychiatrist Alfred Adler once expressed,[3] "If we are truly to understand another person, we must see the problem through his eyes, hear it with his ears, and feel it with his heart." In order to understand the TMJ disorder patient, the clinician should develop an understanding of how the patient views his or her current condition; of what his or her lifestyle, emotional state, and family life is like; and of his or her outlook for the future. Many people suffering from craniomandibular disorders feel that they will never be rid of their pain and that they will always have this condition. Patients often express feelings of helplessness and hopelessness, the two cardinal traits of depression. There is no anticipation of anything that can be done to help.

Patients with TMJ symptoms are found in every type of dental practice. In pedodontics, patients as young as 3 have been found to have TMJ clicking noise. The parents of many patients frequently have TMJ symptoms. When screening for craniomandibular disorders there is usually one or all

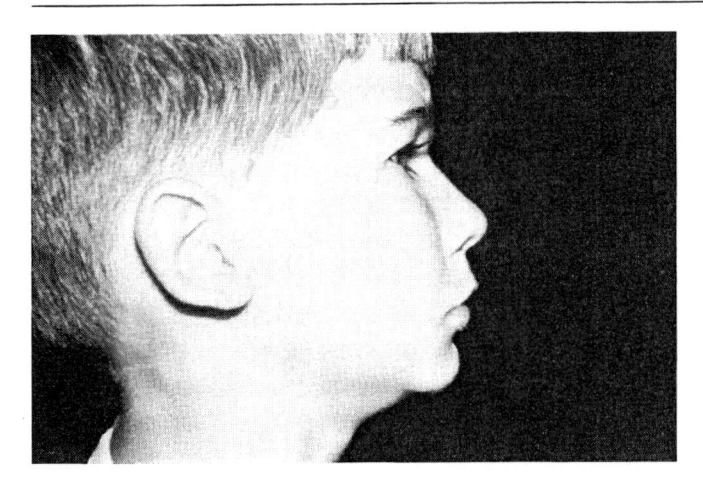

Treatment of Craniomandibular Disorders With Maxillofacial Orthopedic Appliances

Fig. 10-1 This postural relationship of the atlas and occiput could indicate a possible TMJ disorder or a cervical spinal lesion.

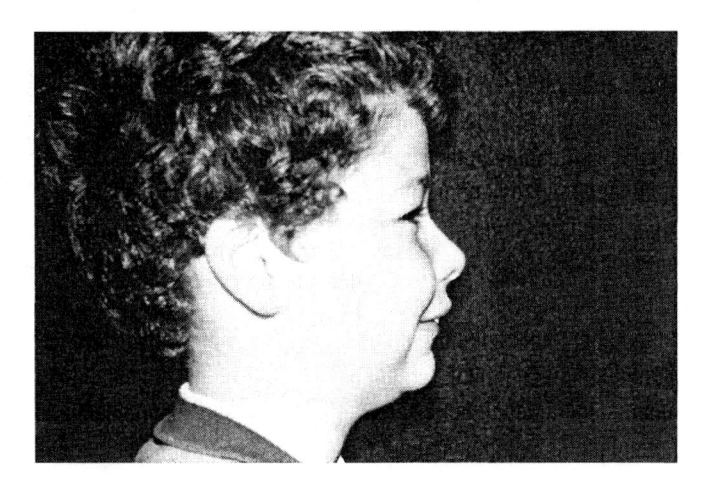

Figs. 10-2a and b Facial profile of a patient with a primary complaint of "pretty bad headaches for two years." A deep mentonian groove is present.

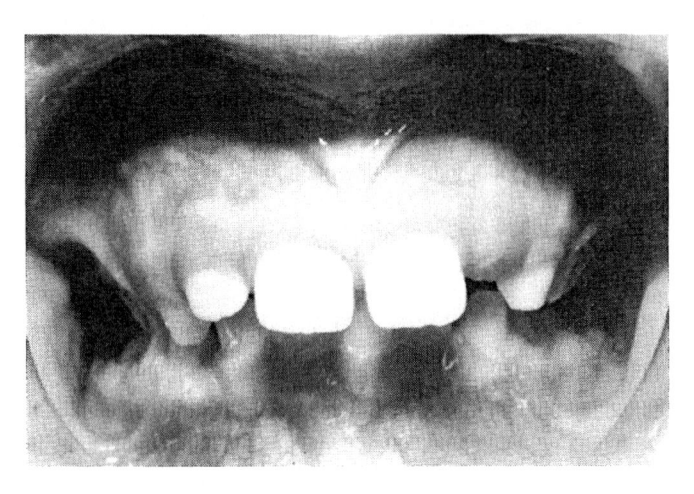

Fig. 10-2b Note the deep bite malocclusion.

218

of the following signs or symptoms: TMJ noise, an aberrant or limited opening and closing articulation, and head, neck, and/or shoulder pain.

Physical profile: posture

Many TMJ disorder patients have a characteristic posture. The head is forward, or forward and hyperextended. The head is also rotated and side bended. The rotation and side bending is the compensatory mechanism the body uses to adjust the right and left condyles. With the head in extension, the atlas is brought into close approximation with the occiput and the chance of peripheral nerve entrapment neuropathy is increased[4] (Fig. 10-1).

The extension of the head and flexion of the neck cause the occiput to roll back into the cervical spine. If there is a deep-bite malocclusion with overjet, a deep mentonian groove and an everted lower lip may also be evident (Fig. 10-2). These individuals usually attain proper posture after the correction of the malocclusion.

The individual should be able to attain a postural relationship in which the different segments of the body (head, neck, shoulders, chest, and abdomen) are balanced one upon the other with the weight born evenly by the bony framework. Funakoshi et al.[5] have studied the relationship of occlusal interference and head position. It was found that balanced muscle response corresponds to a functionally normal occlusion. Moreover, Schwartz[6] has shown that occlusal discrepancies contribute to the onset of masticatory muscle spasm and TMJ disorder.

The size, shape, and angle of the sternocleidomastoid muscle may be diagnostic for an incorrect orthostatic relationship of the head in space. The SCM muscle forms a 45° angle from the tendinous origin on the sternum and the broader origin on the head of the clavicle to its insertion into the lateral surface of the mastoid process and adjoining part of the occipital bone (see Fig. 4-5 in Chapter 4).[7] This angle gives strength to the muscle in much the same way a bridge is given tensile strength by a combination of 45° angle structures.

The SCM muscle becomes shorter and more vertically inclined as the head comes forward. It loses overall length. This shortening induces contraction, then loosening and flabbiness. Patients with TMJ disorder often have bulging sternocleidomastoid muscles (see Fig. 5-8 in Chapter 5).[8]

If the sternocleidomastoid and levator scapula muscles both tighten, three other muscles in the side of the neck, the scalene muscles, will also tighten and undergo hyperactivity.

If there is unilateral contraction of the scalene muscles, the head will turn to that side. If there is bilateral contraction of the scalene muscles, the head comes forward, and the individual has to hyperextend it in order to keep the bipupilar plane parallel to the horizon for visual coordination.

As the scalene muscles go further into contraction, the individual begins to use them as respiratory muscles. Since these muscles attach to the first and second ribs and are accessory muscles of respiration, the first and second ribs are pulled superiorly and the individual becomes an "upper-respiratory breather." When questioned, these patients will complain about being tired all day.

As the head goes into extension, the hyoid bone is brought up and forward by the geniohyoid and digastric muscles; the tongue drops backward. These patients develop a tongue thrust and have trouble breathing deeply and sleeping on the back.

Not all TMJ patients have this characteristic posture (Figs. 10-3a and b), but related signs are usually present: elevated scapulae, forward clavicle, or elevated first rib. The severity and duration of the dysfunction will determine the psychological and postural factors.

Treatment of Craniomandibular Disorders With Maxillofacial Orthopedic Appliances

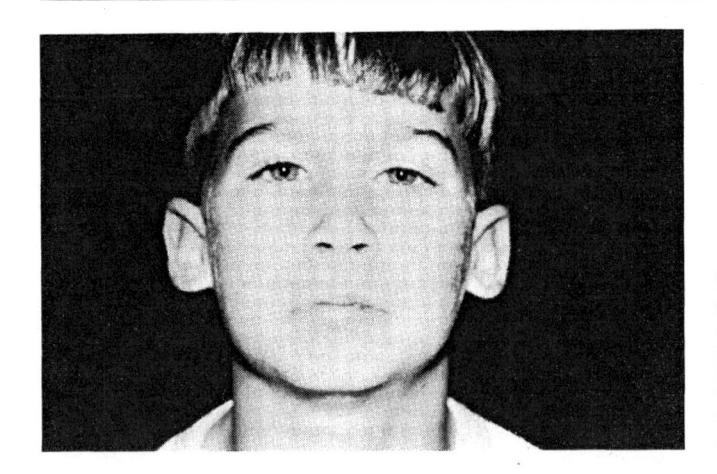

Fig. 10-3a The line of vision is still parallel to the horizon even after the head has adjusted to the pull of the scalene muscles. The neck, shoulder girdle, and upper thorax have all adjusted to the temporomandibular or cervical spine disorder.[10]

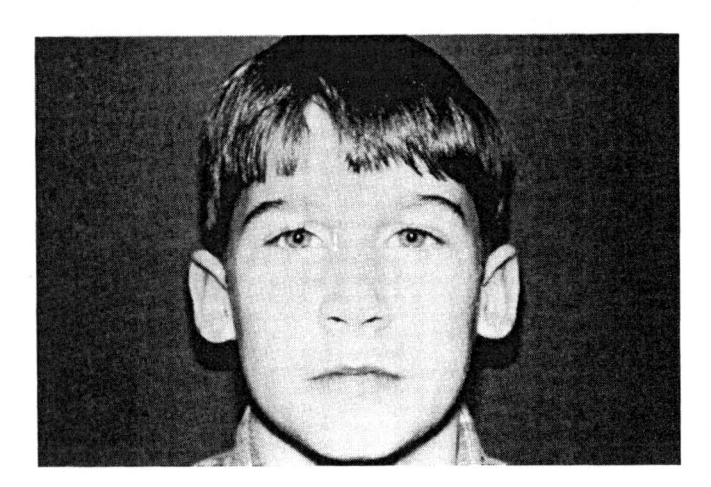

Fig. 10-3b Posttreatment head posture.

Characteristic temporomandibular joint anatomy

Knowledge of the anatomic structure of the temporomandibular joint aids in the clinical examination for functional deviation. Figures 10-4 and 10-5 show normal anatomy of the joint. There is a very strong correlation between its structure and function.[11] The function is by far the most complex of any joint in the human body. It maintains bilateral stability during rotary and translatory movements, even while the mandible is closing forcefully against resistance. Skeletally, the joint appears as two bones articulating one upon the other with a thin fibrous articular disc interposed between the articular surfaces (Fig. 10-6).

An aberrant relationship of the osseous joint tissue may interrupt normal function. If the condylar head is distally or superiorly displaced in the fossa, stress is placed on all anatomical structures of the temporomandibular joint.[12] Details of the skeletal anatomical relationships of the temporomandibular joint are shown in Fig. 10-7.

If the mandible is removed and the zygomatic arch cut away, the superior, medial, anterior, and posterior walls of the infratem-

Characteristic Temporomandibular Joint Anatomy

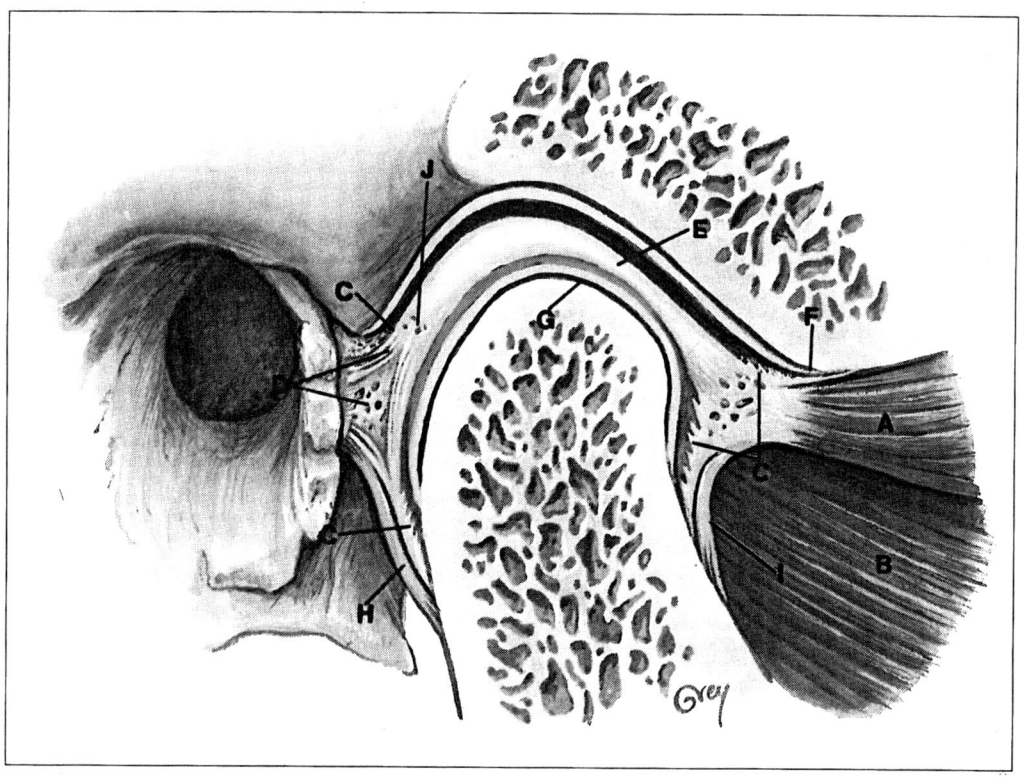

Fig. 10-4 Normal anatomy of the temporomandibular joint, sagittal view: (A) Superior, and (B) inferior head of the lateral pterygoid muscle, (C) synovial villi, (D) bilaminar zone, (E) disc, (F) articular eminence, (G) articular surface of condyle, (H) posterior, and (I) anterior capsule, and (J) genu vasculosa.

poral fossa become visible. Figure 10-7 shows the relationships of structures adjacent to the head of the condyle as it articulates with the disc on the articular surface of the temporal bone.

The posterior and superior medial structures of the infratemporal fossa can be affected adversely by a distally or superiorly located condylar head. Pressure on the tympanic part (plate) of the temporal bone can cause ringing in the ears or a feeling of auditory stuffiness.[13] The lateral part of the anterior surface is the tegmen tympani. This forms the thin roof of the tympanic antrum. Infection may easily reach the temporal lobe of the brain if this thin roof is perforated in the presence of pathogenic bacteria.[7]

Gross clinical evaluation of the TMJ musculature

Clinical evaluation of TMJ musculature is accomplished by gross anatomical inspection and palpation. Without knowledge of the anatomy and function of the TMJ, cranial, cervical, masticatory, and posterior vertebral musculature, a complete diagnostic examination for temporomandibular joint disorder cannot be undertaken. Figures 10-8 to 10-14 demonstrate the primary musculature of the temporomandibular joint: the masseter, temporalis, and medial and lateral pterygoid muscles.

The masseter muscle originates from the zygomatic arch and inserts by way of mus-

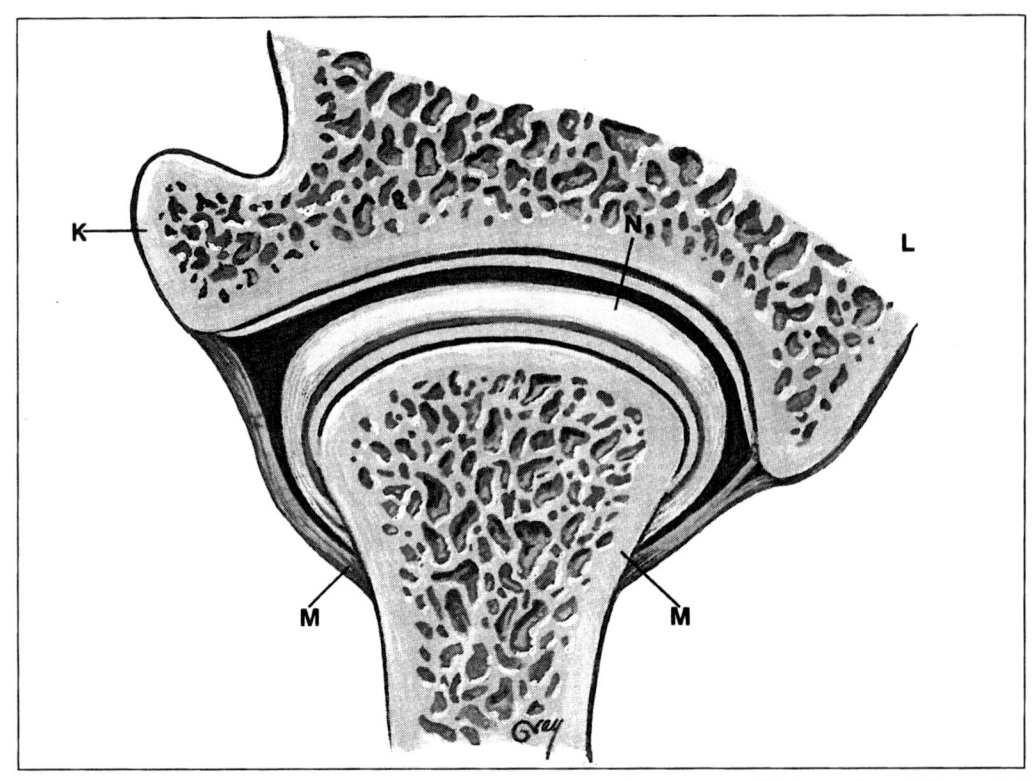

Fig. 10-5 Normal anatomy of the temporomandibular joint, frontal view: (K) Lateral, and (L) medial aspect, (M) capsule, and (N) disc to mandibular condyle.

cular and tendinous fibers into the lateral aspect of the coronoid process, ramus, and angle of the mandible. This muscle can be seen and palpated when the teeth are clenched (Fig. 10-9).

The temporalis muscle originates from the temporal fossa and from the temporal facia covering the muscle. The fanlike origin narrows into a thick, course tendon inserting into the superior and deep aspect of the coronoid process of the mandible. Part of the tendinous insertion extends downward on the anterior border of the ramus toward the third mandibular molar. As the muscle fibers travel from the temporal fossa downward to the coronoid process the tendinous portion passes inferiorly to the zygomatic arch and the lateral pterygoid muscle (Fig. 10-10).

Clinical examination for the temporalis muscle should include bilateral palpation of the anterior, medial, and posterior fibers (Fig. 10-11).

The two pterygoid muscles are separated by the lateral pterygoid plate. The medial pterygoid has four origins. The largest part arises from the inner surface of the lateral pterygoid plate and from the lower part of the pterygoid fossa. Additionally, a portion arises superficially to the lateral pterygoid muscle and from the tuberosity of the maxilla. This quadrilateral muscle joins to insert into the medial aspect of the mandible between the angle and the mylohyoid

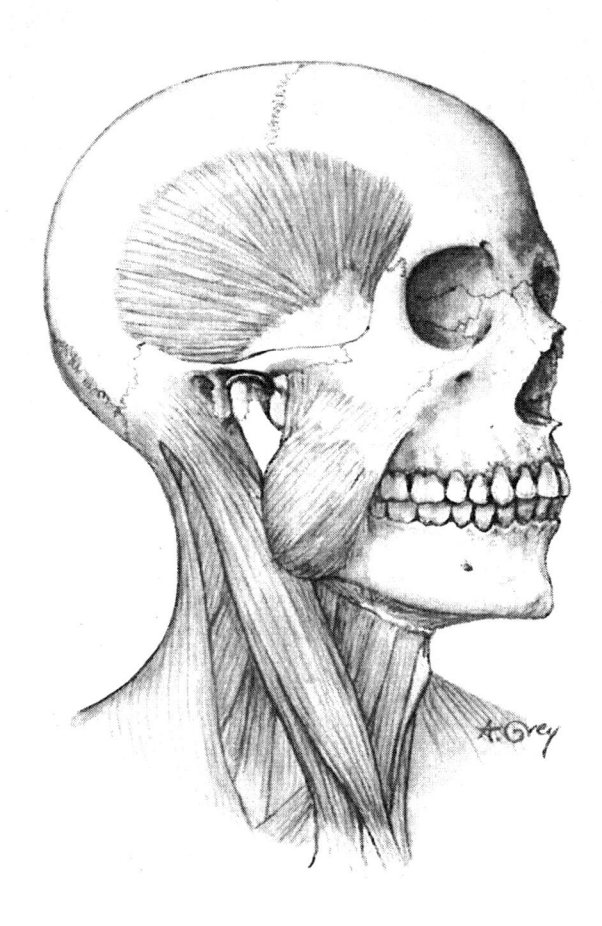

Fig. 10-6 Lateral skull view demonstrating osseous anatomy of the temporomandibular joint.

groove (Fig. 10-12). It acts as an elevator muscle to aid in closing and retracting the mandible.

Tenderness of the medial pterygoid muscle can be checked by palpating laterally to the site normally utilized for an inferior alveolar block anesthetic injection (Fig. 10-13).

The lateral pterygoid muscle arises from two sources. The superior head arises from the floor of the infratemporal fossa. It inserts into the anterior surface of the articular disc and into the deep posterior fibers of the inferior muscle head.

The larger inferior head of the lateral pterygoid muscle arises from the lateral surface of the lateral pterygoid plate and inserts into the anterior portion of the neck of the condyle (Fig. 10-14).

The superior head of the lateral pterygoid muscle acts to balance the articular disc anteriorly from the posterior pull of elastic tension from the posterior disc attachment. This posterior disc attachment is known as the bilaminar zone because it contains two layers of fibers with loose areolar connective tissue between them.[11] The superior fibers of the bilaminar zone are elastic in nature.[14] These fibers are attached to the tympanic plate posteriorly and are counteracted by the anterior pull of the superior

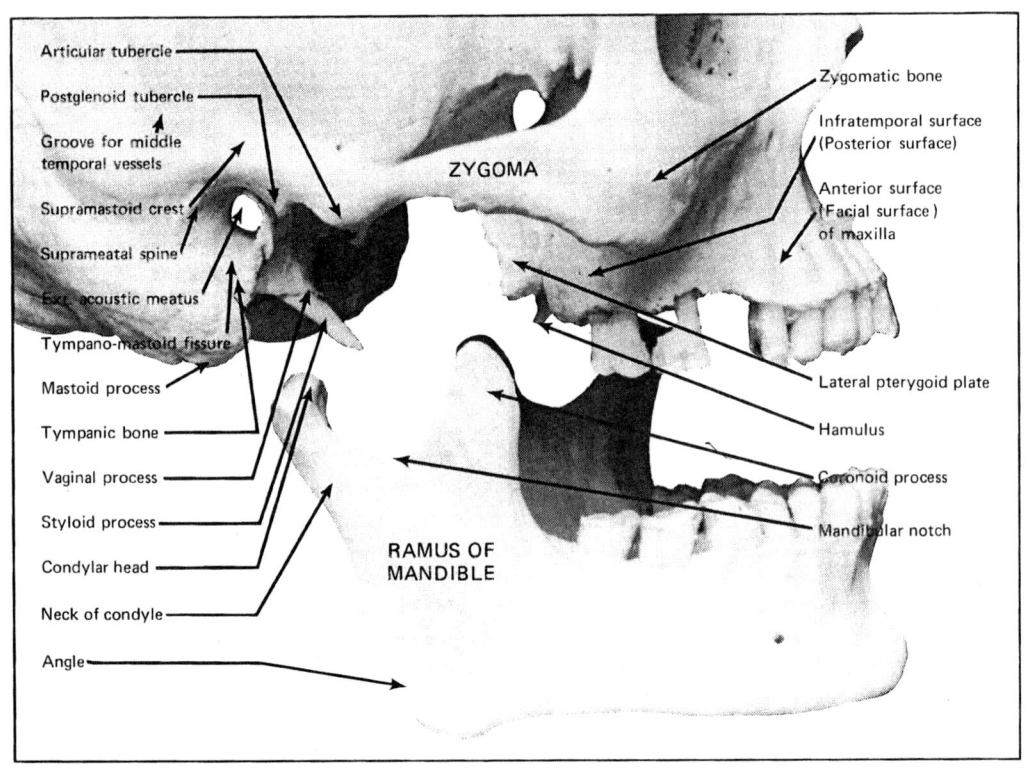

Treatment of Craniomandibular Disorders With Maxillofacial Orthopedic Appliances

Fig. 10-7 Lateral view of infratemporal fossa with skeletal tissue labeled. Osseous structures in close approximation to the head of the mandibular condyle are shown.

head of the lateral pterygoid muscle on mouth closure (Fig. 10-15).

Several authors[11,15,16] have described the action of the superior head of the lateral pterygoid muscle. As the condyle moves downward and forward on opening, the elastic fibers of the superior layers of the bilaminar zone are stretched. On closing, these fibers would pull the disc distal to the condylar head and up into the fossa were it not for the counteraction of the superior head of the lateral pterygoid muscle. This muscle acts together with the elastic superior layer of the bilaminar zone fibers to keep the disc centered between the stress area of the condylar head and the articular surface of the temporal bone.

The lower head of the lateral pterygoid muscle can be palpated by placing the index finger superiorly and distally to the maxillary third molar and pressing medially (Fig. 10-16). The sternocleidomastoid muscle may be palpated bilaterally (Figs. 10-17 and 10-18).

Innervation and vascularity

Innervation and adjacent vascularity are important to consider when treating temporomandibular joint disorders. A posteriorly displaced condyle can place pressure on the tissue between the condylar head and the tympanic plate. The auriculotemporal nerve and superior carotid artery both course near the posterior condylar neck and head area[17] (Fig. 10-19).

Characteristic Temporomandibular Joint Anatomy

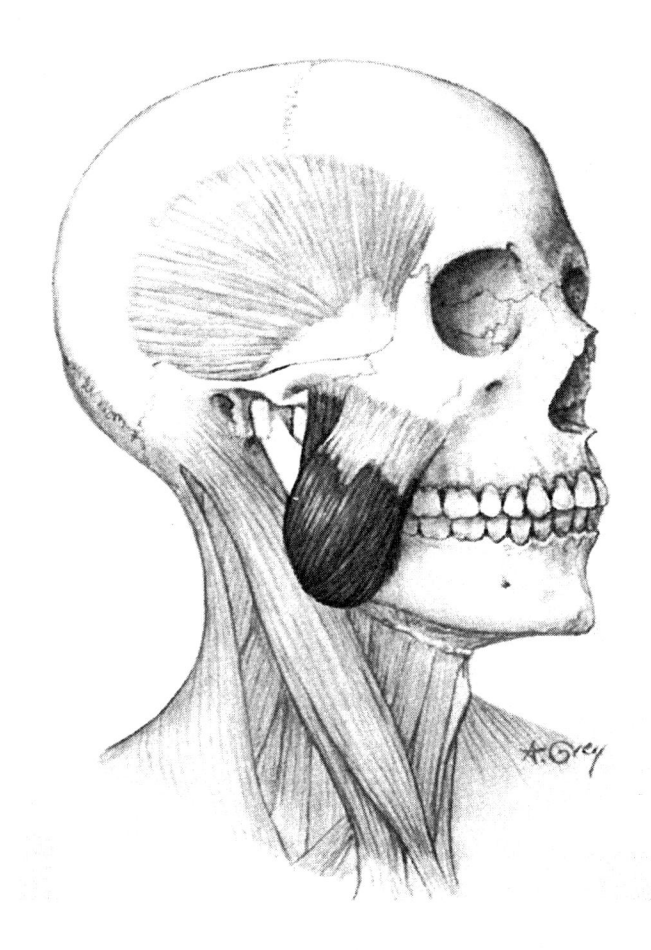

Fig. 10-8 The masseter muscle has a rhomboidal shape; it includes a superficial and a deep head.

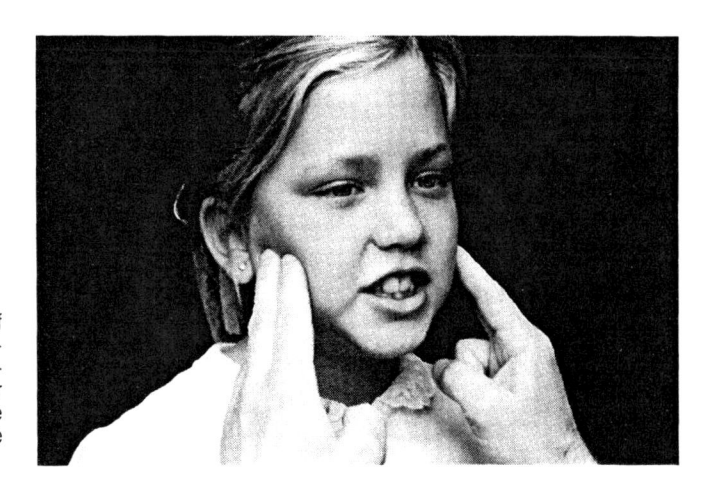

Fig. 10-9 Clinical palpation of the body of the masseter muscles. Palpating these muscles bilaterally can indicate whether one side is more tender than the other. Tenderness may indicate bruxism.

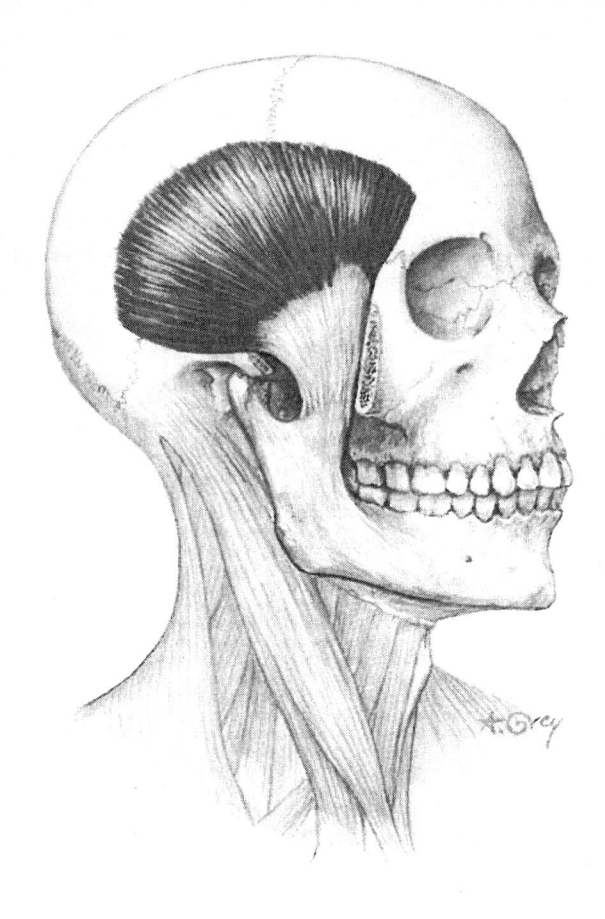

Fig. 10-10 The temporalis muscle origin and insertion with the zygomatic arch removed.

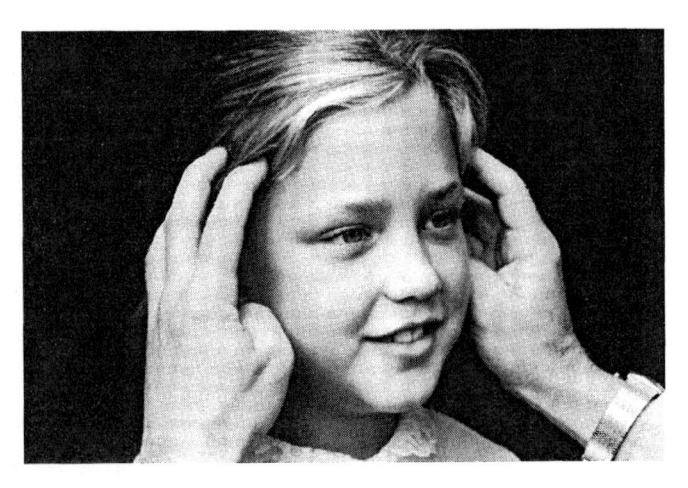

Fig. 10-11 With three fingers spread apart, all aspects of the temporalis muscle can be simultaneously palpated bilaterally. The index finger is placed 1–2 in. posteriorly and superiorly to the lateral wall of the orbit; the third finger stretches posteriorly to reach the posterior fibers.

Characteristic Temporomandibular Joint Anatomy

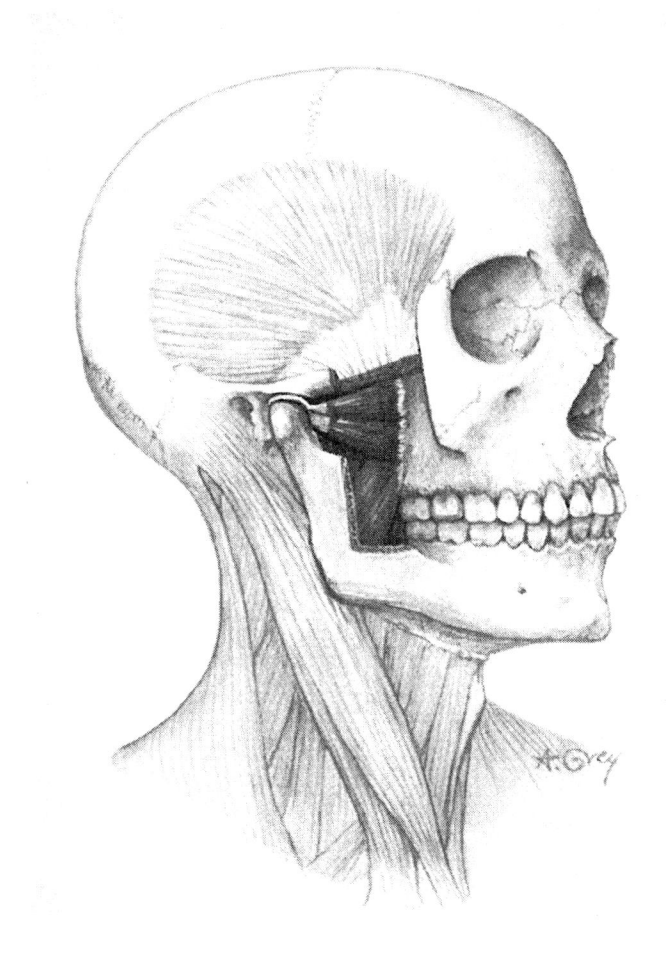

Fig. 10-12 The medial pterygoid takes much the same direction on the medial side of the ramus as the masseter takes on the lateral wall of the ramus.

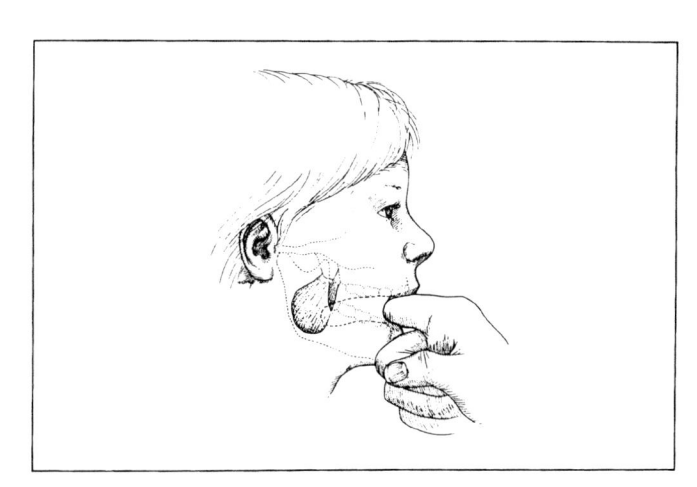

Fig. 10-13 The medial pterygoid muscle palpated from an intraoral position.

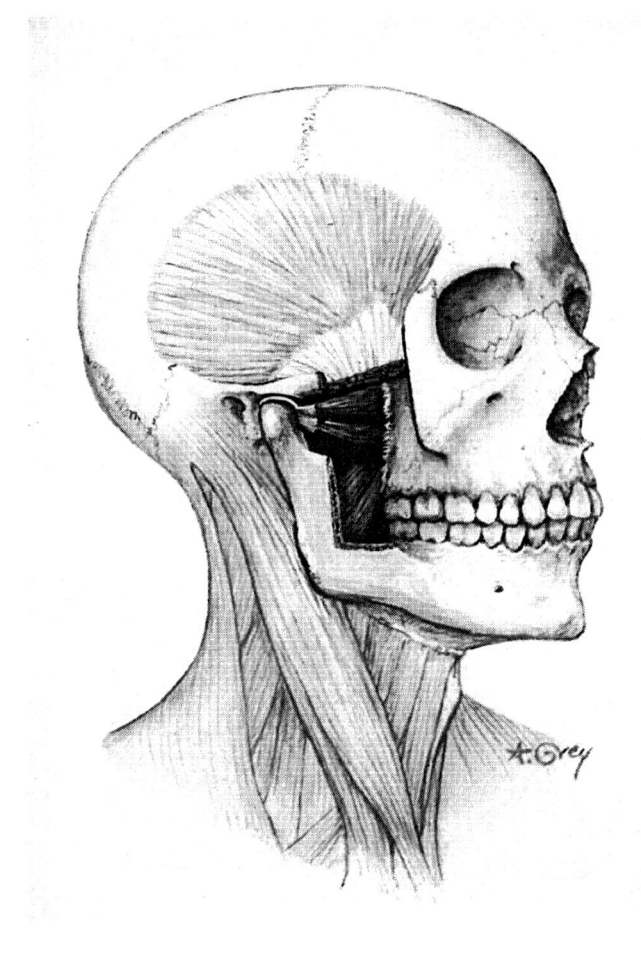

Fig. 10-14 The two heads of the lateral pterygoid muscles function as antagonistic muscles.[15] The inferior head protracts the mandible; it contracts to aid opening of the mouth, the superior head contracting on mandibular closing.

Lockhart[7] describes the pathway of the auriculotemporal nerve after it arises from the large posterior trunk of the mandibular nerve: two roots encircle the middle meningeal artery and pass lateral to the spine of the sphenoid; it then traverses backward between the sphenomandibular ligament and the condylar neck of the mandible, turning superiorly and posteriorly to the temporomandibular joint. Pressure on the auriculotemporal nerve could cause pain or pressure medially or distally to the source of entrapment. After leaving the temporomandibular joint, the auriculotemporal nerve travels through and innervates the parotid gland with a small branch to the tympanic membrane and the anterior wall of the external auditory meatus. After passing behind the superficial temporal artery, the nerve crosses over the zygomatic portion of the temporal bone and sends branches to the skin of the upper anterior and lateral part of the external ear and terminates in the skin on the side over the temporalis muscle.

TMJ ligaments

The ligaments of the temporomandibular

Characteristic Temporomandibular Joint Anatomy

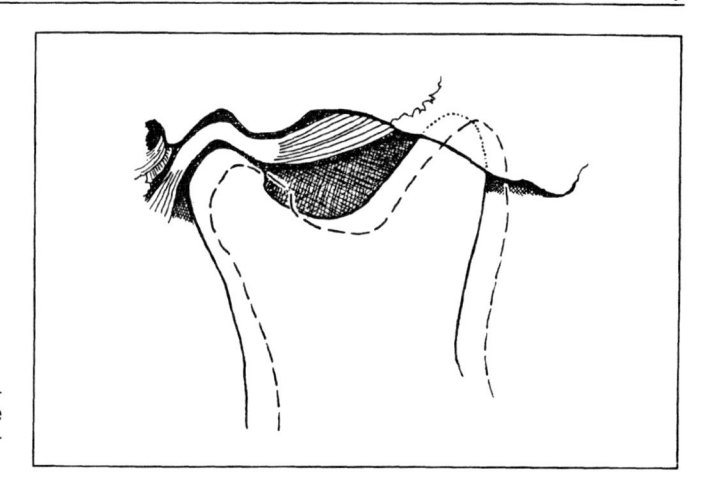

Fig. 10-15 Diagrammatic representation of the function of the superior head of the lateral pterygoid muscle.

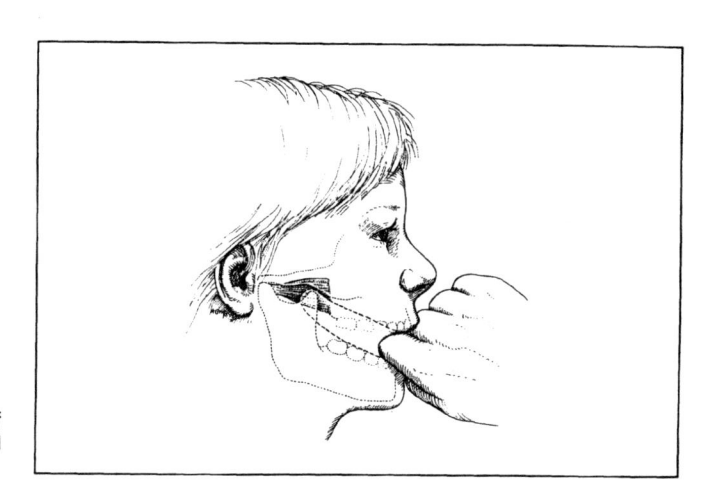

Fig. 10-16 Intraoral palpation of the inferior head of the lateral pterygoid muscle.

joint help keep the functioning articular surfaces in contact. If the ligaments are stretched or damaged, the joint will not function properly and may become hyper- or hypomobile. These ligaments help hold the joint together and help limit TMJ movements.

The collateral ligament or temporomandibular ligament extends from the lateral and inferior surface of the zygomatic arch to the lateral neck of the condyle.

Other fibrous attachments fix the capsule to the medial and lateral poles of the condyle. These attach loosely from the capsule to the lateral lip of the glenoid fossa laterally and medially to the spinous process of the sphenoid bone. The disc is attached tightly to the lateral aspects of the condyle. This tight attachment ensures a smoothness in functioning of the temporomandibular joint. Clicking and popping of the TMJ occur only after these tight attachments are loosened or torn.[11]

Histology of synovial joint tissue

Microscopic examination of the mature condyle and temporal bone reveals a more

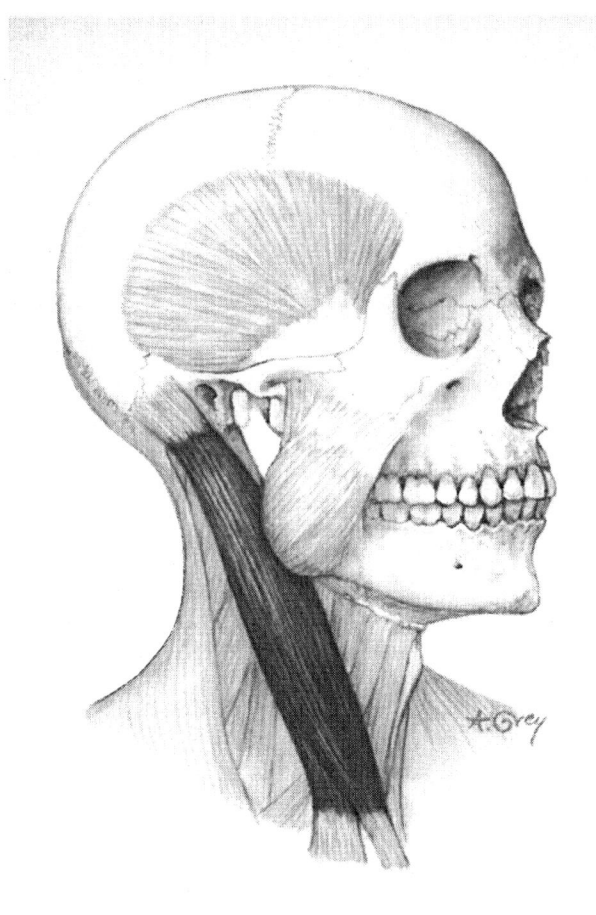

Treatment of Craniomandibular Disorders With Maxillofacial Orthopedic Appliances

Fig. 10-17 The sternocleidomastoid muscle may become painful to palpation when there is a temporomandibular joint disorder.

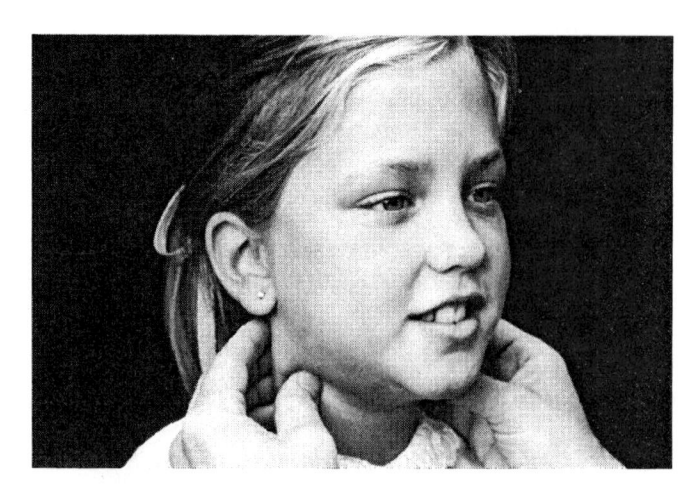

Fig. 10-18 Bilateral palpation of the sternocleidomastoid muscle.

Characteristic Temporomandibular Joint Anatomy

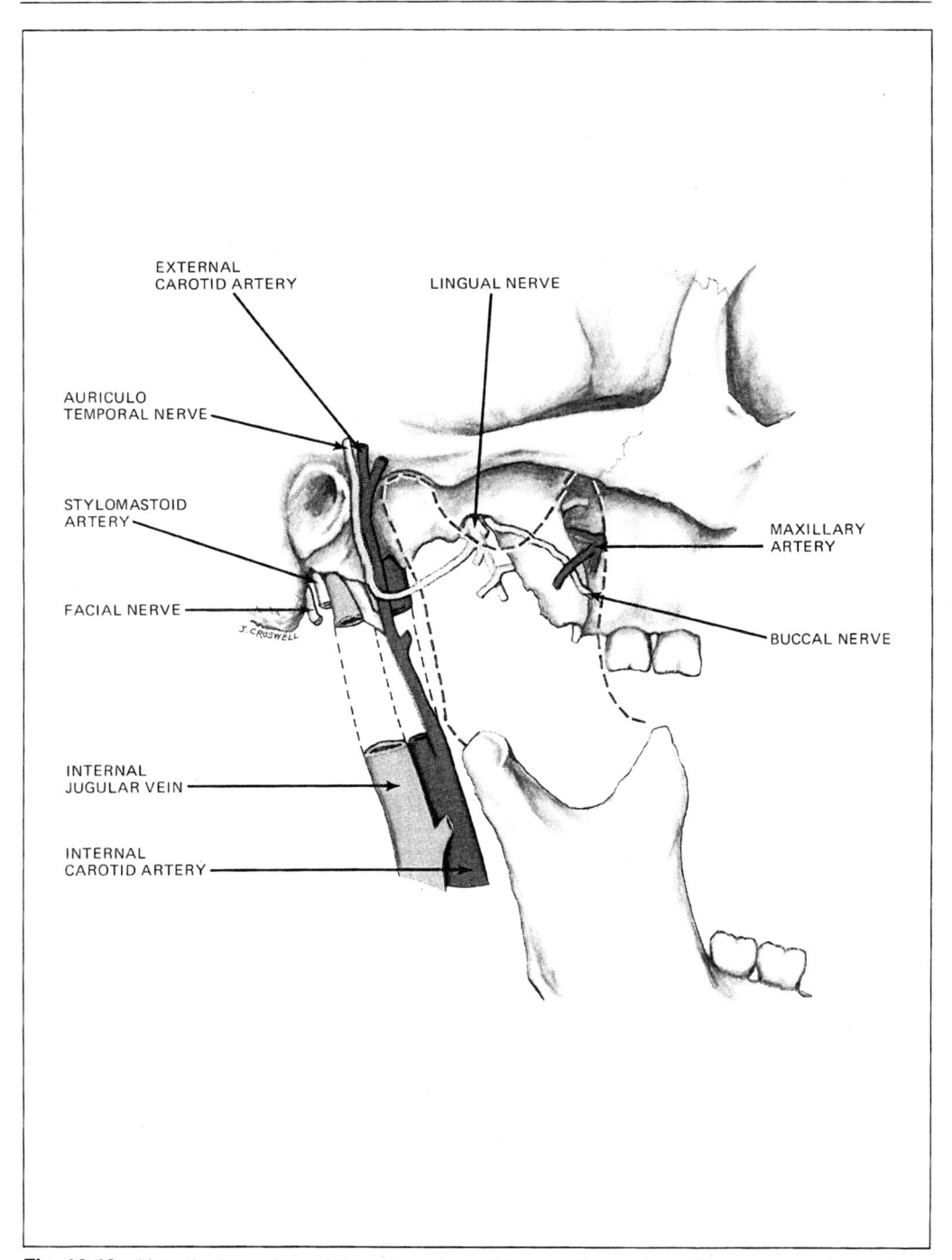

Fig. 10-19 Note the branches of the external carotid artery (internal maxillary artery and superficial temporal artery) and the proximity to the temporomandibular joint. The anterior tympanic artery, corda tympani nerve, and fibroelastic ligament are medially placed in the glenoid fossa.

dense arrangement of osteocytes in the area of the articular surfaces than in other parts of these structures. Ham and Cormack[18] note that the articular cartilage on the surface of synovial joints consists of collagen fibers immeshed in a sulfated amorphous intercellular substance (chondroitin sulfuric acid). These fibers form a densely tangled network which helps to bear the constant stress of synovial joints. Silberberg et al.[19] and their co-workers have studied the electron microscopy of articular cartilage. The intercellular substance appears structureless in the electron microscope.

This sulfated mucopolysaccharide is secreted from the growing chondrocytes and, on gross inspection, gives the articular surfaces of the joint a smooth, glistening appearance.

The nonvascularized dense fibrous tissues of the articular surfaces of the joint help protect the surfaces from susceptibility to degenerative joint disease. The propensity for these surfaces to undergo repair and regeneration readily has significance when planning a treatment regime with maxillofacial orthopedic appliances. In addition Bell[20] has emphasized that condylar growth cartilage responds positively to the demands of function.

Mechanical stress: effect on the craniomandibular articulation

If the mouth is kept wide open for a long period of time (e.g., during prolonged dental treatment), three areas of overt stress are produced:

1. The articular surfaces are in firm contact.
2. The collateral ligaments are stretched.
3. The superior elastic fibers of the bilaminar zone are stretched.

None of these areas of stress is particularly damaging in itself. However, if they are repeated, as in multiple fixed prosthetic procedures, then the individual could well begin to exhibit symptoms of craniomandibular disorder: head, neck, and back pain, ringing in the ears, or limited mobility of the mandible. If the mouth is kept open for prolonged periods of time in the presence of existing TMJ signs or symptoms, the results could be deleterious for the patient. Akeson et al.[21] report that there is significant loss of water (4 to 5%) from the tissue following immobilization of a joint. Immobilizing the TMJ by holding the mouth in a wide open position for periods of one hour or longer should be discouraged. This immobilization causes the tissue of animals to appear dry and less glistening.

By stressing the TMJ with wide opening of the mandible, fluid is squeezed out of joint tissues and fiber movement and elasticity are impaired.[22] Akeson has shown with animals that nine weeks of immobilization will result in a 40% decrease in chondroitin sulfate.[23] Although these studies cannot be directly related to the human temporomandibular joint, some possibilities should be noted. A decrease in the amount of fluid in the joint tissues may cause a loss of elasticity in the collateral ligaments and superior fibers of the bilaminar zone. Also, placing the condylar head, disc, and temporal bone into firm contact with one another may cause stickiness if held together for a prolonged period in the presence of less than ideal lubrication. Stickiness of the disc-temporal bone-condyle relationship can result in reciprocal clicking and stretching of the posterior disc attachment.

The lymphatic capillaries of the synovial villi provide a serumlike synovial fluid for lubrication of the articular surfaces of the TMJ. The synovial fluid itself has been studied qualitatively and quantitatively. Bauer et al.[24] have shown that synovial fluid is an ultrafiltrate of blood plus mucin. The mucin was identified by Meyer et al.[25] as hyal-

QUESTIONNAIRE FOR TMJ PROBLEMS

1. Name _____ Age _____ Phone _____
2. Address _____ City _____ Zip _____
3. Referred by Doctor _____
4. Do you have headaches? _____ Neck pain? _____
   Jaw pain? _____ Ear? _____ Face? _____ Other? _____
   Which side hurts—right? _____ left? _____ both? _____
5. For how long? _____
6. Is the pain constant? _____ Aching? _____
   Burning? _____ Stabbing? _____ Other? _____
   Worse in afternoon? _____ Worse in morning? _____
7. Does it hurt to chew? _____ Open wide? _____
8. Does your jaw make a popping noise? _____
   Clicking? _____ Grinding? _____ Other? _____
9. Has your jaw ever "locked" or slipped out of place? ___
10. Do you ever clench or grind your teeth? _____
    During the day? _____ At night? _____
11. Do you have problems with your ears? _____
    Hearing? _____ Dizziness? _____ Other? _____
12. Is it difficult to swallow? _____ Painful? _____
13. Are your teeth sore or sensitive? _____
14. Are you taking medicine of any kind? _____
    What for? _____
15. Describe the problem in your own words. _____

Fig. 10-20 Screening questionnaire for TMJ patients. (Courtesy of Drs. W. C. Farrar and W. L. McCarty.)

uronic acid. This acid gives a viscous quality to the synovial fluid and aids in the lubrication of the articular surfaces. With hypermobility of the temporomandibular joint, the volume of synovial fluid increases. However, in the healthy TMJ, the superior cavity (between the disc and temporal bone) contains approximately 1.2 ml. The inferior cavity (between the disc and head of the condyle) contains an average of 0.9 ml of synovial fluid.[26]

Salter and Field[27] have found that prolonged compression of articular cartilage can cause degenerative changes in the cartilage. When the articular surfaces are compressed, less than optimal lubrication and nutrition is able to reach these surfaces by way of the synovial fluid. During lengthy dental procedures, care must be taken to allow relaxation of mandibular musuculature. Prolonged mouth opening is not healthy for the temporomandibular joint.

Examination procedure for the patient suffering from craniomandibular disorder

The examination procedure for the patient complaining of temporomandibular joint symptoms includes a history, clinical examination, and necessary radiographs. Much of the examination procedure discussed in Chapter 4 is appropriate for the patient suffering from craniomandibular disorders.

A screening questionnaire similar to one used by Farrar and McCarty[28] is useful for differentiating neuralgia pain (a "burning or shooting" type of pain) from TMJ disc (internal derangement) pain. TMJ-related pain may be intermittent or continuous and is often located retro- or supraorbitally in the area of the anterior fibers of the temporalis muscle. The basic questionnaire also elicits a chief complaint and gives the examiner some insight for the patient's perception of the problem (Fig. 10-20).

The past and present history and clinical examination should focus on symptoms of pain, limitation or deviation of mandibular function, and TMJ noise. Pain is usually in the form of headache, neckache, or backache. The head pain is frequently retroorbital, and young patients are often brought to the optometrist or ophthalmologist for an eye examination for corrective lenses. Bilateral palpation of the temporalis muscle (Fig. 10-11) will often elicit tenderness in the anterior fibers of the muscle. The clinical examination for TMJ disorders includes observation of mandibular function, palpation of the muscles of mastication, and listening for TMJ noise (Figs. 10-21a through e).

Most TMJ history-taking and examination today is directed toward patients with overt symptoms of pain or dysfunction. It is important to recognize signs early so that early diagnosis and treatment can be directed toward minimizing symptoms. TMJ arthropathy is progressive. As symptoms become more serious, treatment becomes more complicated, and successful treatment is more elusive (Figs. 10-22 and 10-23).

Observation of mandibular function

Limited opening and deviate opening are the most obvious clinical signs of TMJ disorder. The velocity and direction of the mandibular midline on opening give clinical indication of internal dislocation (derangement) of the articular disc. Limited opening of the mandible can be due to trismus or an anteriorly displaced (closed-lock) disc.[29] The relationship of the condylar head, disc, and anterior border of the articular eminence of the temporal bone are diagrammed in Fig. 10-24.

The closed-lock condition can be differentiated from trismus by history, radiographs, and attempts to unlock the mandible. When the mandible is mechanically depressed and advanced, the disc may be able to reposition itself. The posterior ligament attachment will reposition the disc posteriorly as long as it is not stretched or torn (Fig. 10-16). Mechanical repositioning of the mandible is the first step in conservative treatment of internal derangement with orthopedic appliances.

Deviation of the mandible on opening is additional clinical evidence of disc-condylar head derangement. In the normal patient—one without TMJ disorder—the condyles move smoothly, without jerking motions, during opening and closing movements of the mandible. However, if the disc on one side is dislocated anteriorly, then lateral movement to the opposite side is limited. The condyle on the dislocated side is prevented from a normal lateral excursion by the disc.[29] On full opening, the mandible will deviate toward the side of the dislocated disc. An increase in velocity of mandibular opening and a click are common if the condyle does snap under the posterior rim of the disc. If the condyle does not snap

Examination Procedure for the Patient Suffering From Craniomandibular Disorder

Patient history forms are on pages 235 to 237 (Figs. 10-21a to c) and clinical examination forms are on pages 238 and 239 (Figs. 10-21d and e).

PATIENT HISTORY PART I 1

Name Mr.____ Mrs.____ Ms.____ _____ Date _____
      Last   First   Middle

Residence _____ Phone _____
          Street   City   State   Zip

Occupation and Employer _____

Business Address _____ Phone _____

Marital Status _____ Age _____ Birthdate _____ Ages of Children _____

Spouse's Name _____ Occupation and Employer _____

Whom may we thank for referring you? _____
                                     Name   Address

On the lines below, please list any physicians, dentists, neurologists, ear, nose or throat specialists, orthodontists, chiropractors, psychiatrists, or clinical teams consulted. Please list their specialty and briefly describe their diagnosis and treatment.

Doctor _____ MD DDS Specialty _____
Address _____
Diagnosis and Treatment _____

Doctor _____ MD DDS Specialty _____
Address _____
Diagnosis and Treatment _____

Doctor _____ MD DDS Specialty _____
Address _____
Diagnosis and Treatment _____

Doctor _____ MD DDS Specialty _____
Address _____
Diagnosis and Treatment _____

Figs. 10-21a to c Individualized patient history.

Treatment of Craniomandibular Disorders With Maxillofacial Orthopedic Appliances

General Health Questions

2

Please answer as many of these general health questions as possible with YES or NO. However, write freely on the discussion questions.
A. Sinus Infection?_____ Ear Infection?_____ Swollen Glands?_____
B. Do you have frequent headaches?_____ What area of the head?_____
   How long do they last?_____
C. Have you ever had a severe blow to the head?_____ What part of the head?_____
   Date?_____
D. Have you ever suffered nutritional deficiencies?_____
E. Do you regularly take any medication?_____ Which?_____
F. Please indicate anything else about yourself which you suspect may be related to your condition. _____

Pain Symptoms

1. Is there pain in the right TMJ joint? _____ Left TMJ joint? _____
2. When did the symptoms start in the right TMJ joint?_____ Left TMJ joint?_____
3. Is the pain constant or intermittent?_____
4. How often do you have pain? _____
5. Does pain start abruptly? _____ Gradually?_____
6. Does pain disappear abruptly?_____ Gradually?_____
7. What time of day or night is pain most severe?_____
8. What is the longest period you have gone without pain? _____
9. What medication, if any, do you take to relieve pain?_____
10. Please describe any method of positioning the jaw that you have found for relieving pain? _____
11. Do any of the following normal daily activities cause pain? If yes, where do you feel pain?
    Yawning_____ Chewing_____ Swallowing_____ Speaking _____
    Brushing teeth_____ Turning head_____ Moving the neck _____
    Moving the shoulders_____
12. Do your teeth hurt? Upper right_____ Lower right_____
    Upper left_____ Lower left_____
    Irregular or raised dental filling_____ Excessive opening of mouth during dental extraction_____ Dental treatment utilizing a head gear_____ Traction for cervical arthritis_____

Fig. 10-21b

Oral Symptoms Other Than Pain

13. Are your jaws clenched when you awaken from sleep? _____
14. Do you grind your teeth when asleep? _____
15. Are your jaw muscles ever tired? _____ When? _____
16. Do you ever feel pressure or tenderness about the right eye? _____ Left eye? _____
17. Do you ever get dizzy? _____ How often? _____
18. Do you ever feel faint? _____
19. In which ear (R or L) do you ever notice: Ringing? (R) _____ , (L) _____ ,
    Popping noises? (R) _____ (L) _____ ,
    Stuffiness? (R) _____ , (L) _____ , Pain? (R) _____ , (L) _____ ,
    A hearing change? (R) _____ (L) _____
20. Is there a family history of temporomandibular joint dysfunction? _____

Finally, by referring back to the names of Doctors on page 1, please answer:

21. Did any of their treatments make you feel better? If so, which helped the most? In what manner? _____

22. Did any of the treatments make you feel worse? Which ones? In what manner? _____

Please Check Yes or No to the Following Questions:

Yes No

☐ ☐ Have lower wisdom teeth been removed?
☐ ☐ Have you ever had orthodontic treatment?
☐ ☐ Were teeth removed for orthodontic treatment?
☐ ☐ Have you ever been treated for a "bad bite"?
☐ ☐ Do you have dental crowns or a bridge?
☐ ☐ Do you have missing back teeth and no replacement?
☐ ☐ Have you ever been treated for problems of your jaw joint, or for facial muscle spasms?
☐ ☐ Do you ever awaken with awareness of your teeth or jaws?
☐ ☐ Do you have any pain or soreness around your eyes, ears or other parts of your face?
☐ ☐ Do you have "tension" headaches?
☐ ☐ Do you frequently have neckaches or stiff neck muscles?
☐ ☐ Do you usually eat breakfast?

☐ ☐ Do you have difficulty in opening your mouth widely?
☐ ☐ Have you ever received a severe blow to the side of the head or jaw?
☐ ☐ Does it cause pain to open your jaw widely?
☐ ☐ Do you ever hear clicking or popping sounds from your jaw joint?
☐ ☐ Are you presently in any pain from your jaw joint or muscles?
☐ ☐ Does pain or discomfort from your jaw joint interfere with your work or other activities?
☐ ☐ Are there times when you notice that this problem or pain is less or gone completely?
☐ ☐ Do you feel you need treatment for this problem?
☐ ☐ Do you take aspirin frequently?
☐ ☐ Are you taking any tranquilizers, muscle relaxants, or anti-depressants?
☐ ☐ Are you afraid your problem is serious?

Fig. 10-21c

Treatment of Craniomandibular Disorders With Maxillofacial Orthopedic Appliances

PART II 4

For Doctor's Use Only

Date_____

Intraoral Findings:
CLASS   I   II   III
( ) Missing Teeth   ( ) Crossbite
( ) Third Molars Present: 1 16 17 32   ( ) Abnormal Wear
( ) Non-Functional Cuspid R L   ( ) Incisal Interference R L

Miscellaneous:
( ) Orthodontics _____
( ) Previous Occlusal Treatment _____
( ) R$_x$ Medications _____
( ) Injury _____

Radiography:
( ) Lateral Transcranials:
   R L
   ☐ ☐ Reduced Joint Space
   ☐ ☐ Flattened Condyle
   ☐ ☐ Bony Lipping Condyle
   ☐ ☐ Essential 3mm Space   LEFT 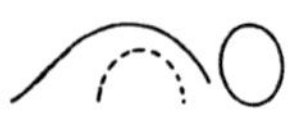   RIGHT
( ) Arthrograms: _____
_____

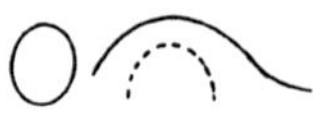

( ) Other: _____
_____

TMJ Noise: Right   Left
Opening Click   Early   Late   Early   Late
Crepitus   _____   _____
Disc Locked Out   _____   _____

Figs. 10-21d and e Clinical examination. An orderly and complete clinical evaluation of intraoral, radiographic, and muscular signs will aid in a correct diagnosis. (Courtesy of European Orthodontic Products, St. Paul, Minn.)

Examination Procedure for the Patient Suffering From Craniomandibular Disorder

X — uncomfortable
O — hurts

1.

1) TMJ
2) Post. TMJ
3) Deep Masseter
4) Superficial Masseter
5) Masseter Body
6) Anterior Temporalis
7) Posterior Temporalis
8) Vertex
9) Posterior Neck
10) Sternocleidomastoid
11) Lateral Pterygoid
12) Temporalis Insertion
13) Medial Pterygoid
14) Posterior Digastric

15) HEADACHES:_____

(Mark Triggers with "T")

2. R ⊢⊢⊢⊢⊢⊢⊢ L
15 10 5 0 5 10 15 mm
DEFLECTION

3. Mandibular Movement:

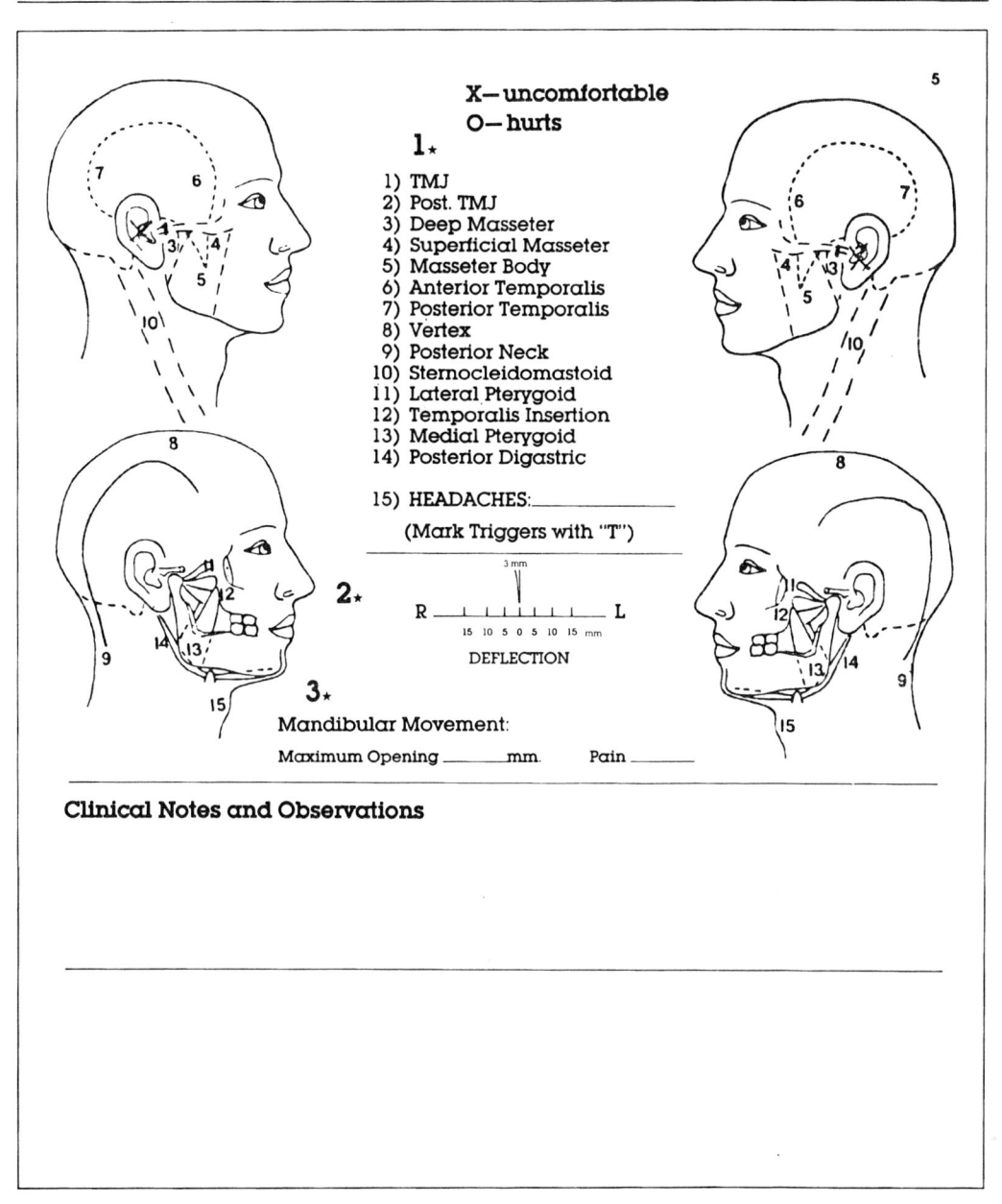

Maximum Opening _____ mm.   Pain _____

Clinical Notes and Observations

Fig. 10-21e

239

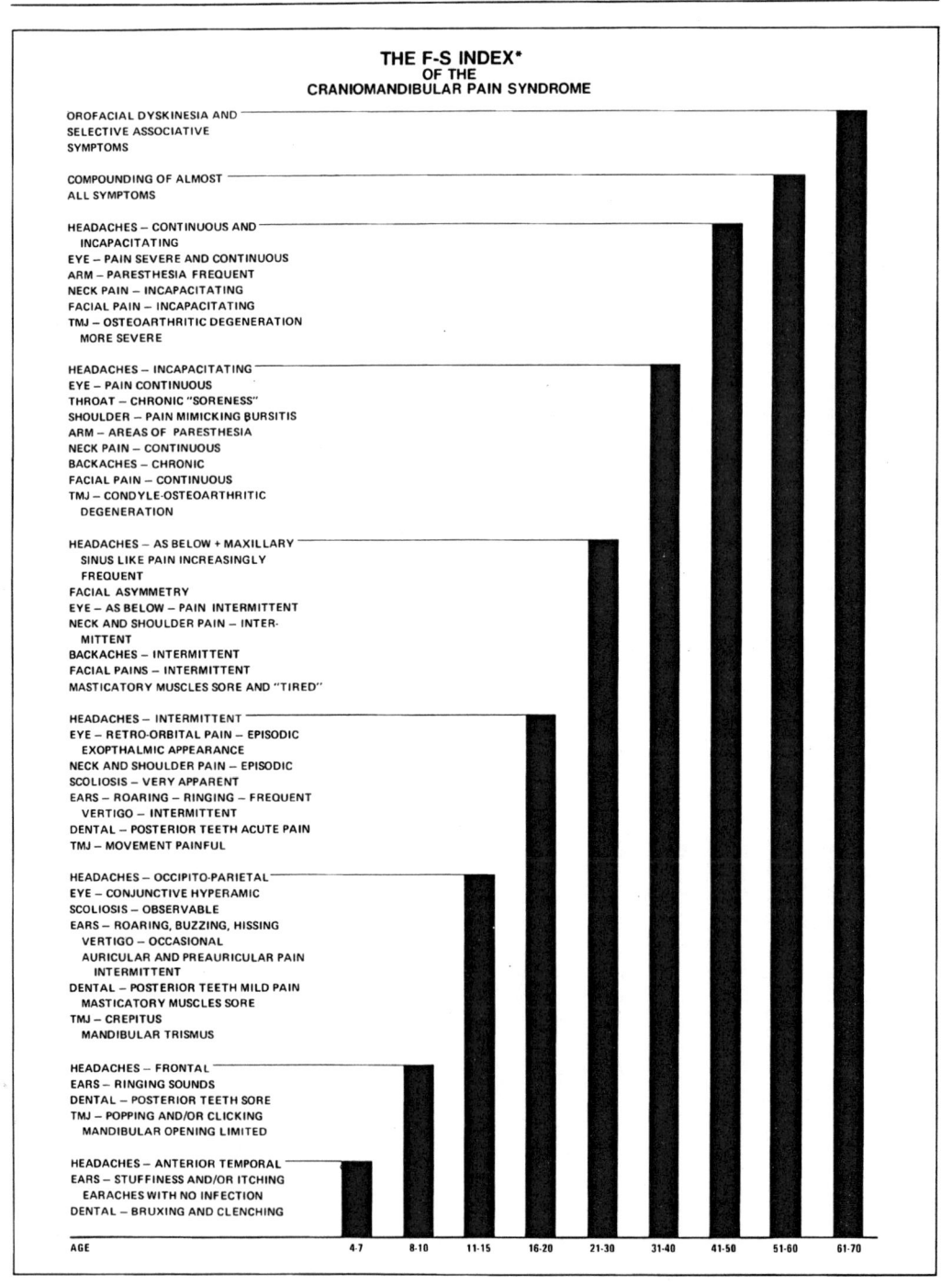

THE F-S INDEX*
OF THE
CRANIOMANDIBULAR PAIN SYNDROME

OROFACIAL DYSKINESIA AND
SELECTIVE ASSOCIATIVE
SYMPTOMS

COMPOUNDING OF ALMOST
ALL SYMPTOMS

HEADACHES – CONTINUOUS AND
  INCAPACITATING
EYE – PAIN SEVERE AND CONTINUOUS
ARM – PARESTHESIA FREQUENT
NECK PAIN – INCAPACITATING
FACIAL PAIN – INCAPACITATING
TMJ – OSTEOARTHRITIC DEGENERATION
  MORE SEVERE

HEADACHES – INCAPACITATING
EYE – PAIN CONTINUOUS
THROAT – CHRONIC "SORENESS"
SHOULDER – PAIN MIMICKING BURSITIS
ARM – AREAS OF PARESTHESIA
NECK PAIN – CONTINUOUS
BACKACHES – CHRONIC
FACIAL PAIN – CONTINUOUS
TMJ – CONDYLE-OSTEOARTHRITIC
  DEGENERATION

HEADACHES – AS BELOW + MAXILLARY
  SINUS LIKE PAIN INCREASINGLY
  FREQUENT
FACIAL ASYMMETRY
EYE – AS BELOW – PAIN INTERMITTENT
NECK AND SHOULDER PAIN – INTER-
  MITTENT
BACKACHES – INTERMITTENT
FACIAL PAINS – INTERMITTENT
MASTICATORY MUSCLES SORE AND "TIRED"

HEADACHES – INTERMITTENT
EYE – RETRO-ORBITAL PAIN – EPISODIC
  EXOPTHALMIC APPEARANCE
NECK AND SHOULDER PAIN – EPISODIC
SCOLIOSIS – VERY APPARENT
EARS – ROARING – RINGING – FREQUENT
VERTIGO – INTERMITTENT
DENTAL – POSTERIOR TEETH ACUTE PAIN
TMJ – MOVEMENT PAINFUL

HEADACHES – OCCIPITO-PARIETAL
EYE – CONJUNCTIVE HYPERAMIC
SCOLIOSIS – OBSERVABLE
EARS – ROARING, BUZZING, HISSING
VERTIGO – OCCASIONAL
  AURICULAR AND PREAURICULAR PAIN
  INTERMITTENT
DENTAL – POSTERIOR TEETH MILD PAIN
MASTICATORY MUSCLES SORE
TMJ – CREPITUS
  MANDIBULAR TRISMUS

HEADACHES – FRONTAL
EARS – RINGING SOUNDS
DENTAL – POSTERIOR TEETH SORE
TMJ – POPPING AND/OR CLICKING
  MANDIBULAR OPENING LIMITED

HEADACHES – ANTERIOR TEMPORAL
EARS – STUFFINESS AND/OR ITCHING
  EARACHES WITH NO INFECTION
DENTAL – BRUXING AND CLENCHING

AGE   4-7   8-10   11-15   16-20   21-30   31-40   41-50   51-60   61-70

Fig. 10-22 An evolutionary, progressive, and cumulative clinical index pattern correlated from symptoms documented in craniomandibular pain patients. (Reprinted with permission of Drs. L. A. Funt and B. C. Stack.)

Examination Procedure for the Patient Suffering From Craniomandibular Disorder

The K·F·S Temporomandibular Joint Visual Index*

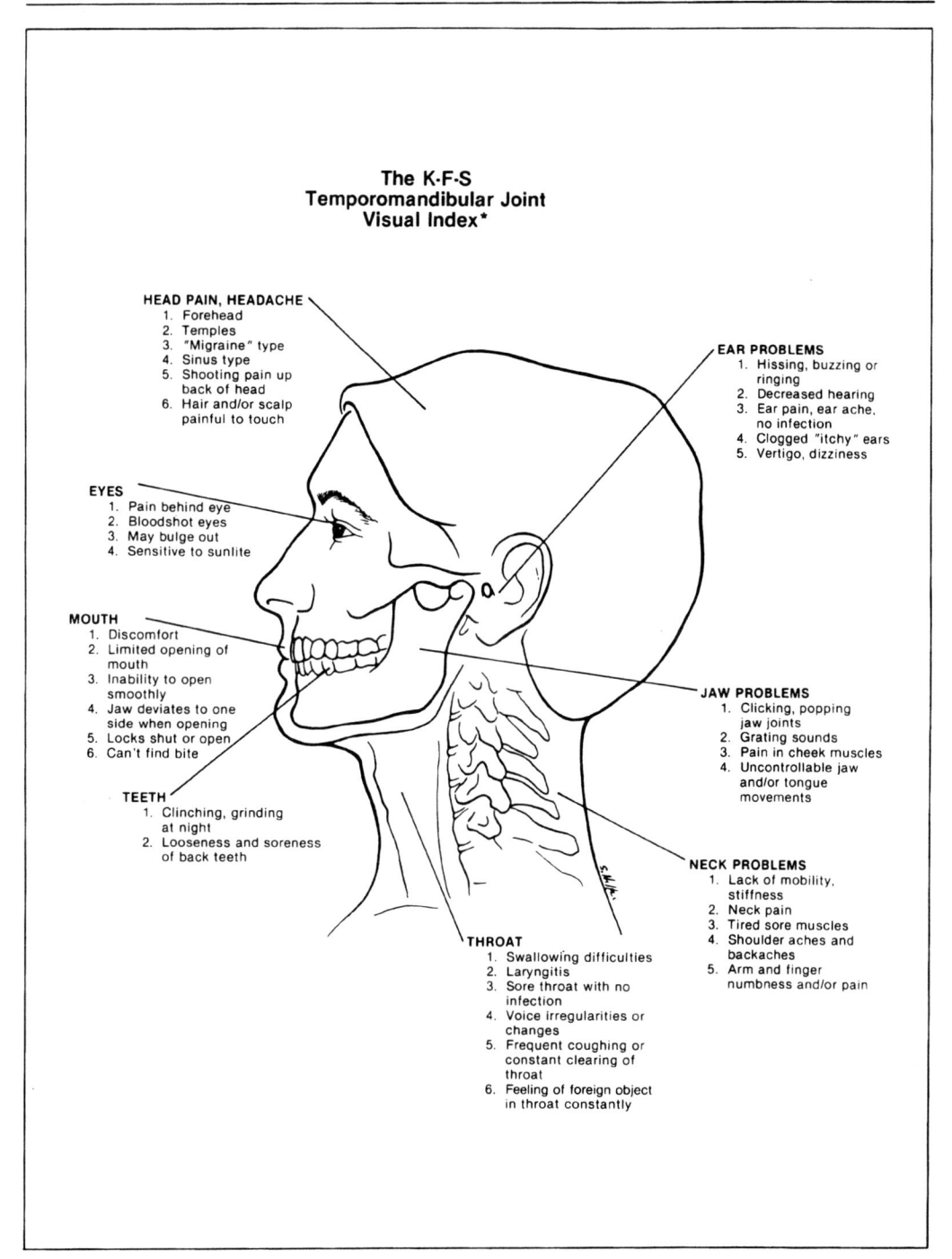

HEAD PAIN, HEADACHE
1. Forehead
2. Temples
3. "Migraine" type
4. Sinus type
5. Shooting pain up back of head
6. Hair and/or scalp painful to touch

EYES
1. Pain behind eye
2. Bloodshot eyes
3. May bulge out
4. Sensitive to sunlite

MOUTH
1. Discomfort
2. Limited opening of mouth
3. Inability to open smoothly
4. Jaw deviates to one side when opening
5. Locks shut or open
6. Can't find bite

TEETH
1. Clinching, grinding at night
2. Looseness and soreness of back teeth

EAR PROBLEMS
1. Hissing, buzzing or ringing
2. Decreased hearing
3. Ear pain, ear ache, no infection
4. Clogged "itchy" ears
5. Vertigo, dizziness

JAW PROBLEMS
1. Clicking, popping jaw joints
2. Grating sounds
3. Pain in cheek muscles
4. Uncontrollable jaw and/or tongue movements

NECK PROBLEMS
1. Lack of mobility, stiffness
2. Neck pain
3. Tired sore muscles
4. Shoulder aches and backaches
5. Arm and finger numbness and/or pain

THROAT
1. Swallowing difficulties
2. Laryngitis
3. Sore throat with no infection
4. Voice irregularities or changes
5. Frequent coughing or constant clearing of throat
6. Feeling of foreign object in throat constantly

Fig. 10-23 A visual, clinical index correlated from the symptoms most documented in craniomandibular pain patients. (Reprinted with permission of Drs. B. H. Kinnie, L. A. Funt, and B. C. Stack.)

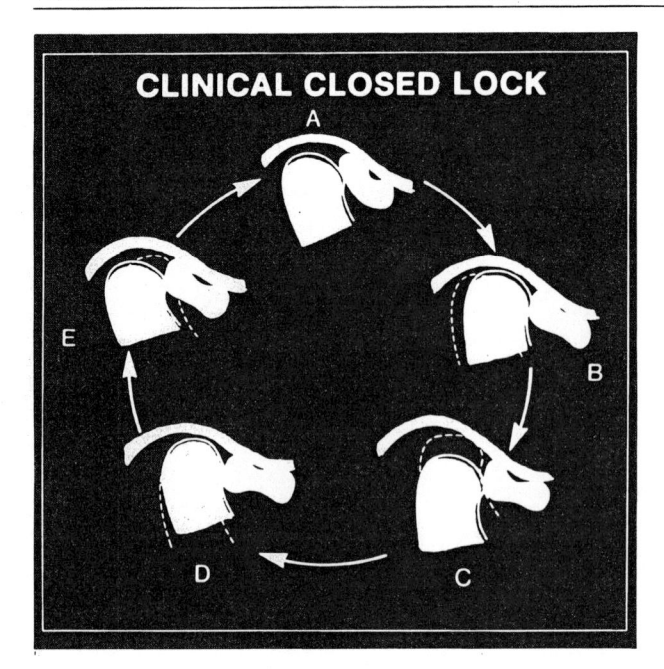

Fig. 10-24 Diagram of the disc relationship in a clinical closed lock condition. Complete anterior displacement of the articular disc will limit mandibular opening. Normal condylar translation is blocked. (Reprinted with permission of Drs. W. B. Farrar and W. L. McCarty.)

under the disc, it will be held back and cause mandibular midline deviation to that side.

Palpation of muscles of mastication

The anatomical landmarks of the temporomandibular joint and the palpation of the masticatory muscles have been described (Figs. 10-6 to 10-18). Placing the fingertips over the temporomandibular joint during mandibular movements will help the clinician "feel" the clicking of the condyle as it snaps over the posterior rim of the disc. The bulge of the lateral pole of the condyle and the deviation of the condylar path is easily felt with the fingertips over the joint.

Patients that are aware of bruxism tend to show tenderness in the masseter muscles on palpation. Solberg, Woo, and Houston[30] have shown that in a young adult population, TMJ-dysfunction subjects with headache had tender masseter and temporalis muscles. In this and other studies,[31] women demonstrated a higher frequency of muscle tenderness than men.

Tenderness in the lateral pterygoid muscle is a common finding in pretreatment orthodontic patients; the medial pterygoid and masseter muscles are second and third in sensitivity.[32] This tenderness in the lateral pterygoid muscles can be explained by the function these muscles perform during mandibular movement. Several studies[33-36] demonstrate that the lateral pterygoids are the muscles most active in opening, forward, and lateral function of the mandible. Williamson[32] has shown that more than 50% of the dysfunctioning adolescent patients examined before orthodontic treatment have had deep overbites. The lateral pterygoid muscles have to function more than normal in order to overcome the deep anterior guidance and make lateral excursion in the presence of a deep overbite. Opening a deep overbite is routinely accomplished with orthopedic appliances. *This ability to reposition the mandible forward and open a deep overbite is* part of the reason for success in treating TMJ disorders with orthopedic appliances. Evaluation of malocclusion type (Chapter 4) will help establish treatment criteria.

Listening for craniomandibular joint noise

Understanding temporomandibular joint noise is essential in formulating a treatment plan. An outline of TMJ noise demonstrates the level of dysfunction:

I. No joint noise
   A. Healthy TMJ. Patient has full range of mandibular movements without deviation or symptoms
   B. Closed lock. Patient has limited opening (25–30 mm or less) with possible symptoms of headache, neckache, backache, and/or ringing in the ears
II. Joint noise
   A. Clicking noise
      1. Opening click
      2. Opening and closing click (reciprocal clicking)
   B. Grinding noise on translation of mandible: degenerative arthritis
   C. Grating or cracking noise on translation of mandible: advanced degenerative arthritis

A stethoscope is useful for listening to joint noise. A healthy temporomandibular joint has a full range of mandibular opening and excursions without joint noise. The closed lock joint does not click because the disc is dislocated anteriorly to the condylar head. There are no grating sounds because the disc mechanically blocks the condyle from going into translation. Grating or grinding noises are seldom heard with condylar head rotation only.[29] In the clinical closed-lock condition, the disc remains displaced anteriorly to the condyle during all mandibular opening and closing movements. With the disc anteriorly displaced, the posterior ligament attachment to the articular disc can be stretched or torn.

An opening click occurs the instant the condyle slips over the posterior border and snaps into the thinner avascular portion of the disc. Figure 10-25 shows drawings from arthrograms that demonstrate disc displacement and a click at different stages of mandibular movement.

A closing click occurs when the condyle slips past the posterior border of the disc and snaps onto the posterior disc attachment (retrodiscal pad). This displaces the disc forward and the condylar head distally and superiorly into the fossa. With the condylar head displaced distally, either pressure on the nerves and blood vessels (Fig. 10-20) distal to the condylar head or the aberrant position of the coronoid process (insertion of the temporalis muscle) may lead to head pain.[37,38]

When clicking occurs during mandibular opening and closing it is called reciprocal clicking; reciprocal clicking is represented in Fig. 10-26.

TMJ radiography

After a thorough history and clinical examination, radiographs of the temporomandibular joint help confirm a diagnosis and determine a prognosis. Oberg suggests TMJ radiographs to aid in the choice of a therapeutic regime, to plan a course of treatment, to evaluate the success of treatment, and to monitor the course of joint pathology.[39] Because of the risk of radiation-induced carcinogenesis,[40] a conservative treatment plan is suggested in children until it is determined that radiographs are essential for making a diagnosis. For any age, and for every radiographic exposure, the question should be asked: "Is this film absolutely necessary?"[41] The history and clinical signs and symptoms help determine the necessity of radiography. If the symp-

Treatment of Craniomandibular Disorders With Maxillofacial Orthopedic Appliances

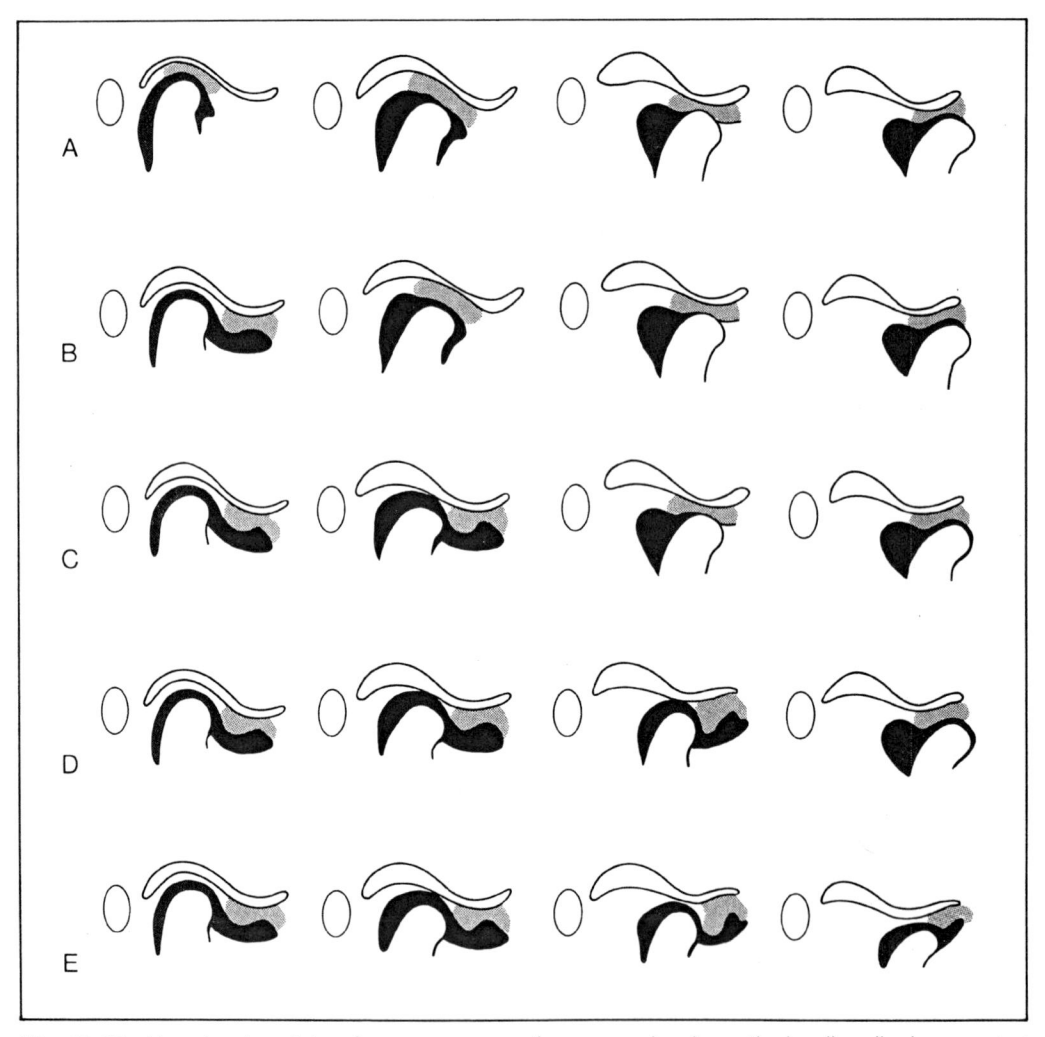

Fig. 10-25 Line drawings taken from numerous arthrograms showing articular disc displacement at various points of condyle movement. *(A)* normal joint. *(B)* early opening click. *(C)* intermediate opening click. *(D)* late opening click. *(E)* complete anterior dislocation of the articular disc or closed lock. (Reprinted with permission of Drs. W. K. Solberg and G. T. Clark.)

toms are not severe, a conservative course of treatment is recommended. When conservative treatment does not bring results after two to four weeks, radiography of the TMJ is required. If symptoms are severe, or of rapid onset, then radiographs and medical-surgical consultations may be necessary for determining a diagnosis.

Four different types of radiographs are currently used to view the temporomandibular joint: the panoramic film, transcranial film, transmaxillary film, and the tomographic film. Each has specific qualities that make it useful in diagnosing craniomandibular disorders.

The temporomandibular joint is the most difficult joint to radiograph in the human body. The challenge for the clinician is first,

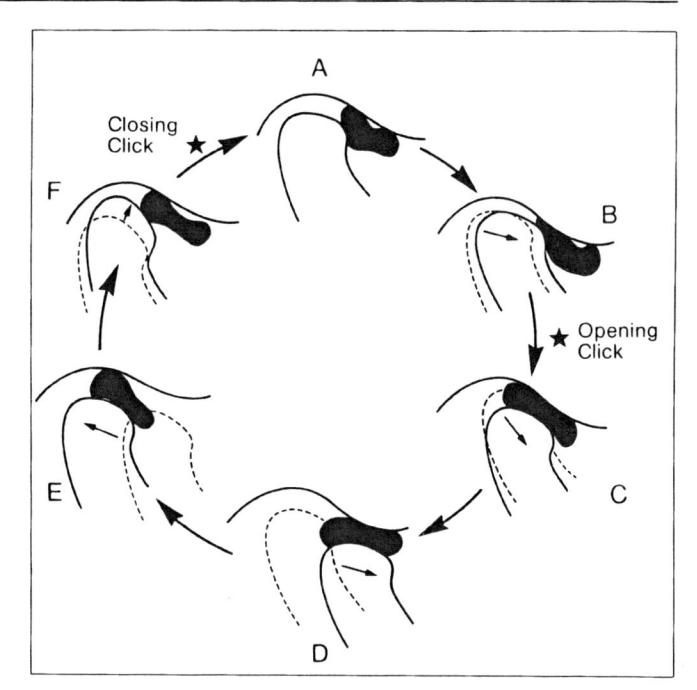

Examination Procedure for the Patient Suffering From Craniomandibular Disorder

Fig. 10-26 Schematic drawing of reciprocal clicking. The asterisk represents the point where the clicking sound occurs on opening and closing. If reciprocal clicking continues, the disc may eventually become permanently displaced forward of the condyle, furthering the chance for stretching or tearing of the posterior ligament attachment. (Reprinted with permission of Drs. W. K. Solberg and G. T. Clark.)

to decide whether TMJ radiographs are necessary, and second, which radiographic projection will justify (in terms of diagnostic yield) the radiation exposure that the patient will undergo.

Panoramic radiography

The panoramic radiograph gives the least reliable view of the TMJ. The head of the condyle is seen in a lateral projection only and its position in the fossa is distorted. Changes in the shape of the condylar head from a rounded, smooth surface can be detected. Traumatic fracture to the mandibular condyle, rami, or body are detectable. There is some evidence that the dosage of radiation to the thyroid gland of young patients makes this film undesirable because of the more superior position of this gland in children.[41]

Transcranial radiography

The transcranial projection is useful for viewing the lateral aspect of the hard tissue components of the temporomandibular joint. Six radiographs of the TMJ are taken (three on each side) with the mandible in three positions: maximum intercuspation, postural rest, and maximum open.

The central ray passes through the longitudinal axis of the condylar head (as directed from 25° above the horizontal) and at a 90° angle to the film (Fig. 10-27). By utilizing a headholder similar to that shown in Fig. 4-7, reproducible projections can be obtained. Figure 10-28 demonstrates an individualized transcranial projection.

Diagnostic yield of transcranial radiography

Although the transcranial projection is the most popular radiograph of the TMJ, the diagnostic yield is limited. The basilar skull

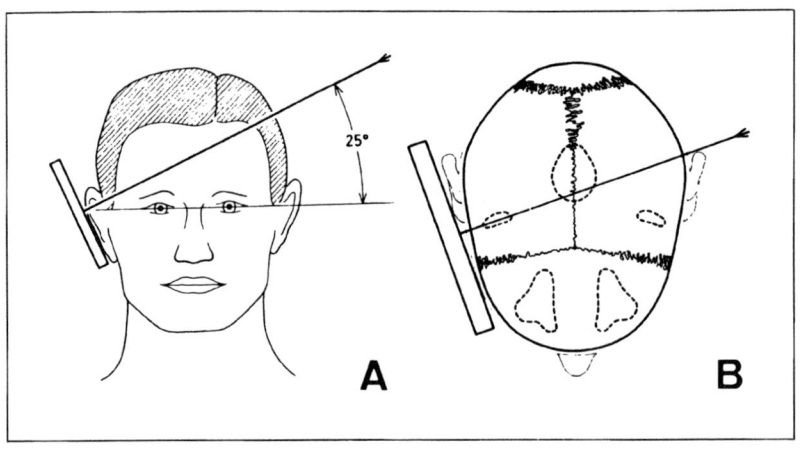

Fig. 10-27 The path of the beam passes through the longitudinal axis of the condylar head (as directed from 25° above the horizontal) and at a 90° angle to the film.

structures obscure the joint on the side that the clinician would like to see. The skull also prevents the radiographic beam from coming into proper alignment with the long axis of the condylar head.

Current techniques were developed to avoid the superimposition of basal skull structures over the TMJ. However, with the transcranial projection, only the superior border of the condylar head and the lateral border of the glenoid fossa are clearly visible. Most of the pathological changes to the head of the condyle occur between the lateral and medial poles on the superior surface. Because of the variability in the shape of the condylar head, transcranial radiography is of value primarily for determining relative condylar position and possible osseous changes in border outline.

Transmaxillary radiography

The transmaxillary projection is taken with the mandible wide open. The central x-ray beam is directed slightly inferiorly to the infraorbital foramen through the mediolateral plane of the condyle in order to intersect the film at a 90° angle (Fig. 10-29).

Transcranial and transmaxillary radiography both show the bony relationship of the condyle to the fossa. The soft tissue elements, including the articular disc, are not seen. The position of the articular disc can be determined with arthrography by the space between the bony structures. Petersson[43] has compared transcranial radiographs with tomographic radiographs with respect to condylar position and radiographic joint space. The joint space was found to be unpredictable in the transcranial radiographs. Tomographic radiography was the most reliable method of viewing joint space.

Tomographic radiography

Tomographic radiography allows a predetermined layer of the condyle and fossa to be displayed clearly on the film. Structures in front of and behind the predetermined layer are blurred or eliminated.[39] Investigators agree that tomographic radiography is the most accurate method of viewing the temporomandibular joint.[39,42-44] Tomography can show structural changes that are missed in conventional radiographs.

Since there is no superimposition of anatomical structures, the tomogram gives a

Fig. 10-28 Notice the configuration of the condylar head in this edentulous 35-year-old female. She has complained of chronic headaches since shortly after getting her dentures 10 years ago. Insertion of a mouthguard-type appliance, worn only at night with her dentures, stopped her headaches within a week. Her dentures were subsequently remade to restore the vertical dimension.

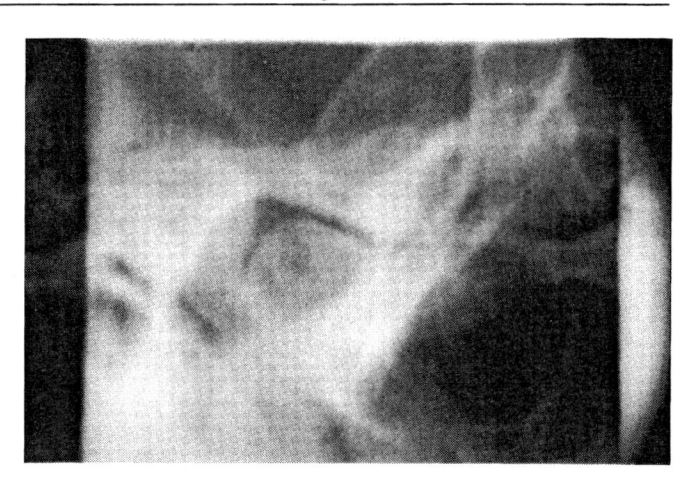

well-defined view of the TMJ. The film and the radiographic source move in opposite directions during the exposure time. The further the beam source moves, the wider the exposure angle and the thinner the section of the TMJ observed. A beam source angle of 40° to 50° would demonstrate an approximately 1.0 mm slice of the TMJ.[45]

Some streaking of the image does occur with tomographic techniques. This "parasitic streaking" is most pronounced when the long axis of the object parallels the path of the tube travel. The streaking is least pronounced when the long axis of the object is perpendicular to the path of tube travel. To reduce parasitic streaking, complex trajectories of tube travel have been devised. An example of this pluridirectional tube movement is seen in Fig. 10-30.

Hypocycloidal tube movement produces a very clear diagnostic image. It significantly improves the "separating capacity," or separation of anatomic structures, through the blur effect on the film.[45]

A combination of radiographic techniques would yield the maximum amount of information. When arthrograms are combined with tomographic radiography, the position of the articular disc can be determined. The literature contains much in-depth discussion of arthrography.[28,46-50]

The technique consists of infusing the lower joint compartment with a water soluble radiographic contrast medium (iodine) and recording condylar head movements during function with tomographic or transcranial films (Fig. 10-25).

Radiographic evidence of TMJ pathology

Evaluation of the fossa

Deviation from the normal size, shape, and form of the glenoid fossa can indicate pathology. Fossa size and shape partially dictate condylar function. For example, a long narrow fossa might have a "locked in" condylar head. The border or outline of the fossa should be free of bone spicules (osteophytes) and be well-defined and radiopaque. Any changes in radiopacity or indications of radiolucent or mottled areas of the fossa outline indicate evidence of osteoarthritic lesions.[51] Irregularity or departure from a smooth contoured fossa surface are visible on a transcranial radiographic projection.

Evaluation of the joint space

The joint space is evaluated with arthro-

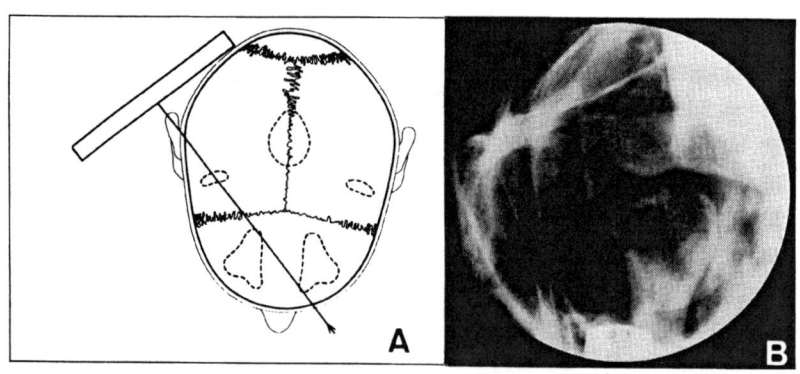

Fig. 10-29 Schematic drawing of the path of the central ray in the transmaxillary projection *(left)*. (From Omnell and Lysell.[42]) Transmaxillary projection radiograph of the right TMJ *(right)* articular tubercle is seen along with the medio-lateral plane of the condyle.

graphic techniques. Since the articular disc is radiolucent, changes in shape or location of a radiopaque medium will define disc location. The thickness and uniformity of joint space and breaks in the integrity of the upper and lower joint compartments are examined in tomographic or transcranial radiographic projections.

Evaluation of the condyle

The relative position of the condyle in the fossa is evaluated in the transcranial projection or tomogram. Anterior, superior, or posterior displacement is noted and correlated with the symptoms of the patient. The size and form of the condyle itself is studied. Irregular surface, shape (e.g., flattening or beaking), osteophytes, and necrotic areas on the condyle can all suggest osteoarthritic degeneration.

carefully listening to the patient and evaluating the signs, symptoms, and related data. The goal is to improve the condition of the patient by definitive treatment or by proper referral.

The chart (Fig. 10-31) is representative of radiographic findings of the condylar head during the three stages of change. The normal condylar head will function smoothly without noise or jerking motion. Stage I degeneration would show beginning radiographic change with a clicking noise on opening, or on opening and closing (reciprocal clicking). Stage II degeneration would show further condylar changes: lipping, osteophytes, and severe flattening of one or more condylar surfaces. A grinding noise on translation of the mandible would indicate a more severe arthritic degeneration and thinning of the neck of the condyle. A grating or cracking noise is heard on mandibular rotation and translation. Advanced degenerative arthritis is common.

Diagnosis and treatment planning

Diagnosis is accomplished after all the historical facts, radiographs, and the differential diagnostic list of problems are established. The diagnosis is defined after

Treatment modalities

Craniomandibular disorders are too complex to propose an all-encompassing treatment regime for every patient suffering from them. Too many peripheral factors affect

Diagnosis and Treatment Planning

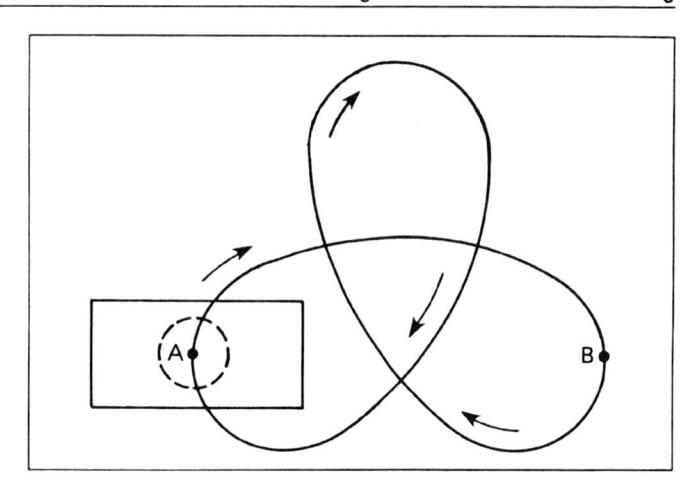

Fig. 10-30 Hypocycloidal tube path for tomographic radiography.

treatment results: some patients complain of headache and neck pain, but have no audible joint noise; others might have a distinct click, with radiographic evidence of condylar flattening, but no symptoms; still others may have pain in the joint area, but no overt pathology shown radiographically. Some of these patients may be helped with adjustment of the dental component (occlusion) with splint appliances, prosthetic replacement of missing teeth, or occlusal equilibration. Other patients may benefit from direct repositioning of the condylar head with orthopedic appliances. A small percentage of patients may need surgical intervention to restore health.

Treatment of disc displacement

Up to 80% of all TMJ problems may be associated with, or caused by, a form of intracapsular dysfunction known as internal derangement (displacement) of the articular disc.[29] It is this disc-related dysfunction that may be helped with orthopedic appliances. Early treatment is encouraged to minimize potentially more serious symptoms that can occur later if the clicking, pain, or occlusal discrepancies are left untreated. Since TMJ symptoms are cumulative and often progressively more severe as the patient matures,[38] early correction of contributory malocclusion and condylar malposition will help alleviate painful symptoms and ensure nonrecurrence.

It has been shown that young patients who develop TMJ-related symptoms often have a deep overbite malocclusion.[32,37] Opening a deep overbite is routinely accomplished with orthopedic appliances. This ability to reposition the mandible forward, stimulate condylar and posterior alveolar growth and remodeling, and open a deep overbite may be part of the reason for success in treating TMJ disorders with orthopedic appliances.

There are two additional considerations. First, as the condyle and the entire mandible are repositioned forward, the coronoid process of the mandible is also brought to a more anterior position. Altering this position of the insertion of the temporalis muscle may help to interrupt some of the painful spasms that are associated with the anterior, medial, and posterior fibers of this muscle. Interrupting the muscle spasms by placing the tendinous temporalis muscle insertion (Fig. 10-10) in a more forward and possibly more physiologically acceptable position may be part of the reason for a diminution or cessation of headache in some patients treated with orthopedic appli-

249

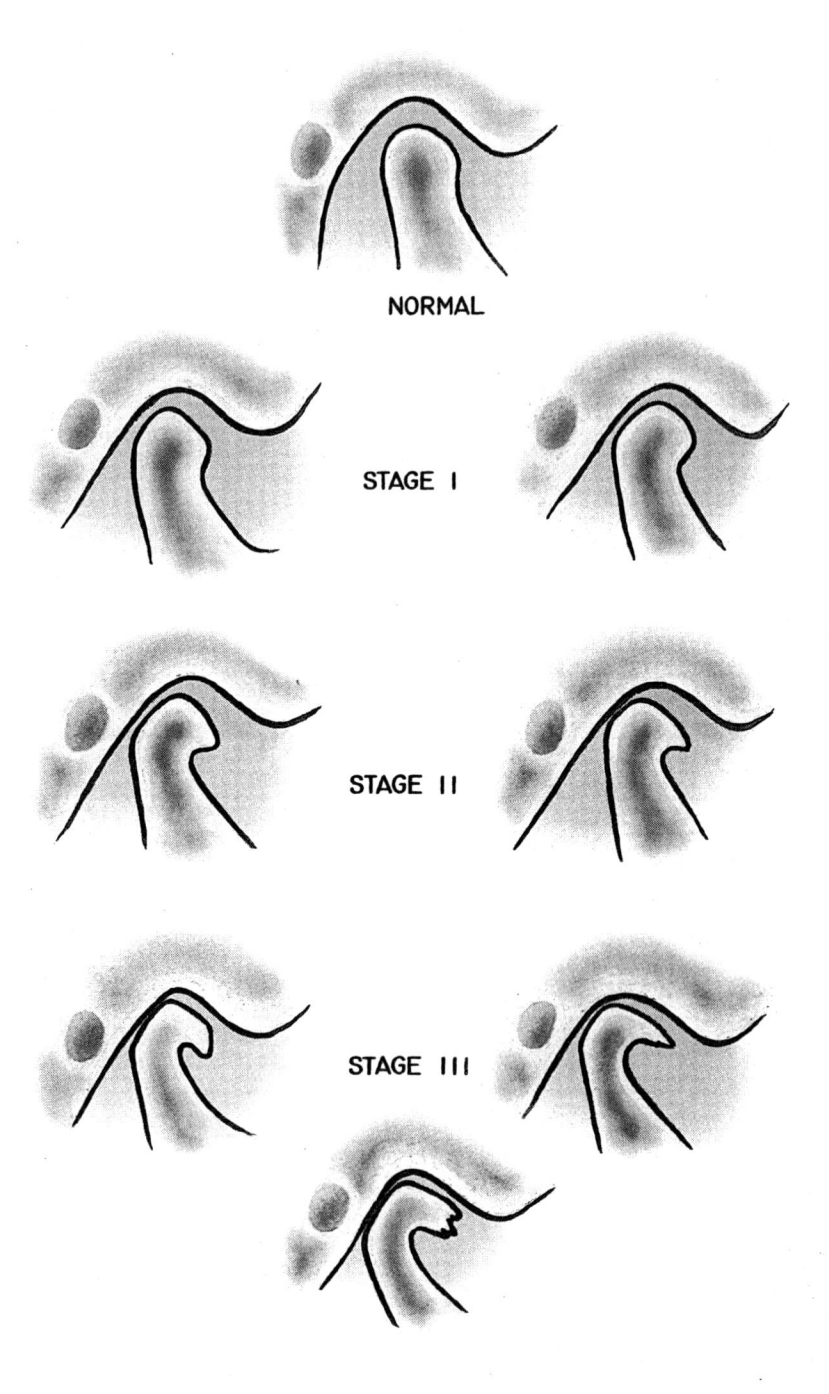

Fig. 10-31 Radiographic findings in normal and early-to-late stages of condylar abnormality associated with internal derangement within the temporomandibular joint.

ances. Facial pain may also be abated because of a more physiological position of the masseter and pterygoid muscles.

Second, and perhaps most important, orthopedic appliances that are constructed to increase the posterior vertical dimension hold the mandible in a slightly forward (protracted) and open position. This position causes an anterior and inferior relocation of the condylar head in the fossa while the appliance is in the mouth. This position of the condylar head allows the elastic fibers of the posterior disc attachment (Fig. 10-15) to retract and reposition the anteriorly dislocated articular disc to a more physiologically acceptable position between the condylar head and the articular surface of the temporal portion of the zygomatic bone.

The success of TMJ treatment with orthopedic appliances is partially age-dependent: the younger the patient, the more rapid the cure. Relief of symptoms can occur independent of age, but correction of a deep overbite or loss of vertical dimension is more time-consuming after ages 18 to 20. Wright and Moffett[52] have shown that before ages 18 to 20, cartilagenous and osseous growth of the condyle and fossa will result in permanent repositioning of the condylar head. After this age, condylar repositioning is the result of fossa and condylar remodeling.[53]

Physiologic condylar position

Careful evaluation of patient history, TMJ radiographs, joint noise, and other pertinent data may indicate mandibular (condylar) repositioning as a treatment option. The problem for the clinician is twofold: How far forward should the mandible be repositioned, and how far should it be opened?

The mandible is brought forward and opened to a position that allows opening and closing without (or with diminished) grating, popping, or clicking. This nonclick position usually indicates a more forward, inferior condylar position in the fossa. If there is very little overjet and overbite and the nonclick position is an edge-to-edge incisal occlusion, then the mandible is placed (and the appliance constructed) for this position. When the nonclick position is attained, two additional factors must be considered before taking the construction bite: the age of the patient and esthetics. With patients under 12 years, a forward position, even slightly past an edge-to-edge incisal relationship, is well-tolerated by the mandibular musculature. After age 12, more consideration should be given to muscle tolerance and esthetics. A less protrusive position is used for constructing appliances for older patients. A patient 40 or 50 years old cannot tolerate the forward muscular position that a patient under 12 years can tolerate.

The orthopedic corrector appliance (Figs. 1-10 and 10-32) is very useful for older patients with TMJ disorders. Frequently, the mandible cannot initially be repositioned forward sufficiently because of pain and inflammation in the temporomandibular joint. As the musculature becomes tolerant of the new mandibular position, the lateral screws can be opened to advance the mandible forward.

The 10 mm rule is an approximate guideline that works for most younger patients. If the mandible is brought forward 8 mm, the vertical dimension could be opened 2 mm. If the bite is to be opened 4 mm, then the mandible should be brought forward 6 mm. The anterior and vertical distances add up to a maximum of 10 mm. This general guideline is not successful for patients more than 20 to 25 years old. The sagittal and vertical repositioned distance cannot approach 10 mm in the older patient.

Taking dental impressions for appliance treatment of patients with a closed-lock condyle-disc relationship and limited opening may be difficult. The remoldable craniomandibular appliance (RCM) (Fig. 10-33) has been used successfully for patients suffering from disorders of the cranioman-

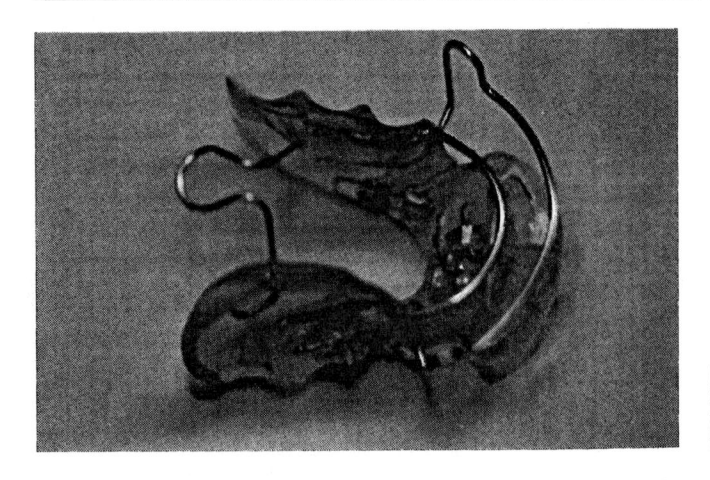

Fig. 10-32 Orthopedic corrector. Screws lateral to the premolar teeth reposition the mandible forward.

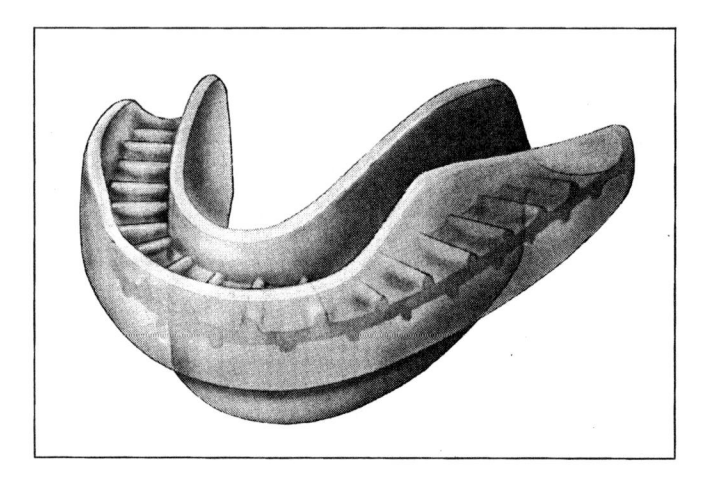

Fig. 10-33 The RCM appliance.

dibular articulation. Since the appliance is part of stock inventory, the patient receives the condylar repositioning at that visit without waiting for a laboratory fabricated device. A differential diagnosis may be hastened and radiation to the patient minimized. Boiling water is required to soften the appliance so that the patient can close into the construction bite.

Recommendations for TMJ patients

There are several suggestions that help minimize pain for TMJ patients: *(1)* do not use chewing gum, *(2)* try to minimize external stress in your life, *(3)* eat a well-balanced, nutritious diet, *(4)* get routine daily exercise, and *(5)* sleep on the back with a small pillow under the neck to let the platisma muscle hold the mandible in a slightly open position. Sleeping on the side or stomach may stimulate clenching or bruxism.

Pharmacologic considerations

There is an effort in treatment to minimize the use of pharmacologic methods of alleviating head, neck, face, and back pain that is common with TMJ patients. Several anal-

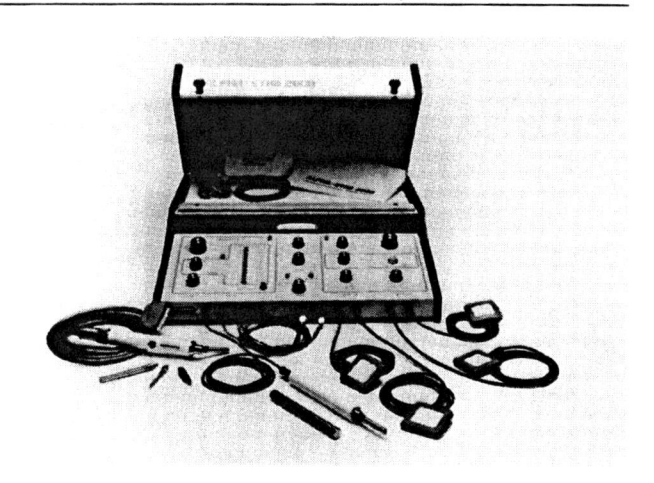

Fig. 10-34 The Alpha-Stim 2000, one type of multimodality transcutaneous electrical nerve stimulation (TENS) unit. (Courtesy of Dyna-Flex, Ltd., St. Louis, Mo.)

gesic medications have been used successfully in the beginning stages of TMJ therapy when headache has been the most common complaint.[54] It is important for long-term results to minimize and eliminate drug-related therapy as quickly as possible. Drugs only mask and do not cure TMJ-related headache. The prescribed dosage of the medication can vary widely with the weight and physical condition of the patient. Each drug dosage should be individualized according to patient response. Medical consultation will aid in a differential diagnosis.

Electrical physical therapy

Electrical physical therapy is useful for abating acute pain symptoms at the initiation of diagnostic procedures. High voltage electrogalvanic stimulation (HVGS), transcutaneous electric nerve stimulation (TENS) (Fig. 10-34), and ultrasound are the three most effective electrical physical therapy modalities.

High-voltage electrogalvanic stimulation can be used for locating and treating pain trigger points and muscle spasm and for pain reduction. The HVGS and TENS modalities submit the tissues to a flow of electrons. As the thermal and physiochemical effects of the electrons are recognized and controlled, therapeutic and diagnostic benefit may ensue.[55]

Transcutaneous electric nerve stimulation can cause acute and chronic pain reduction by two theoretic routes: short-circuiting the normal pain transmission mechanism or by the production of natural body opiates—endorphins and enkephalins.

Ultrasound utilizes the production of acoustical energy or mechanical vibration to cause a temperature increase and cavitation (vibration) of the deeper tissues. Pain relief can be accomplished by increasing the temperature, which increases the pain threshold of peripheral nerves, or by transmitting medication through the tissues (phonophoresis).

Expectations for success

Several variables will affect treatment success: correct diagnosis, patient attitude and cooperation, amount of time the appliance is worn, and appliance construction. Each variable can be controlled by either the patient or the clinician. If the diagnosis is incorrect, little positive treatment will be accomplished, pain and suffering may be prolonged, and the clinician might then be in legal jeopardy.

A positive attitude and enthusiastic clinical approach can effect patient cooperation. Good patient cooperation is needed: if the appliance is not worn, positive results are not possible. Patients less than 30 years old are encouraged to wear the appliance as much as possible. Patients over 30 are asked to wear the appliance while sleeping and as much as possible during the day. Patients older than 45 to 50 are asked to wear the appliance one hour out of six and gradually work up to half time. Good appliance construction without overextended borders or thick, bulky acrylic encourages longer wearing time.

Common sense will prevent many TMJ disorder patients from getting worse. If a patient with tenderness in the masticatory muscles requires extensive restorative treatment, treatment should begin gradually. The clinician should have a keen awareness of condylar position. A patient with pterygoid muscles that are painful to palpation should not be scheduled for a long appointment with the mandible in an open position. Akeson[23] has shown that keeping the mouth open for prolonged dental treatment can compress and damage retrocondylar tissue. After essential restorative treatment, it would be wise to ensure a functionally stable temporomandibular joint before additional restorative treatment is undertaken.

Patient histories

Specific patient histories can demonstrate the effectiveness of TMJ treatment with orthopedic appliances.

K.H., age 29 (Figs. 10-35a to h)

Chief complaint: One-sided (R) or bilateral headache almost every day for the past 18 months. Headache was noticed even on wakening in the morning.

History: Medical consultation in ophthalmology, internal medicine, and gynecology could find no organic cause for the headache. The pain had been intermittent for approximately 12 months and had been more frequent during the previous six months. There was no family history of headache.

Oral examination: The temporalis and external pterygoid muscles were sensitive to palpation on the right side. The following posterior teeth were missing: 3, 13, 14, 19, and all third molars. Mandibular movement was equal bilaterally with some TMJ clicking on opening on the right side. Overjet was 4 mm with an overbite 6.5 mm deep.

Treatment plan: A treatment regime that would minimize patient radiation exposure was instituted. Treatment included condylar and occlusal repositioning via a mandibular repositioning appliance and fixed prosthodontic replacement of missing teeth.

Treatment: A panoramic radiograph and intraoral and facial photographs were taken to document and complete the dental and TMJ examination. Transcranial films were scheduled if no relief of symptoms was noted within the first month of treatment.

Orthopedic treatment included mandibular repositioning with a bionator and orthopedic corrector appliance over an 18-month period, and fixed prosthodontic replacement of missing posterior teeth.

A diminution of headache pain was noticed by the patient within one week. Cessation of headache, including waking headache was noticed within one month. The patient also noticed an improvement in facial esthetics as documented in Figs. 10-35a to h.

Expectations for Success

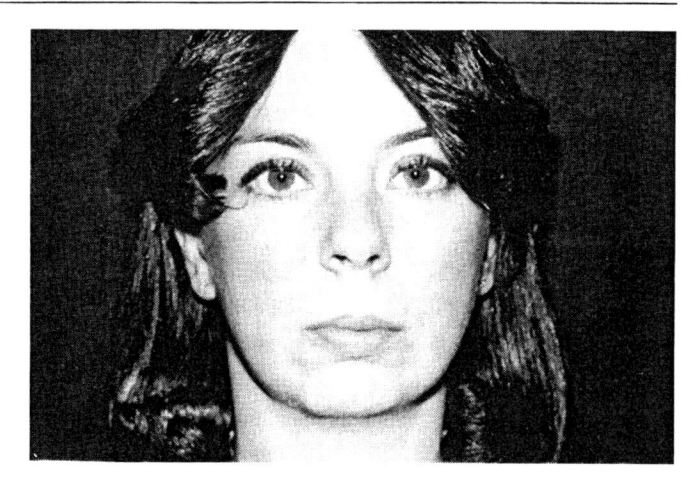

Fig. 10-35a K. H. Facial front view on the day she presented for treatment of bilateral temporomandibular joint-related headache.

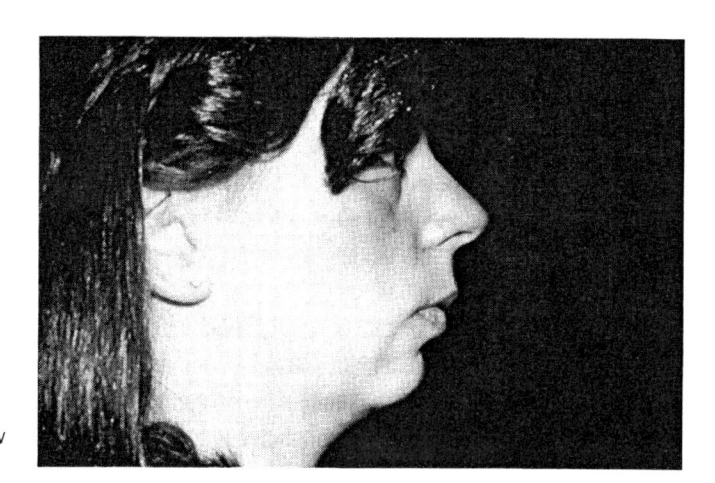

Fig. 10-35b Facial profile view at first appointment.

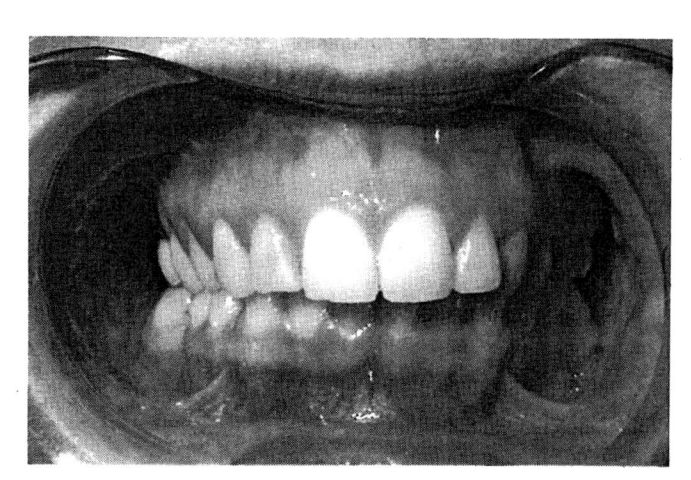

Fig. 10-35c Frontal view of occlusion showing a 6.5 mm deep overbite as K. H. presented for treatment.

Treatment of Craniomandibular Disorders With Maxillofacial Orthopedic Appliances

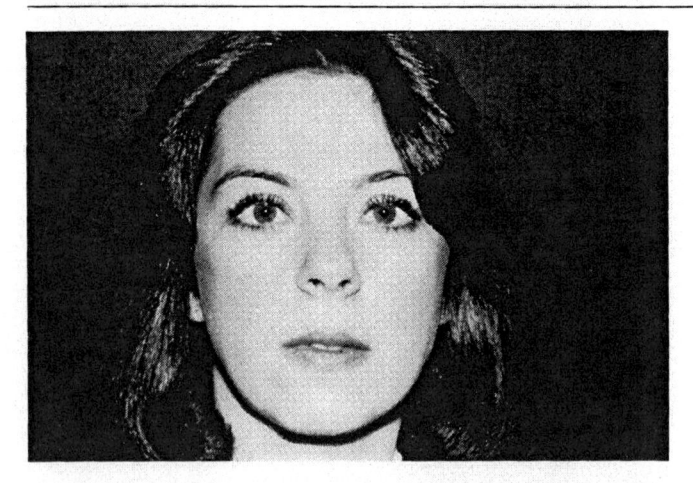

Fig. 10-35d Facial front view after 10 months of treatment with a bionator appliance. An increase in lower face height and improved facial esthetics are evident.

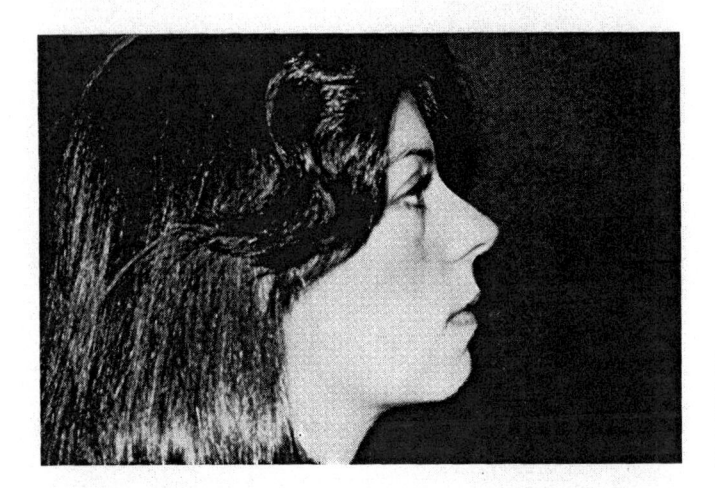

Fig. 10-35e Facial profile view after 10 months of continuous bionator treatment. Both lip and chin positions and entire facial profile have been improved.

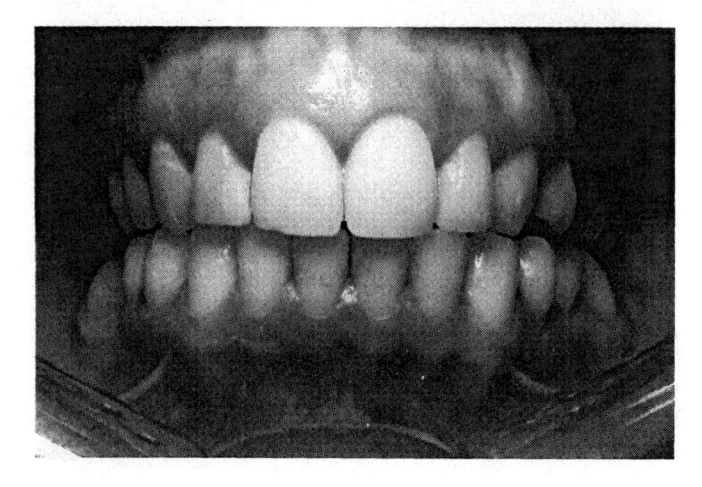

Fig. 10-35f Frontal view of occlusion after 10 months of continuous treatment with a bionator appliance. The deep overbite has been reduced.

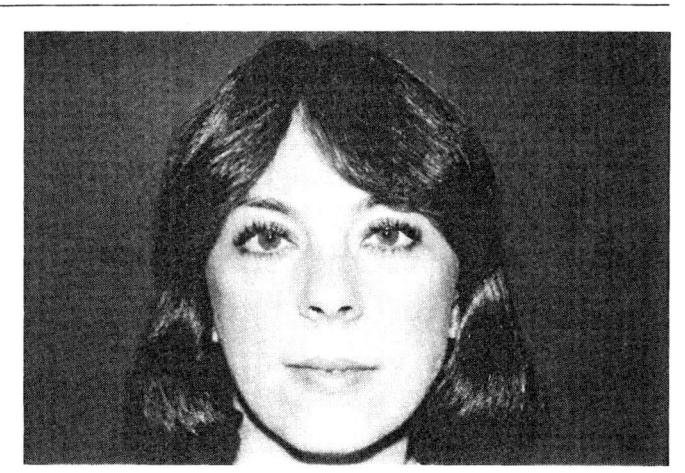

Fig. 10-35g Facial frontal view after bionator and four months of orthopedic corrector treatment.

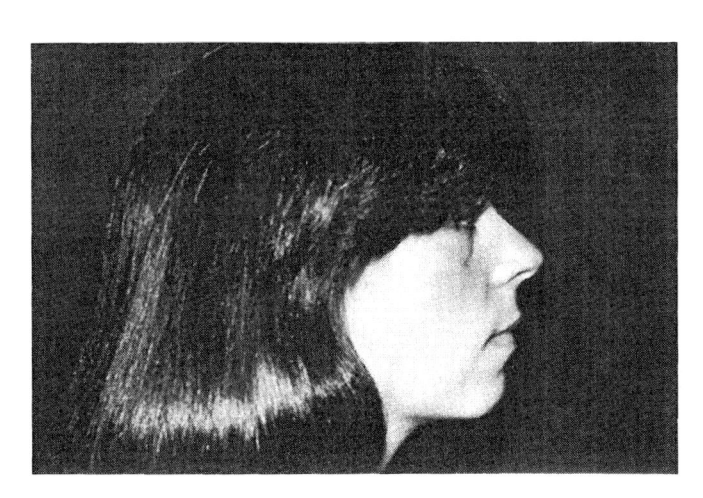

Fig. 10-35h Facial profile view after 14 months of treatment, comprised of 10 months of bionator therapy and four months of orthopedic corrector treatment. Mandible could not be forced distally. Patient referred for fixed prosthetic treatment.

R.G., age 53 (Figs. 10-36a to g)

Chief complaint: Facial pain, inability to chew solid food, inability to swallow food without difficulty, and limited mouth opening.

History: This patient had previously been treated for extensive fixed prosthodontic restoration of the posterior occlusion. The onset of symptoms began after prolonged mouth opening for endodontic and prosthodontic treatment. The symptoms became so severe that multiple dental, medical, and legal consultations were sought. Nutritional deficiency was complicating the clinical symptoms. Multiple TMJ splints had been fabricated for the patient and several series of TMJ and dental radiographs had been taken.

Oral examination: The temporalis, external and internal pterygoid, and masseter muscles were painful to palpation bilaterally; tooth #31 and all third molars were missing. Lateral mandibular movements were restricted, as was mouth opening. Crepitus and grating were present bilaterally. Overjet was 5 mm with an overbite 6 mm deep.

Treatment plan: A treatment goal that would restore condylar and disc position

Treatment of Craniomandibular Disorders With Maxillofacial Orthopedic Appliances

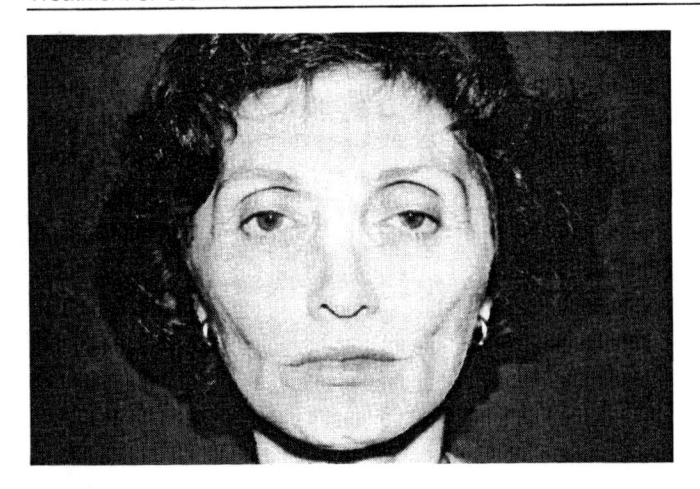

Fig. 10-36a R. G. Facial front view on day she presented for treatment of TMJ disorder with limited bite opening. Patient could eat only pureed food.

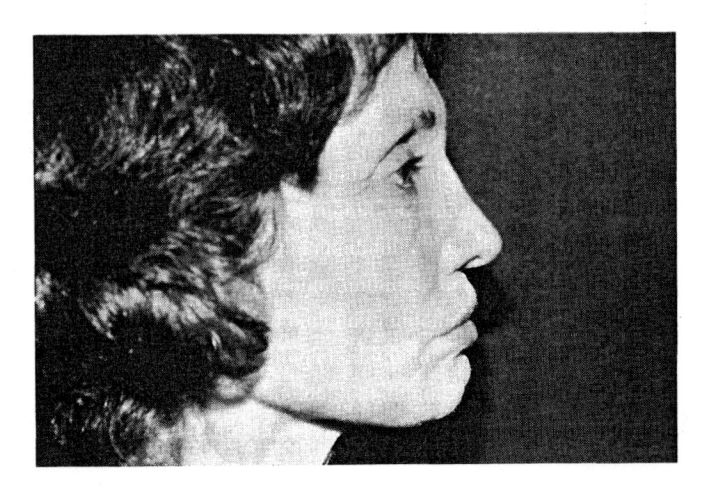

Fig. 10-36b Facial profile view at first appointment.

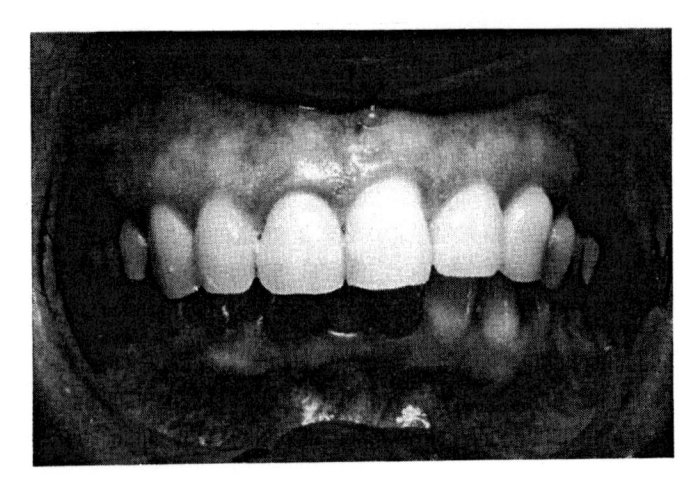

Fig. 10-36c Frontal view of occlusion showing a 6 mm deep overbite as R. G. presented for treatment.

Expectations for Success

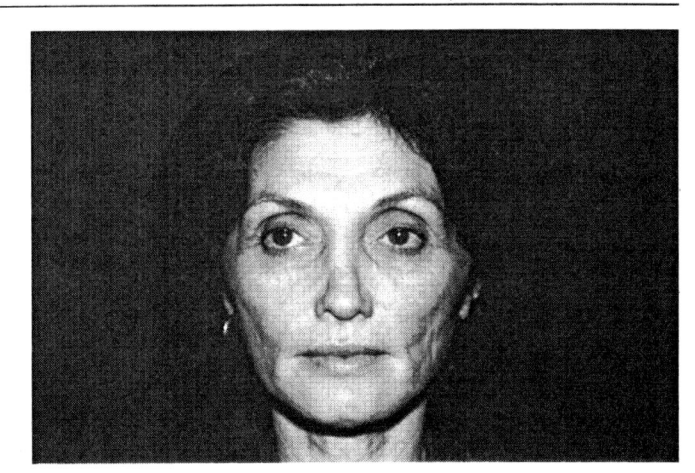

Fig. 10-36d Facial front view after 10 months of treatment with a bionator appliance.

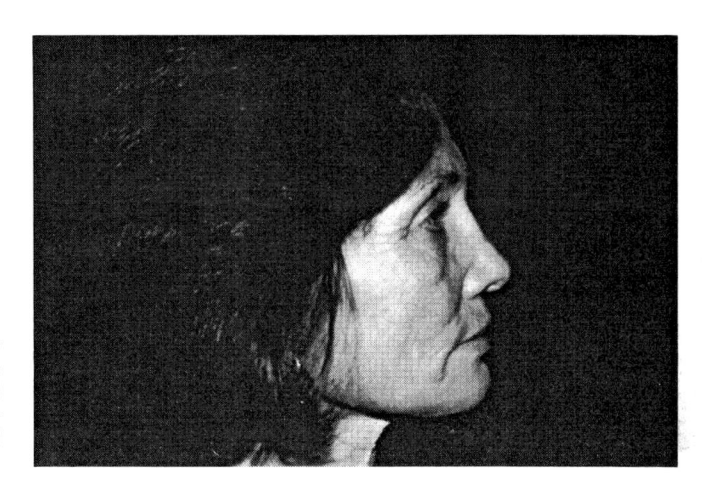

Fig. 10-36e Facial profile view after 10 months of bionator treatment. Both the lip and the facial profiles have been improved. Patient is able to eat semisolid food.

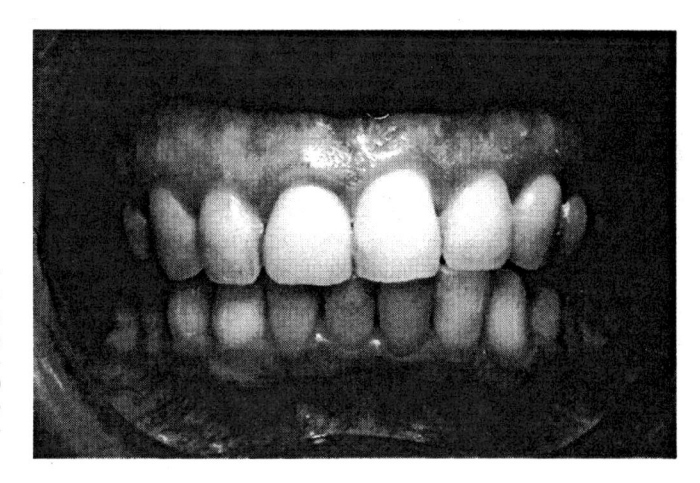

Fig. 10-36f Frontal view of occlusion after 10 months of bionator treatment. The deep overbite has been reduced. Care must be taken when making the construction bite. Patients more than 40 years old should not have the mandible repositioned too far forward.

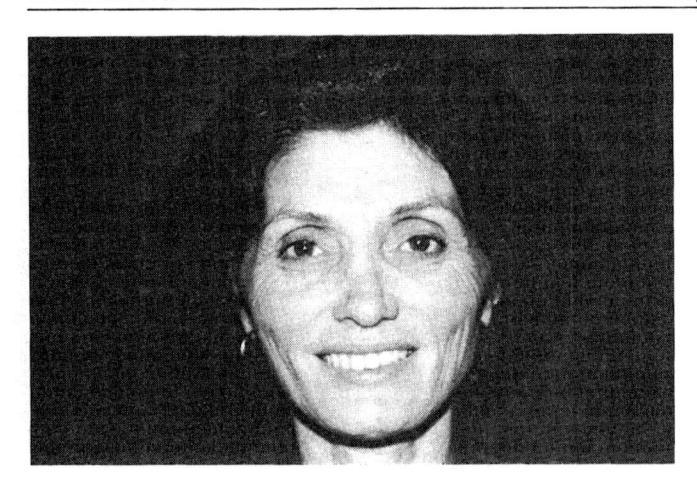

Fig. 10-36g Full smile and improved facial features.

was suggested for this patient. Further dental treatment was not recommended until restoration of normal TMJ function. Nutritional supplementation was recommended in order to restore any deficiency that may have resulted from the inability to eat solid food. Condylar repositioning was required in order to let the elastic fibers of the posterior disc attachment reapproximate the disc from an anteriorly dislocated position to a position between the articulating surfaces of the condylar head and the articular surfaces of the zygomatic portion of the temporal bone.

Treatment: Previously exposed recent radiographs along with intraoral and facial photographs were used to complete the documentation of the oral and TMJ examination.

Orthopedic treatment with a bionator appliance to reposition the mandible forward was used for one hour out of six during the day and continuously while sleeping. A mandibular splint was worn the remaining time and during meals. Physical therapy was instituted to help reduce the amount of time needed for bionator treatment, and to restore full mandibular movement.

A diminution of facial pain and an improvement in facial esthetics were noticed within 30 days. The ability to chew solid food had not improved significantly until after six months of treatment. Esthetic improvement is documented in Figs. 36a to g.

Anatomical considerations

Surgical intervention may be unavoidable if the patient has had a rupture of the capsule, a torn posterior disc attachment, or a degenerative articular surface of the condyle with osteophyte formation or anterior lipping.[56]

McNamara et al.[57] have found limited histologic evidence of condylar and fossa tissue response to orthopedic repositioning in young adult animals. Although this study demonstrates some adaptive capability of the young adult TMJ, the amount of tissue response is limited and variable.

Schneiderman and Carlson[58] have shown, in a cephalometric study of adult female monkeys, that a bite opening device resulted in the deposition of an average of 1.5 mm of new bone along the posterosuperior aspect of the condyle after 48 weeks of appliance usage.

The potential for adaptive growth in the temporomandibular joint of young adult and adult patients should not be ignored. Although the primary occlusal changes in adults treated with maxillofacial orthopedic technique are from dentoalveolar and muscle adaptation to a new, more physiologically acceptable anatomical position, the potential for positive clinical results requires consideration, examination, and trial before a surgical procedure is suggested. Gelb and Bernstein[59] point out that although many TMJ problems are associated with a loss of posterior vertical dimension, a more likely explanation may be unrealized vertical dimension. Woodside et al.[60] have shown extensive condylar remodeling and change in mandibular size using occlusal altering appliances in monkeys. Their experiments clearly demonstrate that changing the muscle activity will affect bone morphology.

TMJ litigation

The plethora of lawsuits arising from people with TMJ disorders underscores the need for careful evaluation of all patients. Careful record gathering, treatment planning, and a conservative regime of treatment are directed toward optimal results. Patient expectations should be kept within realistic goals.

Why are there so many lawsuits? The primary reason is misdiagnosis or no diagnosis of preexisting TMJ disorder. The clinician may begin restorative, prosthetic, or orthodontic treatment on an apparently healthy individual, when suddenly the patient complains of pain in the temporomandibular joint area, temporalis muscle, neck, back, or ear. The propensity for TMJ disorder should have been well-established before dental treatment was initiated.

If the history does not include questions about TMJ pain or clicking noise and the clinical examination does not include palpation of the masticatory musculature, then the clinician is leaving the door to legal recourse wide open.[61]

Summary

A thorough examination for possible TMJ disorder will ensure optimal treatment for the patient. A painful response to palpation of the musculature can define an area of spasm and poor circulation. Muscle examination (palpation) and an awareness of correct structural symmetry and condylar position aid in treatment planning. Maxillofacial orthopedic appliance technique can aid in correcting the position of superiorly and distally displaced condyles and can prevent and facilitate treatment of temporomandibular joint capsular disorder.

The human organism is designed to heal itself. Treatment should be directed toward nutritionally, emotionally, and therapeutically attaining maximum health with minimal pharmacological or splint support.

References

1. Richards, L. C., and Brown, T. Dental attrition and degenerative arthritis of the temporomandibular joint. J. Oral Rehabil. 8:293–307, 1981.
2. Funt, L. A. A new approach to chronic headache. The female patient. Vol. 5, no. 5, 1980.
3. Adler, A. Problems of neurosis. New York: Harper Torchbooks, 1964.
4. Rocabado, M. Biomechanical relationship of the cranial, cervical, and hyoid regions. J. Craniomandib. Prac. 1 (3):61–66, 1983.
5. Funakoshi, M., Fujita, N., and Takehana, S. Relations between occlusal interference and jaw muscle activities in response to changes in head position. J. Dent. Res. 55:684–690, 1976.
6. Schwartz, L. Disorders of the Temporomandibular Joint. Philadelphia: W. B. Saunders Co., 1966.

7. Lockhart, R. D., Hamilton, G. F., and Fyfe, F. W. Anatomy of the Human Body. Philadelphia: Lippincott, 1965.
8. Gelb, H. (ed.) Clinical Management of Head, Neck and TMJ Pain and Dysfunction. Philadelphia: W. B. Saunders Co., 1977.
9. Cohen, L. A. Role of eye and neck propioceptive mechanisms in body orientation and motor coordination. J. Neurophysiol. 24:1–11, 1961.
10. Wyke, B. Neurology of the cervical spinal joints. Physiotherapy 65:72–76, 1979.
11. Mahan, P. E. The temporomandibular joint in function and pathofunction. In W. K. Solberg, and G. T. Clark (eds.) Temporomandibular Joint Problems. Chicago: Quintessence Publ. Co., 1980.
12. Standlee, J. P., Caputo, A. A., and Ralph, J. P. The condyle as a stress-distributing component of the temporomandibular joint. J. Oral Rehabil. 8:391–400, 1981.
13. Kreutziger, K. L., and Mahan, P. E. Temporomandibular degenerative joint disease, part II: diagnostic procedure and comprehensive management. J. Oral Surg. 40:297–319, 1975.
14. Griffin, C. J., and Sharpe, C. J. The structure of the adult human temporomandibular meniscus. Aust. Dent. J. 5:190–195, 1960.
15. McNamara, J. A., Jr. The independent functions of the two heads of the lateral pterygoid muscle. Am. J. Anat. 138:197–205, 1973.
16. Lipke, D. P., et al. An electromyographic study of the human lateral pterygoid muscle. J. Dent. Res. 56(Special Issue B): B230, (abstr. no. 713), 1977.
17. Thilander, B. Innervation of the temporomandibular joint capsule in man. Trans. R. Sch. Stoch. Umea No. 7:1, 1961
18. Ham, A. W., and Cormack, D. H. Histology. 8th ed. Philadelphia: Lippincott, 1979.
19. Silberberg, R., Silberberg, M., and Feir, D. Life cycle of articular cartilage cells: an electron microscope study of the hip joint of the mouse. Am. J. Anat. 114:17, 1964.
20. Bell, W. E. Understanding temporomandibular biomechanics. J. Craniomandib. Prac. 1(2):27–33, 1983.
21. Akeson, W. H., Amiel, D., and Woo, S. L-Y. Immobility effects of synovial joints. The pathomechanics of joint contracture. Biorheol. 17:95–110, 1980.
22. Swann, D. A., et al. Role of hyaluronic acid in joint lubrication. Ann. Rheum. Dis. 33:318–326, 1974.
23. Akeson, W. Collagen crosslinking alterations in joint contractures: changes in the reducible crosslinks in periarticular connective tissue collagen after nine weeks of immobilization. Connect. Tissue Res. 5:15–19, 1977.
24. Bauer, W., Ropes, M. W., and Waine, H. The physiology of articular structure. Physiol. Rev. 20:272–312, 1940.
25. Meyer, K., Smith, E. M., and Dawson, M. H. The nature of the mucopolysaccharide of synovial fluid. Science 88:129, 1938.
26. Toller, P. A. Opaque arthrography of the temporomandibular joint. Int. J. Oral Surg. 3:17–28, 1974.
27. Salter, R. B., and Field, P. The effects of continuous compression on living articular cartilage. J. Bone Joint Surg. 42-A:31–49, 76, 90, 1960.
28. Farrar, W. B., and McCarty, W. L., Jr. Outline of temporomandibular joint diagnosis and treatment. The Normandie Study Group, Montgomery, Alabama, Feb. 1980.
29. McCarty, W. L., Jr. Diagnosis and treatment of internal derangements of the articular disc and mandibular condyle. In W. K. Solberg and G. T. Clark (eds.) Temporomandibular Joint Problems. Chicago: Quintessence Publ. Co., 1980.
30. Solberg, W. K., Woo, M. W., and Houston, J. B. Prevalence of mandibular dysfunction in young adults. J. Am. Dent. Assoc. 98:25–34, 1979.
31. Agerberg, G., and Carlsson, G. E. Functional disorders of the masticatory system. Acta Odontol. Scand. 30:597–613, 1972.
32. Williamson, E. H. Temporomandibular dysfunction in pretreatment adolescent patients. Am. J. Orthod. 72:429–433, 1977.
33. Moyers, R. E. An electromyographic analysis of certain muscles involved in temporomandibular movement. Am. J. Orthod. 36:481–515, 1950.
34. Woelfel, J. B., Hickey, J. C., and Rinear, L. L. Electromyographic evidence supporting the mandibular hinge axis theory. J. Prosthet. Dent. 7:361–367, 1957.
35. Moller, E. The chewing apparatus: an electromyographic study of the action of the muscles of mastication and its correlation to facial morphology. Acta Physiol. Scand. 69(suppl. 280):216, 1966.
36. McNamara, J. A., Jr. Neuromuscular and Skeletal Adaptations to Altered Orofacial Function. Monogr. no. 1, Craniofacial Growth Series. Ann Arbor: Center for Human Growth and Development, Univ. of Michigan, 1972.
37. Ahlin, J. H., and Ramos-Gómez, F. J. Treatment of temporomandibular joint-related headaches in the pedodontic patient: a preliminary report. J. Pedod. 6:164–175, 1982.
38. Stack, B. C., and Funt, L. A. Temporomandibular joint dysfunctions in children. J. Pedod. 1:240–247, 1977.
39. Oberg, T. Radiology of the temporomandibular joint. In W. K. Solberg and G. T. Clark (eds.) Temporomandibular Joint Problems. Chicago: Quintessence Publ. Co., 1980.
40. Valachovic, R. W., and Lurie, A. G. Risk-benefit considerations in pedodontic radiology. Pediatr. Dent. 2:128–146, 1980.
41. Lurie, A. G., and Brandt, S. Risk-benefit considerations in orthodontic radiology. J. Clin. Orthod. 15:469–475, 478–484, 1981.
42. Omnell, K. A., and Lysell, L. Rontgendianostik. In W. Krogh-Poulsen and O. Carlsen (eds.) Bidfunktion/Bettysiologi II. Copenhagen: Mundsgaard, 1974.
43. Petersson, A. Radiography of the temporomandibular joint: a comparison of information obtained from different radiographic techniques. Thesis,

References

University of Lund, Malmö, Sweden, 1976.
44. Faivovich, G., and Omnell, K. A. Axial tomography of the temporomandibular joint using hypocycloidal movement of the tube and film. Dentomaxillofac. Radiol. 6:7–16, 1977.
45. Rosenberg, H. M., and Silha, R. E. TMJ radiology with emphasis on tomography. Dent. Radiog. Photog. 55:1–24, 1982.
46. Wilkes, C. H. Structural and functional alterations of the temporomandibular joint. Northwest Dent. 57:287–294, 1978.
47. Wilkes, C. H. Arthrography of the temporomandibular joint. Minn. Med. 61:645–652, 1978.
48. Norgaard, F. Arthrography of the mandibular joint. Acta Radiol. 25:679–685, 1944.
49. Agerberg, G., and Lundberg, M. Changes in the temporomandibular joint after surgical treatment. Oral Surg. 32:865–875, 1971.
50. Toller, P. A. Opaque arthrography of the temporomandibular joint. Int. J. Oral Surg. 3:17–28, 1974.
51. Worth, H. M. Radiology of the temporomandibular joint. *In* G. A. Zarb and G. E. Carlsson (eds.) Temporomandibular Joint Function and Dysfunction. St. Louis: The C. V. Mosby Co., 1979.
52. Wright, D. M., and Moffett, B. C., Jr. The postnatal development of the human temporomandibular joint. Am. J. Anat. 141:235–249, 1974.
53. Moffett, B. C., Jr., Johnson, L. C., McCabe, J. B., and Askew, H. C. Articular remodeling in the adult human temporomandibular joint. Am. J. Anat. 115:119–142, 1964.
54. Barrett-Griesemer, P., Meisel, S., and Rate, R. A guide to headaches and how to relieve their pain. Nursing 11:50–57, 1981.
55. Murphy, G. J. Electrical physical therapy in treating TMJ patients. J. Craniomandib. Prac. 1(2):67–73, 1983.
56. Kreutziger, K. L. Microsurgical approach to the temporomandibular joint: a new horizon. Arch. Otolaryngol. 108:422–428, 1982.
57. McNamara, J. A., Jr., Hinton, R. J., and Hoffman, D. L. Histologic analysis of temporomandibular joint adaptation to protrusive function in young adult rhesus monkeys. Am. J. Orthod. 82:288–298, 1982.
58. Schneiderman, E. D., and Carlson, D. S. Growth and remodeling of the mandible following alteration of function in adult rhesus monkeys (abstr.). Am. J. Phys. Anthropol. 54:275, 1981.
59. Gelb, H., and Bernstein, I. Clinical evaluation of two hundred patients with temporomandibular joint syndrome. J. Prosthet. Dent. 49:234–243, 1983.
60. Woodside, D. G., et al. Primate experiments in malocclusion and bone induction. Am. J. Orthod. 83:460–468, 1983.
61. Leib, M. A cloud—larger than a man's hand. Int. J. Orthod. 18:17–19, 1980.

Part 4

Special Considerations

Chapter 11

Extraction for Treatment of Malocclusion

Removal of primary and permanent teeth has long been an accepted method of improving malocclusion. The two basic questions confronted by the clinician are: which teeth to extract, and at what stage of the patient's development to extract them. Most extractions to improve malocclusion are initiated because of dental crowding. Occasionally, teeth will be removed because of overdevelopment of the maxilla[1] or mandible.[2]

Extraction of primary teeth for treatment of malocclusion

In the primary dentition, overretained and ankylosed teeth are frequently removed to stimulate or allow the proper eruption of the succedaneous permanent teeth. Overretained teeth can cause buccal, lingual, or delayed eruption of the permanent successor (Fig. 11-1). If overretention of a primary tooth is causing a deflection of the normal eruption of the permanent tooth, extraction is indicated (Fig. 11-2). If an ankylosed primary tooth has not become mobile within six to 12 months of normal exfoliation, or if there is abnormal primary root resorption, then extraction is indicated as long as there is radiographic evidence of a succeeding permanent tooth (Fig. 11-3).

Occasionally, primary teeth are extracted because of crowding. Primary canines are sometimes extracted when the four permanent incisors erupt in a crowded condition (Figs. 11-4a to c). Primary canines and primary first molars are extracted in crowded dental conditions, often at the beginning of serial extraction treatment.[3] Most serial extraction should be discouraged.[4] Mandibular permanent canines can be blocked out by the ill-planned removal of a primary cuspid.[5] Helm and Siersback-Nielsen[6] have found that crowding was most common after early loss of the maxillary primary canine. In this study, the early loss of primary teeth increased the risk of dental crowding. The possible surgical trauma to the young patient does not justify the short-term uncrowding that may result. There are two possible exceptions:

1. Premature unilateral exfoliation of a primary canine, with a resulting midline drift to the affected side. Extraction of the contralateral primary canine may help to spontaneously reapproximate the dental midlines. The extraction, however, would mean certain further loss of arch circumference.

2. Dental crowding so severe that a lateral incisor is prevented from erupting or that periodontal pathology (gingival stripping) of the erupted incisors is occurring. The danger here is that, without proper space maintenance, the extrac-

Extraction for Treatment of Malocclusion

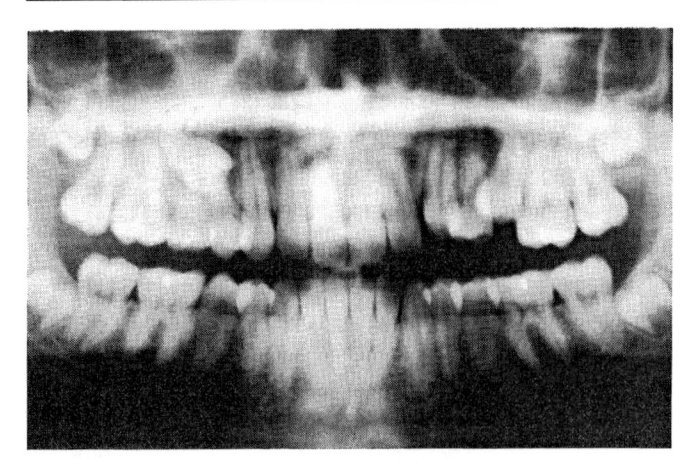

Fig. 11-1 Dilaceration and lingual eruption of the maxillary second premolars in a 15-year-old female. Primary teeth should be removed within 12 to 18 months of normal exfoliation if there is radiographic evidence of a succeeding permanent tooth with more than two-thirds of the root formed.

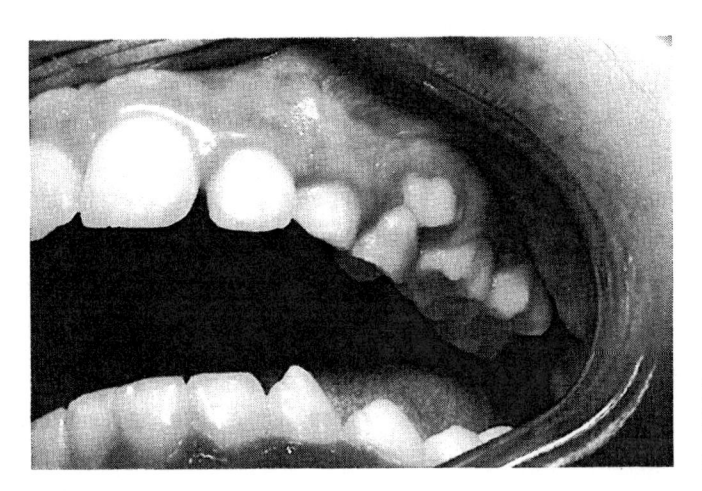

Fig. 11-2 Clinical evidence of overretention of a primary tooth. The primary tooth is removed to allow a normal path of eruption.

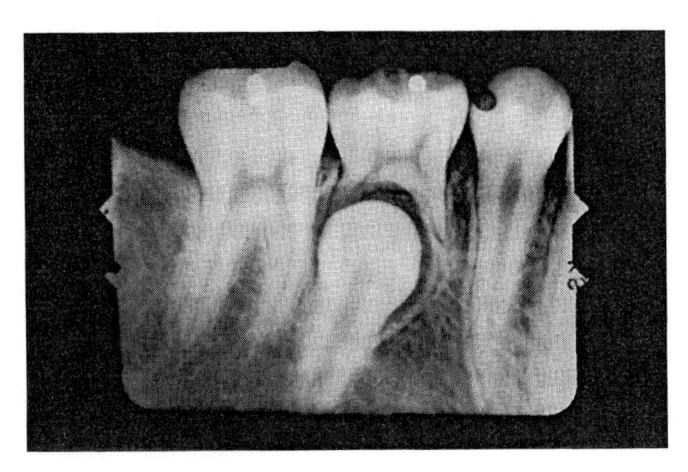

Fig. 11-3 The contralateral second primary molar was lost 12 months ago. The second molars have been removed in order to facilitate treatment of anterior crowding. This overretained second primary molar should also be removed.

Extraction of Primary Teeth for Treatment of Malocclusion

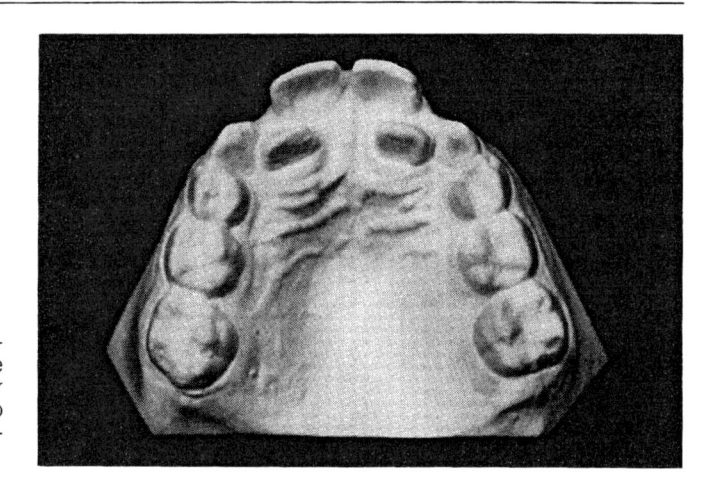

Fig. 11-4a The maxillary permanent lateral incisors have been crowded out of the proper arch contour. The temptation to remove the maxillary primary canines should be avoided.

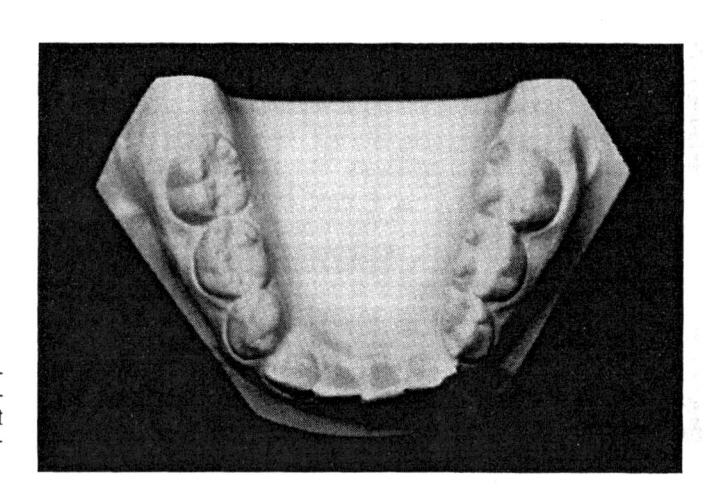

Fig. 11-4b The mandibular primary canines were removed, resulting in acceptable alignment of the mandibular central and lateral incisors.

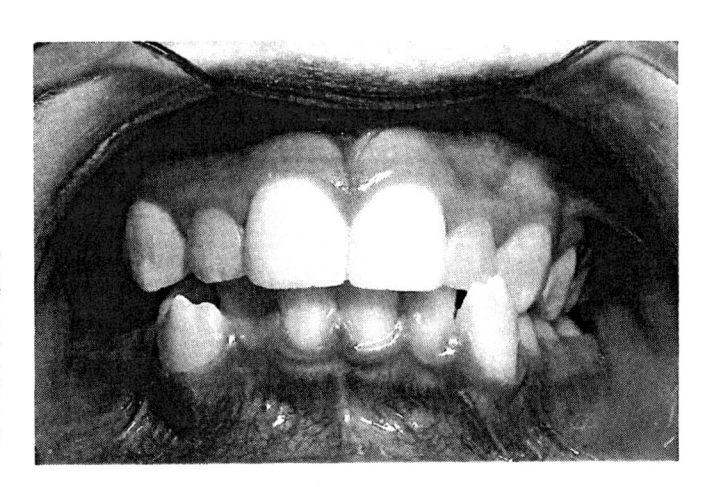

Fig. 11-4c The approach to correcting dental alignment was shortsighted, resulting in loss of arch length and buccal eruption of the mandibular permanent canines. A maxillary sagittal appliance aided in the correction of the maxillary crowding. This patient is congenitally missing the third molars.

Extraction for Treatment of Malocclusion

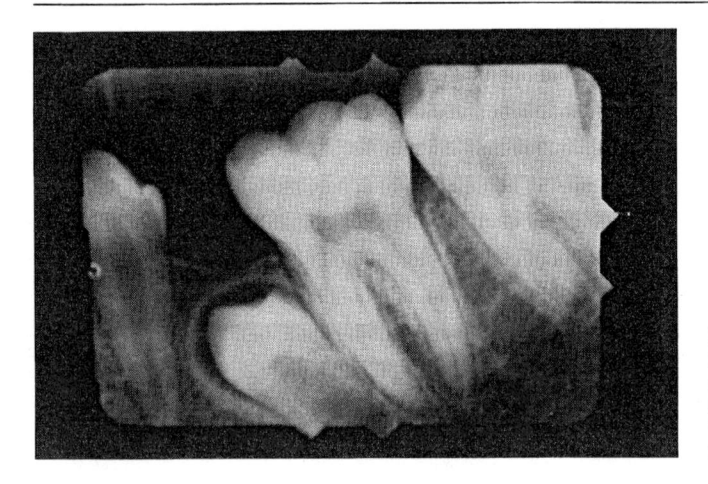

Fig. 11-5 Early loss of the second primary molar has resulted in space loss and bone formation over the second premolar; root formation has also been arrested.

tion of the primary canines would encourage further distolingual repositioning of the incisors and might exacerbate the periodontal problem. Space maintenance and interdental stripping should be accomplished before dental extraction is attempted.

Atkinson[7] encourages early evaluation and treatment planning because of untoward sequelae that consistently occur when primary mandibular canines are prematurely removed:

1. lingual and distal migration of mandibular incisors
2. loss of vertical dimension
3. an increase in the horizontal overjet
4. an increase in the facial convexity

The damage resulting from unwarranted primary canine extraction to the facial-skeletal profile will only compound the problem of dental crowding. The resulting loss of arch length can deepen the bite and may adversely affect the temporomandibular joint articulation. Extraction of primary canines is not usually beneficial to the overall dental health of the patient and is to be discouraged.

Consideration should always be given to the effect any extraction may have on alveolar bone formation or resorption and to its effect on the development of the neuromuscular component. Premature extraction of a primary tooth may cause delayed eruption of the permanent succeeding tooth. Bone may reform and gingival tissue may become fibrotic over the permanent tooth and inhibit normal eruption (Fig. 11-5). Extraction of the primary tooth close to the time of its normal exfoliation will cause an earlier eruption of the permanent tooth because of the opening of the gubernaculum canal.

Primary tooth extraction may be indicated when there is a lack of development or a congenitally missing permanent incisor or premolar. Consideration must be given to esthetic results and the developing bilateral tooth position. Extraction of any primary tooth should not be carried out if the buccal and lingual segments of bone will be severely compressed after extraction. Tooth movement is more difficult if it must take place through a compressed, more dense alveolar bone.

Extraction of permanent teeth for treatment of malocclusion

An ideal occlusion would include all the permanent teeth in a physiologically well-balanced relationship that enhanced facial esthetics and provided stability in the temporomandibular joint. Incidence of dental crowding renders ideal occlusion a rare phenomenon.

Two methods of treatment for dental crowding are expansion and extraction. Expansion in the lateral and/or sagittal direction can benefit a crowded dental condition. Severe crowding in which one or more teeth per quadrant is forced out of the normal arch contour may require removal of tooth structure to achieve a physiologically balanced and uncrowded occlusion. Extraction of any tooth from the permanent or primary dentition requires careful evaluation of the diagnostic data. The decision for tooth removal based on a desire to use a particular appliance system can no longer be tolerated. Integrity of the temporomandibular joint and facial esthetics are more important than dental alignment.

Premolar extraction

Premolar teeth are the most often-extracted permanent teeth for correction of malocclusion. The position of the first premolar in the arch and in the eruption sequence makes it a convenient candidate for extraction. In addition, anterior crowding and blocked-out canines can often be corrected quickly when the tooth just distal to the crowded or blocked-out canine is removed (Figs. 11-6a to c). The planned (serial) extraction of crowded primary canines, primary first molars, and permanent premolars has been a popular and effective method of minimizing appliance usage and shortening active treatment time. It has been shown[8,9] that the advantages of this technique often are outweighed by the potentially deleterious effect that a reduction in tooth structure may have on the stability of facial esthetics, occlusion, periodontium, and stability of the condylar relationship to the disc and fossa in the temporomandibular joint.

Effects of premolar extraction on facial esthetics

Disadvantages of premolar extraction include the effect that the loss of premolars has on facial esthetics. Facial form, fullness, and profile are dependent on the integrity of the facial musculature and underlying dental structural component. When the dental component is reduced through extraction of premolars, subsequent osseous resorption and reduction of arch fullness can affect facial form and profile. Mechanical distalization of the arch with headgear treatment can exacerbate a lack of facial fullness. Patients that have undergone premolar extraction and headgear treatment often complain of a "dished-in" facial appearance. The nose and chin of the patient are in the correct anatomical position but look prominent because of the distalization of the dental component. Loss of vertical dimension is common after premolar extraction.[8,9] This loss of lower facial height coupled with a "dished-in" facial appearance can be disconcerting for the patient and is to be avoided (Figs. 11-7a and b).

Effects of premolar extraction on occlusion

A frequent effect of first premolar extraction on the occlusal component is an open contact area between the canine and second premolar teeth.[10] Spacing in the arch can lead to instability of the dental component and food impaction areas between the teeth (Fig. 11-7b). Premolar extraction can also result in tipping of adjacent teeth and a lingual tipping of the lower incisor teeth. The lower lip tends to fall back on the lingually inclined incisors and to emphasize a

Extraction for Treatment of Malocclusion

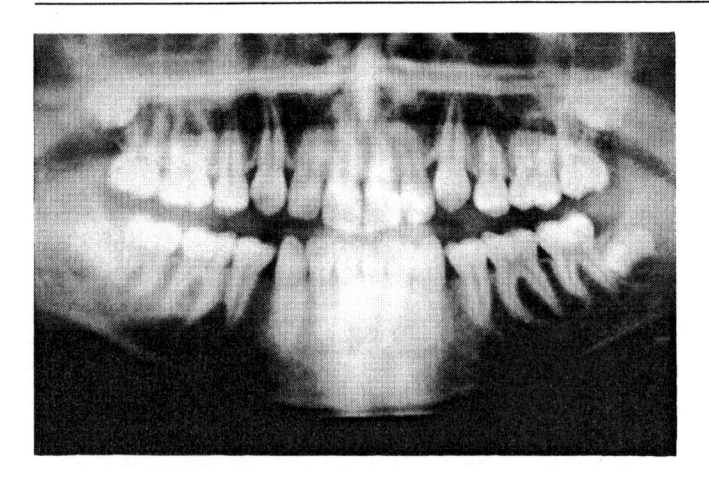

Figs. 11-6a to c Patient D. K. three years posttreatment.

Fig. 11-6a Unacceptable root parallelism and fair crown contact areas with a four-premolar extraction technique. Third molars may yet have to be extracted.

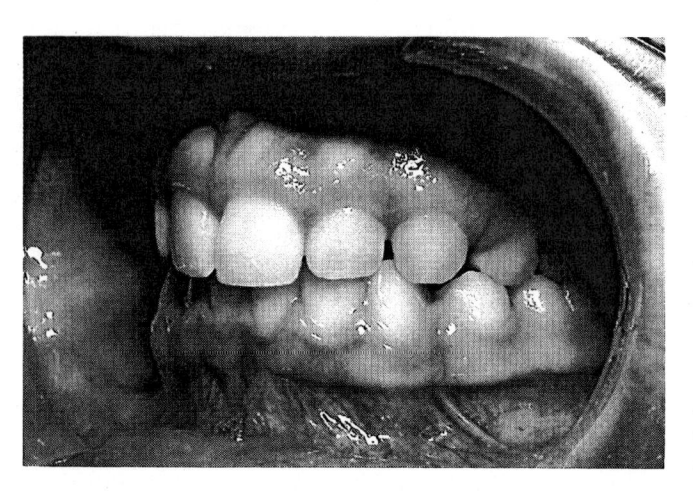

Fig. 11-6b Unacceptable dental results with fair canine position. Overjet and overbite show some relapse.

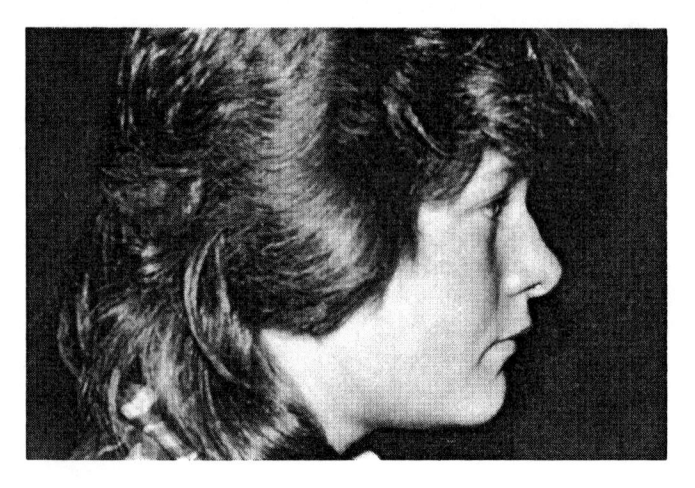

Fig. 11-6c Acceptable facial contour, although a more forward chin position may be desirable. Head posture is somewhat forward of a correct anatomical position. Slight clicking is evident bilaterally in the temporomandibular joint.

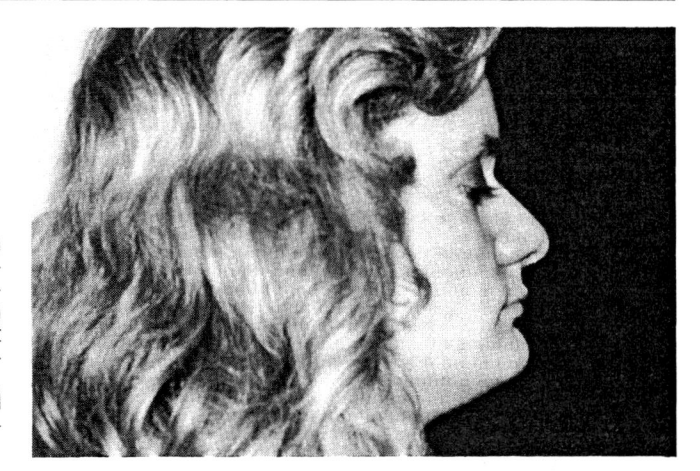

Fig. 11-7a Twenty-five-year-old patient as she presented at an oral diagnosis clinic. Chief complaint: bilateral temporalis muscle headaches so severe that on several occasions she could not work. This patient wore fixed appliances from ages 8 to 18 years. Loss of vertical dimension and dished-in facial contour are evident.

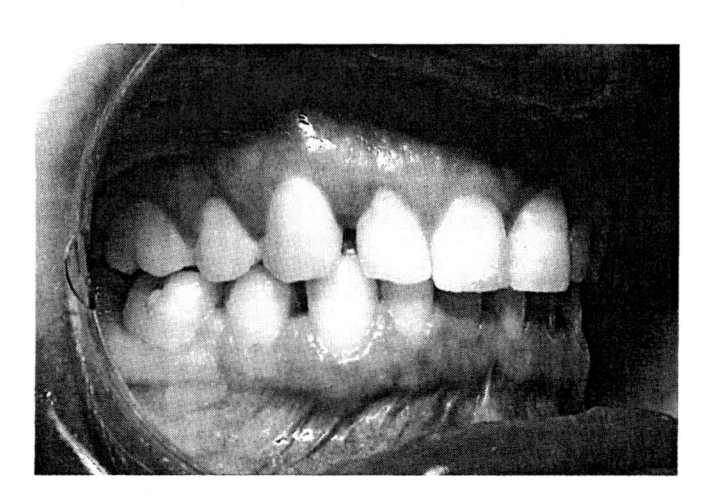

Fig. 11-7b The dental result is also unacceptable. Interdental spacing with complete lack of crown contact is evident. The deep bite is excessive.

concave facial profile (Figs. 11-8a and b). Extraction of premolar teeth and the resulting loss of osseous alveolar tissue can lead to underdevelopment of the arch or segment.[1,2] The lack of full development of the dental arch can result in molar, premolar, canine, or incisor crossbite or ectopic eruption.

Wilkinson[10] suggests that advocates of premolar extraction might not utilize the technique so frequently after a review of cases completed five to 10 years out of retention. Little et al.,[11] in a study of 65 patients treated with first premolar extraction, found long-term alignment to be "variable and unpredictable" with this technique. The authors found a *decrease* in length and width of arch dimension and an *increase* in dental crowding. The prediction for long-term success of mandibular anterior alignment was less than 30%. Almost 20% of the patients treated demonstrated marked crowding many years after removal of retainers.

Effects of premolar extraction on the periodontium

Premolar extraction and a fixed banded-bonded technique for correction of maloc-

Extraction for Treatment of Malocclusion

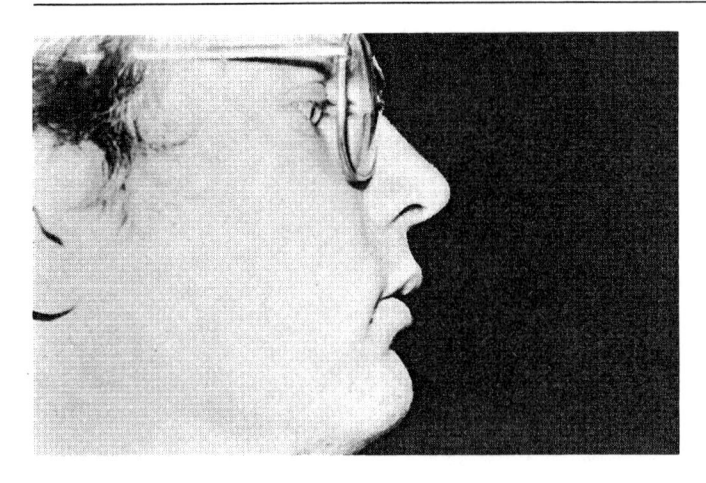

Fig. 11-8a This 28-year-old male complained of pain and clicking in the temporomandibular joint. Note the deep mentonian groove and retroclined lower lip.

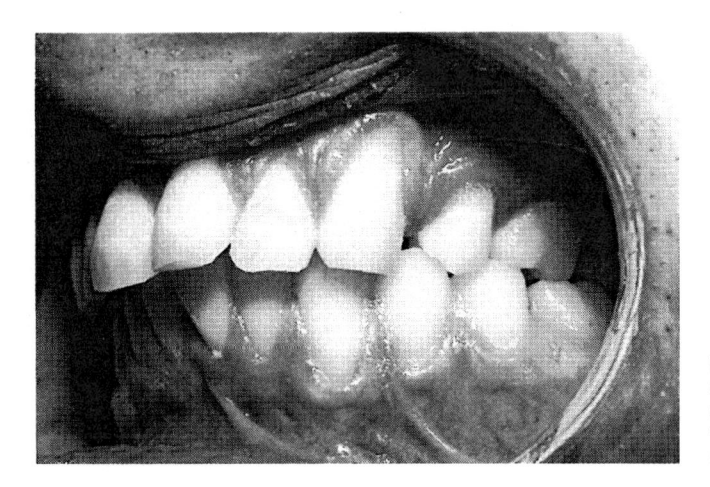

Fig. 11-8b The occlusion is unacceptable. The molar is in crossbite; interdental spacing with poor crown contact is evident.

clusion can cause an adverse response from gingival and osseous tissue.[12,13] Gingival recession, periodontal pockets, osseous recession, and root resorption are possible as teeth are moved through bone to close extraction sites. Gingival invaginations commonly occur during orthodontic treatment that involves first premolar extraction and space closure. They can persist for years after treatment, especially in the mandibular arch, and can impair gingival health in the extraction site area.[14] Tooth enamel can become decalcified with poor oral hygiene if metal orthodontic bands are not cemented properly, or if a stannous fluoride cement is not used (Fig. 11-9).[15,16,17] The use of bonded brackets reduces the chance of plaque accumulation. However, plaque formation does occur, particularly around the gingival border of the bracket.[18] Root parallelism and correct interproximal tooth contact can be difficult to achieve when premolars have been extracted (Fig. 11-10). Proper fixed appliance therapy would have prevented the poor coronal contacts.

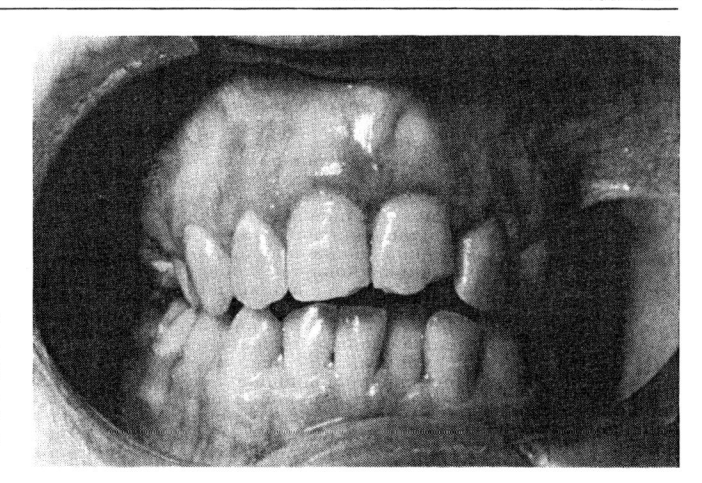

Extraction of Permanent Teeth for Treatment of Malocclusion

Fig. 11-9 This patient's mother is concerned about her 17-year-old son's "bleeding gums" and about "white marks" on his teeth. The patient has had considerable dental relapse after three years of fixed orthodontic care.

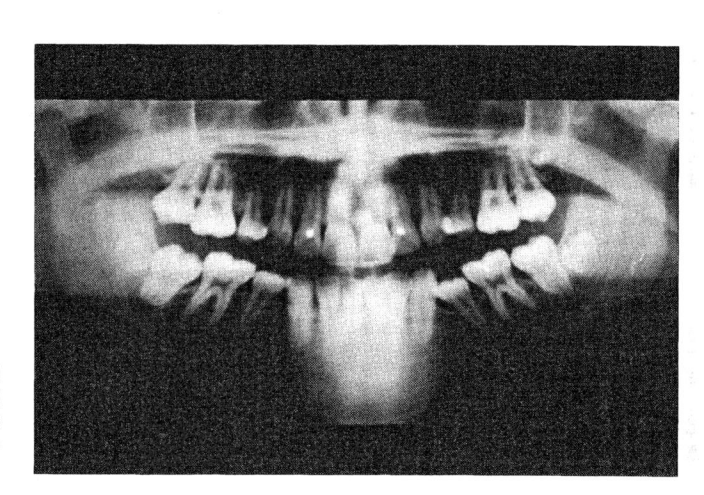

Fig. 11-10 Root parallelism and proper interproximal coronal contact areas can be difficult to achieve after premolar extraction.

Effects of premolar extraction on the temporomandibular joint

Investigators[8,9] have shown that the loss of premolars can reduce vertical dimension and deepen the bite. The effects of a reduction of vertical dimension may be harmful to the physiological stability of the temporomandibular joint. If the vertical dimension is reduced, the head of the condyle may tend to achieve a more distal and superior position in the fossa.[19] This retruded, superior position can force the disc to a position anterior to the condylar head and cause stretching of the posterior ligament attachment of the disc to the tympanic bone. Clicking, grating, and the host of other TMJ symptoms discussed in Chapter 10 can ensue. *Protection of the vertical dimension and the physiological relationship of the condylar head to the disc and fossa in the temporomandibular joint is essential for optimal treatment results.*

Occasionally, in order to retract the anterior dental component and close an excessive overjet, only the maxillary premolars are removed. In many instances this may give excellent occlusal and esthetic results.

273

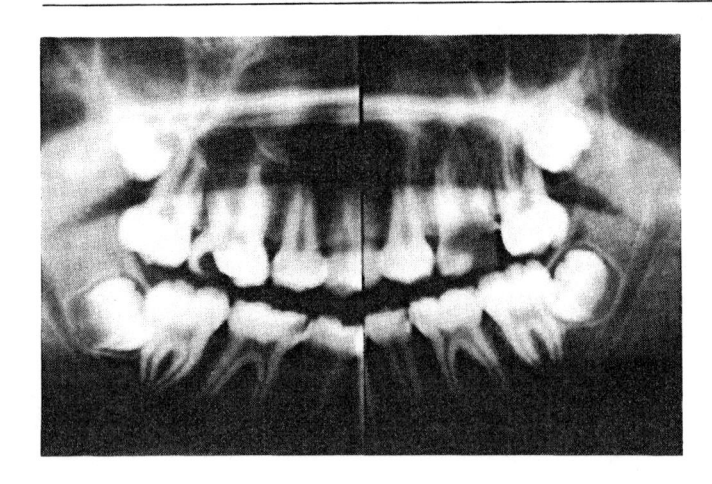

Fig. 11-11a If the prognosis for the maxillary first molars is poor, extraction may be the best alternative for the patient. A fixed appliance would be required for proper tip, torque, and in/out dental occlusal relationships.

The danger is that the mandible may get locked or trapped in a retruded position by the maxillary retruded incisors. With the condyle retropositioned, untoward TMJ symptoms can develop.

Watson[20] has summarized the attitude of many clinicians toward removal of premolar teeth:

> The removal of four premolars for the purpose of aligning a slight irregularity of lower incisors, uprighting aligned incisors to a particular angle over basal bone, or for the sake of having a Class I molar relation cannot always be construed as a beneficial procedure when you are considering the gingiva, bone, root structure, and psyche of the individual.

Incisor extraction

Occasionally, when anterior dental crowding is extreme, an incisor is extracted in the mandibular arch. In this way, the time for mandibular incisor alignment can be shortened, and the dental crowding is alleviated. The noncoincidental dental midlines do not affect esthetics or condylar position. The periodontium can be improved when the teeth can be more easily kept free of plaque and calculus. The periodontium would be adversely affected if spaces or clefts resulted after incisor alignment. Care must be taken to ensure that the vertical dimension is not reduced or that the mesial-distal tooth-size ratio between the arches is not compromised.[21]

Bolton[22] has emphasized that good dental alignment and stability of both arches is dependent on approximately equivalent mesial-distal size in both arches. An excessive dental mesial-distal size in one arch may require reduction for tooth alignment stability in both of the maxillary and mandibular arches.

Bahreman[23] considers mandibular incisor extraction to be a "last resort" measure since it involves an important stabilizing area of the occlusion. *Mandibular incisor extraction is not a routine orthodontic procedure.* It should be avoided when the patient exhibits a concomitant deep overbite. Mandibular incisor extraction yields the best results in Class I malocclusions with severe mandibular incisor crowding and good buccal intercuspation in the posterior segment. Single mandibular incisor extraction should be considered as a compromise treatment only, if the end result is a healthier periodontium and a functionally stable occlusion.

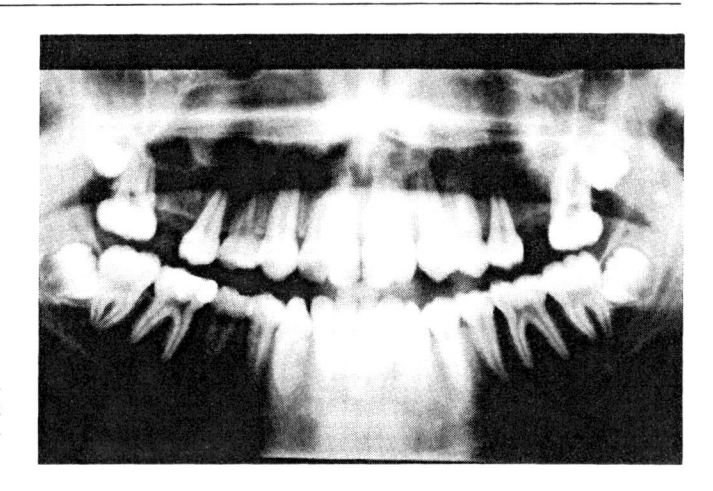

Fig. 11-11b Some spontaneous space closure will occur as shown three months post-extraction.

First molar extraction

Extraction of a first permanent molar is considered if dental caries has jeopardized the prognosis for the tooth and dental crowding facilitates space closure (Figs. 11-11a and b). The chance for space closure without tilting of the second permanent molar is improved if the first molar is removed before the second molar has erupted through the gingival tissue.[24]

When the mandibular first molar is extracted in order to avoid the problem of distal migration of the unerupted mandibular second premolar, careful periodic radiographic monitoring is required in the mandibular arch.[25] Distal migration of the mandibular second premolar occurs frequently enough to require careful consideration before making the decision to extract, and careful monitoring following extraction. However, distal migration of the maxillary second premolar is rare after extraction of the maxillary first molar.

Occasionally, in cases of severe skeletal open bite, first molars are considered for extraction. The patient with skeletal open bite demonstrates some or all of the following characteristics:[26] a high mandibular plane-angle with a distally rotated mandible, excessive lower anterior facial height, anteriorly tipped-up palatal plane, and a large Y-axis angle. Reduction of tooth structure in the first molar region may be effective in reducing a severe skeletal open bite. However, consideration must be given to condylar position before the first molars are removed.

Nasal airway impedance can also influence craniofacial growth and exacerbate an open bite tendency.[27,28] Airway problems are determined during the diagnosis of skeletal open bite malocclusion (see Chapter 13).

Second molar extraction

Second molar extraction and third molar replacement is increasing in importance as a method of reducing dental crowding. Canine, premolar, and third molar crowding are effectively reduced with second molar replacement. Appliance therapy combined with second molar replacement can minimize anterior crowding (see Chapters 7 and 8).

The two primary advantages of second molar extraction are: stability of the condylar position in the temporomandibular joint, and stability of facial esthetics. Removal of second molars does not cause a reduction

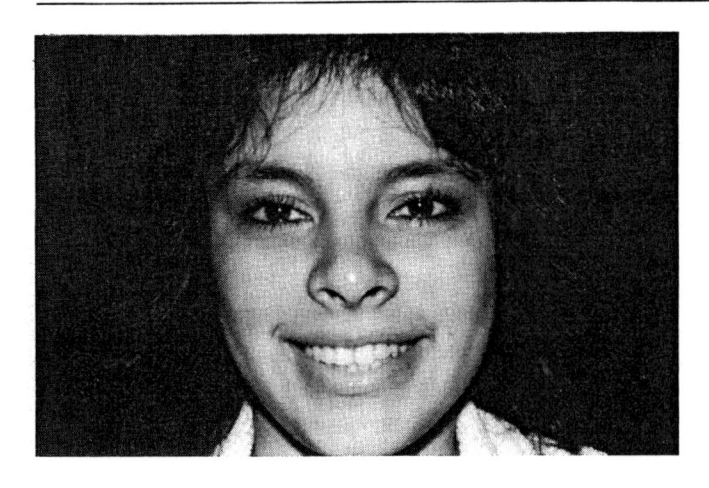

Fig. 11-12 The second molars were replaced with third molars. Full facial features and full smile are the results.

in the vertical dimension,[29] so the condyle-disc-fossa relationship does not change. The second molars are the most posterior teeth in the arch at the time of extraction; therefore, the spaces created are not apparent when the patient smiles. Since there are no spaces to close, treatment time is shortened. If treatment is interrupted or stopped for any reason, the periodontal health of the patient is not compromised. Halting treatment before completion when utilizing a premolar extraction technique can result in poor interdental contact and food impaction areas.

The stable esthetic results with second molar extraction ensure that there will be a full broad smile with no sunken lips (Fig. 11-12). In cases of severe crowding and premolar extraction, the necessity often arises of later removing third molars because of their impaction or partial impaction. Second molar removal makes this additional surgical procedure unnecessary.[30] When premolars are removed, the arch length and tongue space are diminished. Unless retention is continued, the unbalancing of the muscular component that results from diminishing the normal space for the tongue will cause an unstable occlusal relationship and eventual relapse after treatment is completed. Second molar replacement does not interfere with tongue space; hence, posttreatment retention is reduced or eliminated. Minimizing posttreatment retention helps to shorten total treatment time and lower the overall treatment expense for the patient. Pleasantly satisfied patients are an excellent source for referral of new patients.

Removal of second molars creates more mesial-distal space for the teeth in the arch than does extraction of premolars. Ten to 12 mm of space are created with second molar extraction,[31] as opposed to only 7 to 9 mm of space when premolars are extracted.

The second molar space is closed with the natural eruption of the third molar and the posterior uprighting of the first molar. The iatrogenic periodontal problems caused by premolar extraction and mechanical space closure[32] do not arise when second molars are replaced by third molars.

Timing is important in implementing treatment via second molar removal. Children 10 to 14 years old with dental crowding and developing third molars may be considered for second molar replacement. Maxillary second molars can be extracted as late as age 18 or 19 with good occlusal results (Figs. 11-13a to c). The optimal time for sec-

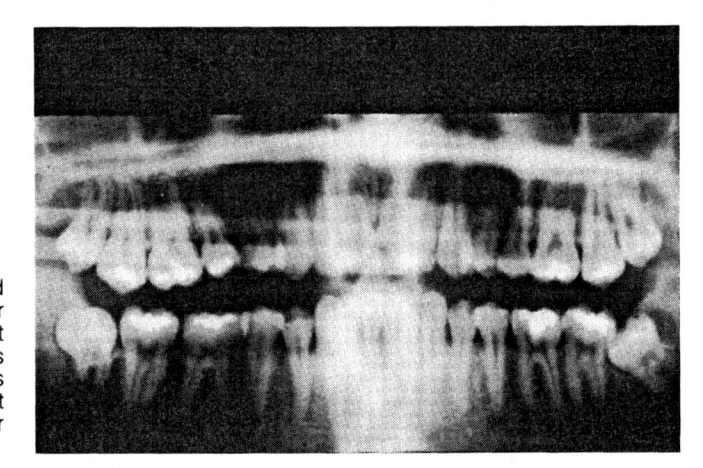

Extraction of Permanent Teeth for Treatment of Malocclusion

Fig. 11-13a This 19-year-old patient desired treatment for dental crowding but did not want "metal bands or wires" on his teeth. Maxillary second molars were removed. Earlier treatment could have included mandibular second molar replacement.

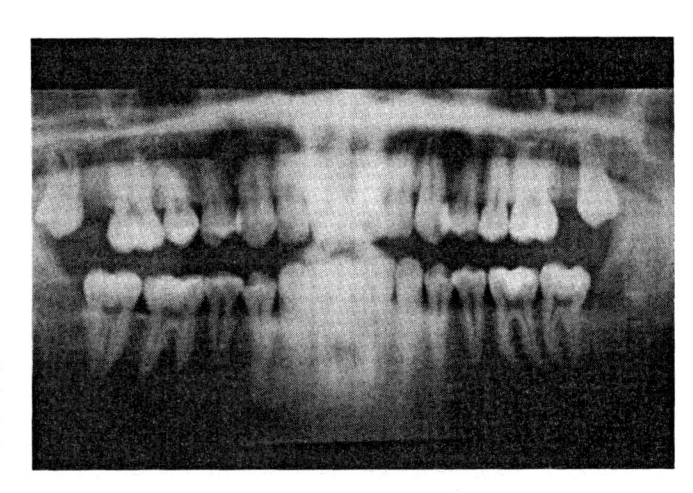

Fig. 11-13b Three months after maxillary second and mandibular third molars were removed. The patient would not wear the maxillary sagittal appliance.

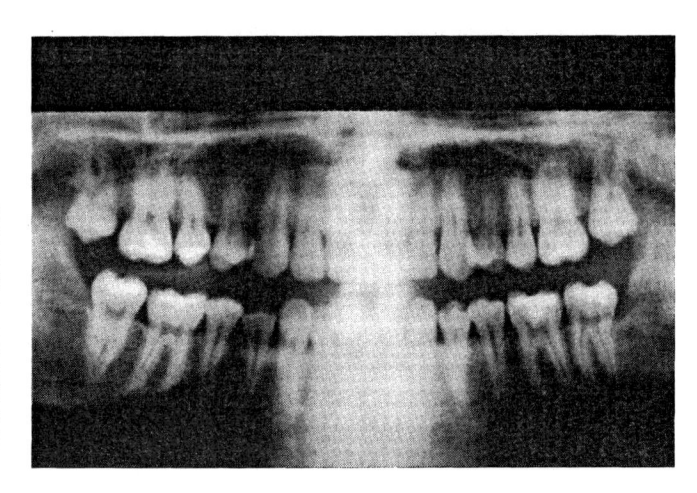

Fig. 11-13c One year after the molar extractions. No appliances have been worn, yet the maxillary molars have uprighted and the maxillary anterior crowding is improved by approximately 50%. Bonding the mandibular first to the mandibular second molars would prevent super-eruption of the mandibular second molars in patients that refuse the maxillary sagittal appliance.

277

Extraction for Treatment of Malocclusion

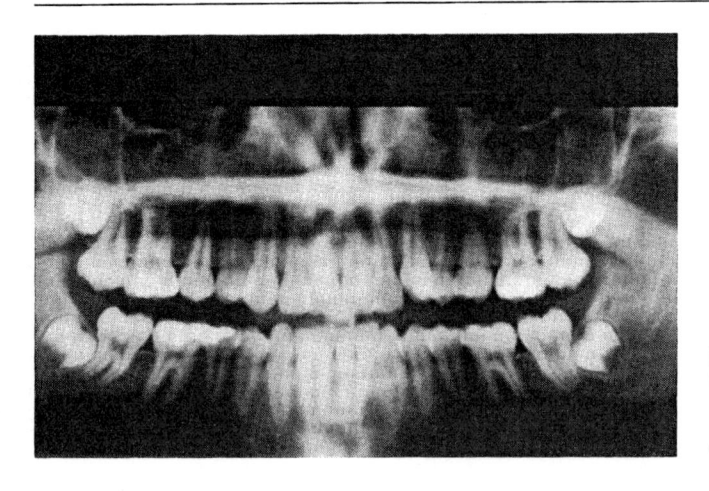

Fig. 11-14a With dental crowding and the third molars in good position to erupt, this 12-year-old patient was considered for second molar replacement.

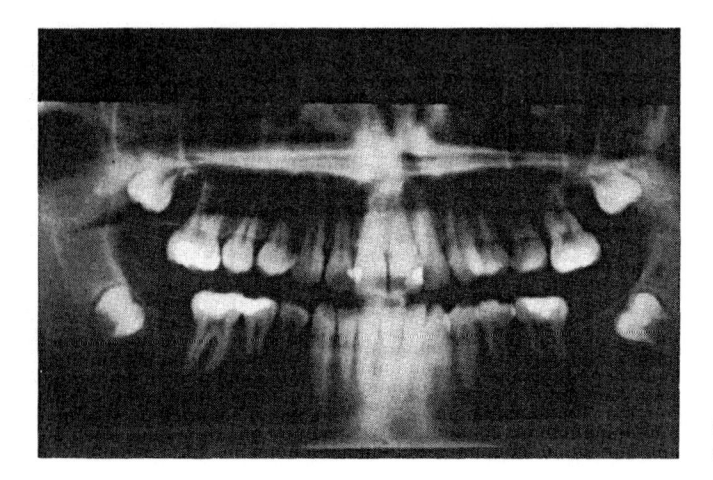

Fig. 11-14b Six months after second molar removal.

ond molar removal would be the time at which the dental crowding occurs, before the furcation of the third molar begins root formation (Fig. 11-14). Frequently, crowding occurs as the second molars begin to erupt. Lawlor[33] recommends that second molar extraction only be undertaken when the third molar is in a favorable position to erupt. Second molar extraction is not considered if the dentition is not crowded or if there is excessive spacing between the second molar and the third molar tooth bud. If a midline discrepancy exists, only one second molar in the arch is removed. The remaining second molar is utilized for reciprocal force resistance until the midlines are corrected.

Extracting *second molars* after age 16 may result in tipping of third molars, especially in the mandible, where the bone is more dense. Another disadvantage of this technique is that some patients (fewer than 10% of cases) are congenitally missing one or more third molars. Trisovic et al.[34] found great variability in the formation and calcification timing of lower third molars. In a study of 3,852 orthodontic patients aged 5 to 15 years the authors found signs of third molar formation as early as 5 years 4 months and as late as 15 years. It is sug-

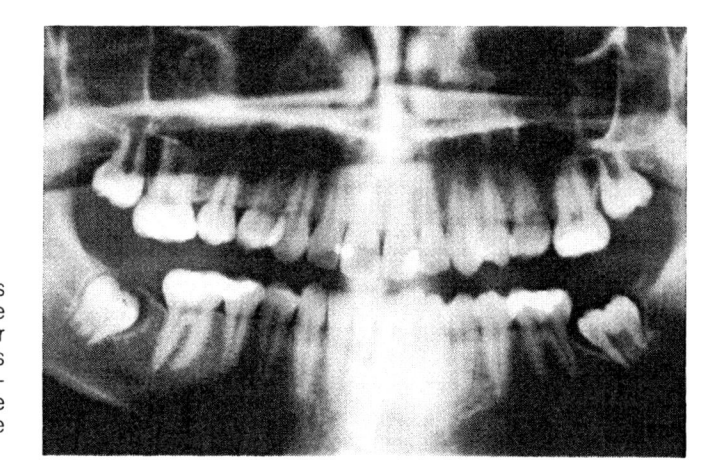

Extraction of Permanent Teeth for Treatment of Malocclusion

Fig. 11-14c Eighteen months after second molar removal. Note the migration of the mandibular third molars. All lower molars should be sectioned before extraction in order to prevent undue lateral torque and strain on the articular disc.

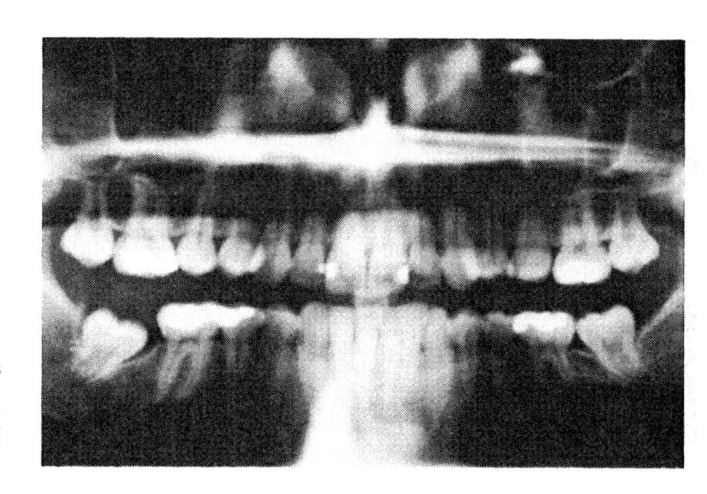

Fig. 11-14d Thirty-six months after second molar removal. All third molars are treated with occlusal sealant after eruption of the clinical crown.

gested that initiation of third molar tooth germs can occur as late as the eighth or ninth years.

The excellent occlusal results obtained with extraction of second molars, along with simplification of treatment and disimpaction of third molars,[35-39] justifies serious consideration for this technique in dental crowded malocclusion.

Huggins and McBride[38] summarize some additional *advantages* of second molar extraction:

1. Mild premolar crowding is corrected without mechanotherapy.
2. The natural contact areas from canine to first molar are retained.
3. Surgical removal of third molar impactions are avoided.
4. Facial esthetics is not compromised by sunken, dished-in lips.
5. Condylar position in the temporomandibular joint is not altered.
6. The dental result is more stable because tongue space has not been compromised and teeth have not been tipped.
7. Since the third molars are allowed to erupt and the premolars are not removed, more teeth are available for chewing and digestion.

The three principal *disadvantages* are summarized below:

1. Third molars may erupt tipped if second molars are extracted late.
2. Some people (fewer than 10% of cases) are congenitally missing one or more third molars.
3. Patients may object to having a second molar removed if there are no third molars present. Treatment must be based on what is best for the individual.

Second molar replacement by third molar eruption does much to diminish the chances of pathology developing from the impacted third molar (Fig. 11-13a). Extraction of second molars is less costly than surgical removal of impacted third molars. The proximity of the second molar to the dental crowding results in more rapid resolution of the crowding than with third molar extraction.

Third molar extraction

Third molars have been considered for early extraction to avoid dental crowding.[40] Some clinicians recommend early enucleation of these teeth to avoid possible future crowding. The effectiveness of early enucleation of third molars to prevent lower incisor crowding has not been proven by scientific study. Because of the danger of facial or inferior alveolar nerve damage or damage to the developing second molar, this technique has not gained acceptance and is to be discouraged.[41]

A definite health hazard exists when impacted third molars are allowed to remain in the older patient.[42-46] As the patient ages, the chances for surgical morbidity from third molar removal increases.[46] Most investigators encourage extraction of third molars in young adulthood if pathological signs or symptoms exist: infection, tumors, cysts (Fig. 11-13a), nonrestorable carious lesions, or destruction of adjacent teeth and bone. Further studies are needed to recommend extraction of asymptomatic impacted teeth.

Summary

Orthopedic repositioning of the maxilla and mandible and cautious use of dental extraction can enhance facial esthetics and condylar position and can reduce or eliminate dental crowding.

No set of cephalometric rules will precisely indicate either the necessity of extraction or dictate which teeth to extract. More and more of our patients are maturing with crowded dental arches. Each individual patient requires careful clinical, radiographic, and photographic evaluation before any teeth are removed. A careful diagnostic evaluation will help ensure a successful course of treatment.

References

1. Chapin, W. C. The extraction of maxillary second molars to reduce growth stimulation. Am. J. Orthod. Oral Surg. 25:1072–1078, 1939.
2. Bassani, S. Treatment of Class III malocclusion in the permanent dentition. Trans. Eur. Orthod. Soc. 191–212, 1970.
3. Dewel, B. F. A critical analysis of serial extraction in orthodontic treatment. Am. J. Orthod. 45:424–455, 1959.
4. Kerr, W. J. S. The effect of the premature loss of deciduous canines and molars on the eruption of their permanent successors. Eur. J. Orthod. 2:123 128, 1980.
5. Moyers, R. E. Handbook of Orthodontics for the Student and General Practitioner. 3rd ed. Chicago: Year Book Medical Publishers, Inc., 1973, p. 264.
6. Helm, S., and Siersback-Nielsen, S. Crowding in the permanent dentition after early loss of deciduous molars or canines. Trans. Eur. Orthod. Soc. 137–149, 1973.
7. Atkinson, C. D. The case against early extraction of mandibular primary canines. J. Am. Dent. Assoc. 104:302–304, 1982.
8. Eirew, H. L. An orthodontic challenge. Br. Dent. J. 3:96–99, 140, 1976.
9. Prichard, J. F. Four bicuspid extractions in orthodontic treatment—is it the treatment of choice? Lecture before the American Academy of Gnathologic Orthopedics. Fort Worth, Texas, Sept., 1974.
10. Wilkinson, L. C. Some things to keep in mind when treating a four bicuspid extraction case. Angle Orthod. 22:47–52, 1952.
11. Little, R. M., Wallen, T. R., and Riedel, R. A. Stability and relapse of mandibular anterior alignment—first premolar extraction cases treated by traditional edgewise orthodontics. Am. J. Orthod. 80:349–365, 1981.
12. Kaswiner, L. M. Hard and soft tissue damage accompanying orthodontic therapy. Clin. Prevent. Dent. 3:9–13, 1981.
13. Baer, P. N., and Coccaro, P. J. Gingival enlargement coincident to orthodontic therapy. J. Periodontol. 35:436–439, 1964.
14. Rivera Circuns, A. L., and Tulloch, J. F. C. Gingival invagination in extraction sites of orthodontic patients: their incidence, effects on periodontal health, and orthodontic treatment. Am. J. Orthod. 83:469–476, 1983.
15. Sniff, R. W. Enamel surface change caused by oxyphosphate cement. Am. J. Orthod. 48:219–220, 1962.
16. Lefkowitz, W. Histological evidence of the harmful effect of cement under orthodontic bands. J. Dent. Res. 19:47–55, 1940.
17. Gurson, A. V. Study of the effect of stannous fluoride incorporated in dental cement. J. Oral Ther. Pharmacol. 1:630–636, 1965.
18. Gwinnett, A. J., and Ceen, R. T. Plaque distribution on bonded brackets: a scanning microscope study. Am. J. Orthod. 75:667–677, 1979.
19. Weinberg, L. Posterior bilateral condylar displacement: its diagnosis and treatment. J. Prosthet. Dent. 36:426–440, 1976.
20. Watson, W. G. An individual compass for extraction. Am. J. Orthod. 78:111–113, 1980.
21. Bolton, W. A. Disharmony in tooth size and its relation to the analysis and treatment of malocclusion. Angle Orthod. 28:113–130, 1958.
22. Bolton, W. A. The clinical application of a tooth-size analysis. Am. J. Orthod. 48:504–529, 1962.
23. Bahreman, A. Lower incisor extracting in orthodontic treatment. Am. J. Orthod. 72:560–568, 1977.
24. Finn, S. B. Clinical Pedodontics. 4th ed. Philadelphia: W. B. Saunders Co., 1973, p. 393.
25. Matteson, S. R., Kantor, M. L., and Proffit, W. R. Extreme distal migration of the mandibular second bicuspid. Angle Orthod. 52:11–18, 1982.
26. Ackerman, R. I., and Klapper, L. Tongue position and open bite: the key roles of growth and nasopharyngeal airway. J. Dent. Child. 48:339–345, 1981.
27. Linder-Aronson, S. Adenoids: their effect on mode of breathing and nasal airflow and their relationship to characteristics of the facial skeleton and the dentition. Acta Otolaryng. (suppl.) 265:1–132, 1970.
28. McNamara, J. A., Jr. Influence of respiratory pattern on craniofacial growth. Angle Orthod. 51:269–300, 1981.
29. Wilson, W. L. The development of a treatment plan in the light of one's concept of treatment objectives. Am. J. Orthod. 45:561–573, 1959.
30. Richardson, M. E. The relative effects of the extraction of various teeth on the development of mandibular third molars. Trans. Eur. Orthod. Soc. 79–85, 1975.
31. Liddle, D. W. Second molar extraction in orthodontic treatment. Am. J. Orthod. 72:599–616, 1977.
32. Prichard, J. F. The Diagnosis and Treatment of Periodontal Disease. Philadelphia: W. B. Saunders Co., 1979.
33. Lawlor, J. The effects on the lower third molar of the extraction of the lower second molar. Br. J. Orthod. 5:99–103, 1978.
34. Trisovic, D., Markovic, M., and Starcevic, M. Observations of the development of third mandibular molars. Trans. Eur. Orthod. Soc. 147–157, 1977.
35. Smith, D. I. The eruption of third molars following extraction of second molars. Trans. Br. Soc. Orthod. 55–57, 1957.
36. Cryer, B. S. Third molar eruption and the effect of extraction of adjacent teeth. Dent. Pract. 17:405–416, 1967.
37. Wilson, H. E. Long-term observation of the extraction of second molars. Trans. Eur. Orthod. Soc. 215–221, 1974.
38. Huggins, D. G., and McBride, L. J. The eruption of lower third molars following the loss of second molars: a longitudinal cephalometric study. Br. J. Orthod. 5:13–20, 1978.

39. Lehman, R. A consideration of the advantages of second molar extractions in orthodontics. Eur. J. Orthod. 1:119–124, 1979.
40. Lindquist, B., and Thilander, B. Extraction of third molars in cases of anticipated crowding in the lower jaw. Am. J. Orthod. 81:130–139, 1982.
41. NIH consensus development conference for removal of third molars. J. Oral Surg. 3:235–236, 1980.
42. Laskin, D. M. Indications and contraindications for removal of impacted third molars. Dent. Clin. North Am. 13:919, 1969.
43. Lytle, J. J. The case for third molar removal. Trans. 117th Annual Session of the American Dental Association. Chicago: ADA, 1977.
44. Hinds, E. C., and Frey, K. F. Hazards of retained third molars in older persons: report of 15 cases. J. Am. Dent. Assoc. 101:246–250, 1980.
45. Amler, M. H. The age factor in human extraction wound healing. J. Oral Surg. 35:193–197, 1977.
46. Bruce, R. A., Frederickson, G. C., and Small, G. S. Age of patients and morbidity associated with mandibular third molar surgery. J. Am. Dent. Assoc. 101:240–245, 1980.

Chapter 12

Special Problems in Treatment of Malocclusion

An ideal orthopedic result can be summarized as a full complement of 32 teeth in a physiologically well-balanced occlusal relationship. The occlusion resulting from treatment should enhance facial esthetics and provide for stability of the temporomandibular joint. Since most patients treated for malocclusion are growing children, knowledge of the growth, physiology, and biological shaping of the craniofacial complex (see Chapter 2) are essential in treatment planning.

There are several special considerations of growth and development that can interfere with attainment of ideal facial esthetics and occlusal results. Hyper- or hypodevelopment of the maxilla or mandible can lead to an unesthetic nose or chin as seen from the facial profile view (Fig. 12-1a). Mandibular hypodevelopment may also lead to lower-incisor crowding (Fig. 12-1b). A poor condylar relationship to the articular disc and fossa may result in temporomandibular joint disorder and limitation of mandibular opening (Figs. 12-2a to d).

Record gathering, diagnosis, and treatment planning prompt many questions: for example, which appliance technique to employ, which teeth (if any) to extract, and when to institute each stage of treatment. Three primary variables determine the end result: growth, patient cooperation, and the skill of the clinician. Between initial record gathering and final end result are several special problems that must be resolved in the treatment of malocclusion. This section analytically evaluates patient cooperation, lower incisor crowding, the maxillary midline diastema, the missing lateral incisor, and the impacted maxillary canine.

Patient cooperation

Without full cooperation from the patient, results with maxillofacial orthopedic appliances are elusive. Month after month of treatment will achieve minimal or no results unless the patient is enthusiastic, cooperative in following instructions, and positively motivated to follow the treatment plan. Participation is a key element in patient motivation. The patient must believe that his or her active participation will determine the results. If the patient is imbued with a sense of desire and responsibility, the most difficult treatment obstacle is overcome.

Participatory motivation is achieved through the initial color photograph, the orthodontic progress report, and bimonthly comparison with the initial study models. When the initial color transparencies are taken, a full face view with the patient smiling is included. This slide is made into a standard 3- by 5-inch color print and given to the patient so that progress can be monitored at home. Mounted in an inexpensive

Special Problems in Treatment of Malocclusion

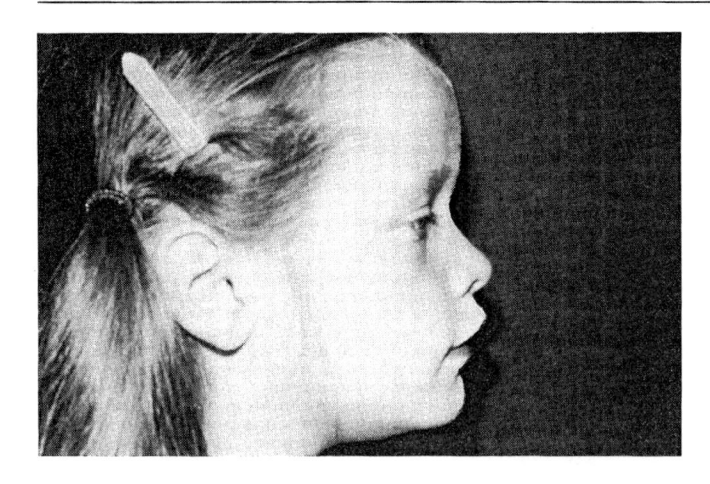

Fig. 12-1a Patient K. D. A poorly developed maxilla or mandible may result in unesthetic aberrations of facial profile.

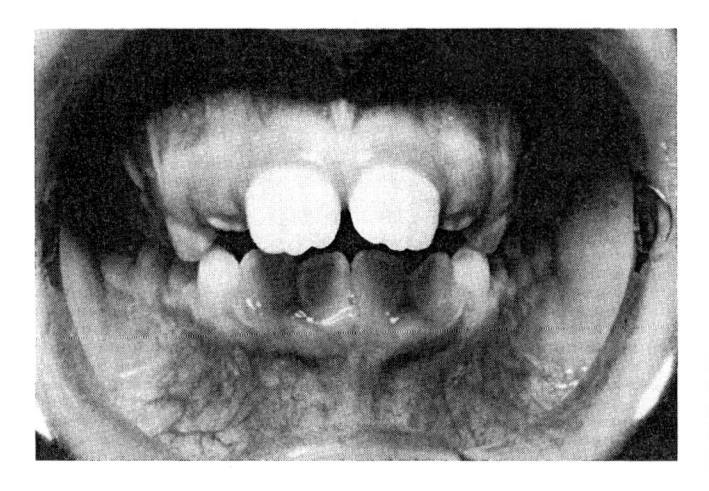

Fig. 12-1b Patient K. D. The dental crowding is a result of a skeletally hypodeveloped mandible and constricted maxilla with protruding central incisors.

frame, it has the effect of positively motivating friends of the patient to inquire about their own malocclusion. The gift is also a symbol of good faith and trust between doctor and patient. Once the transition is made from patient to friend, cooperation, trust, and successful treatment are all but assured.

The orthodontic progress report (Fig. 12-3) includes a calendar with the home and office telephone numbers of the doctor and the home phone number of the assistant written on the inside cover. This calendar acts as a daily record of appliance wear. The patient is instructed to write down, each day, the number of hours the appliance is not worn. Periodic days of the week that specific instructions are to be followed (e.g., turn expansion screw) are noted in the diary. The patient is instructed to personally call the doctor or the assistant, at the office or residence, anytime the appliance is painful and cannot be worn. This diary of appliance progress is checked at each appointment and praise is given for positive results. Too much praise for patient progress can never be given. Both children and adults enjoy hearing their name associated with a task well-completed and with progress toward positive esthetic results.

Patient Cooperation

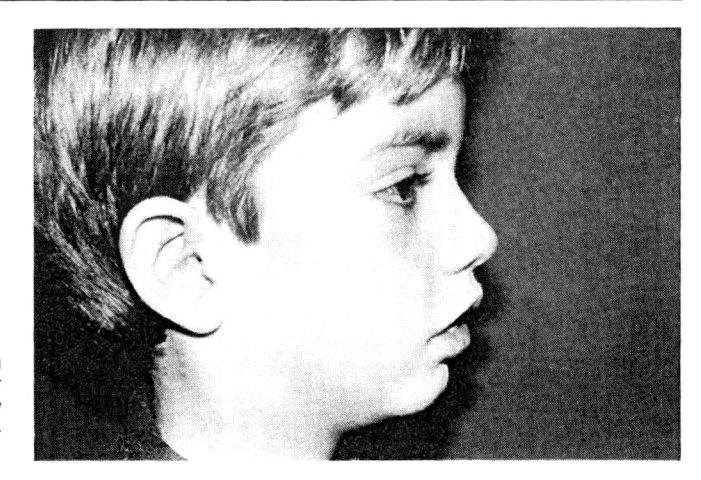

Fig. 12-2a Patient C. K. On mandibular closure, the condylar head was palpable bilaterally through the external auditory canal.

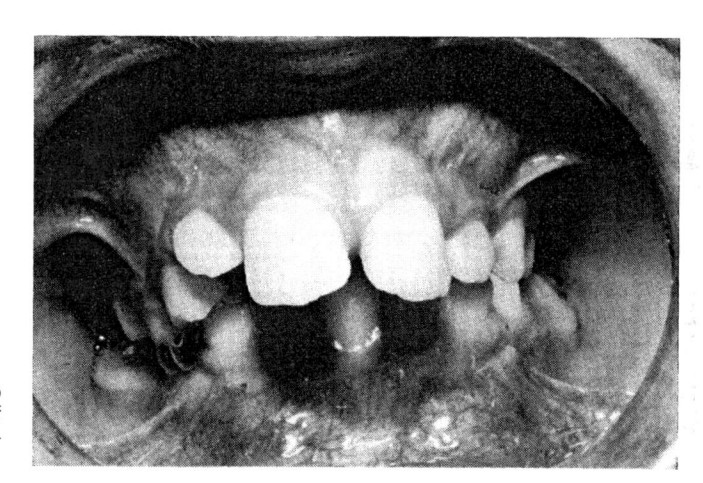

Fig. 12-2b Patient C. K. Deep bite malocclusion is typical of many patients with TMJ disorder.

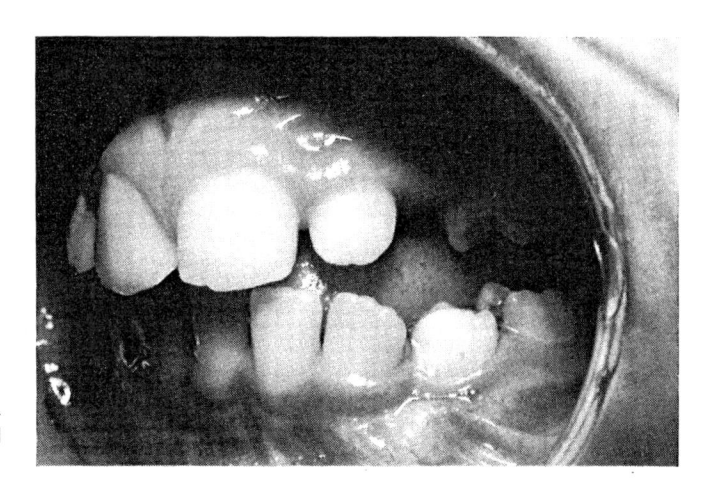

Fig. 12-2c Note the improvement in the overbite, overjet, and maxillary incisal angle.

285

Special Problems in Treatment of Malocclusion

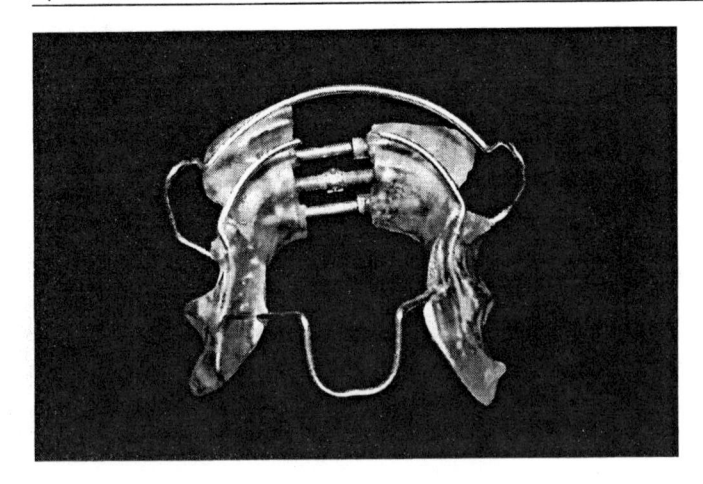

Figs. 12-2d Activation of the midline screw and coffin spring has increased the arch length. The posterior interocclusal space indicates that growth and skeletal changes are taking place. The patient noted an amelioration of headache after two weeks of bionator treatment, and complete cessation after one month. The lingual wire is cut for improved interarch expansion after one month. After breakage the appliance is repaired or replaced.

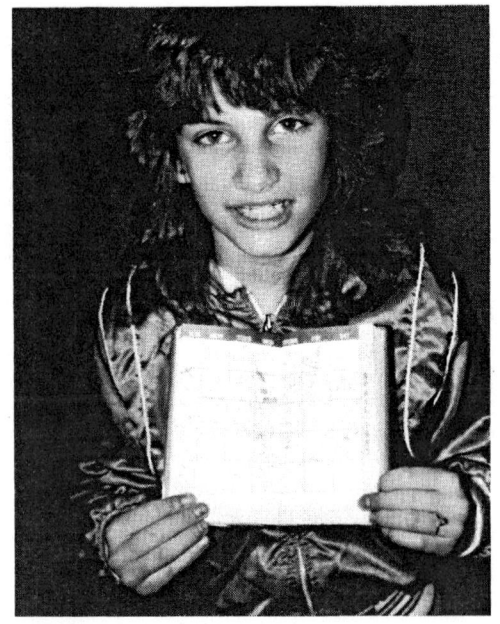

Fig. 12-3 The patient is proudly dedicated to correction of her malocclusion. The number of hours or minutes that the appliance is *out* of the mouth is recorded daily.

Three or four times each year, for the benefit of the patient and/or parent, the study models and colored slides of the original malocclusion are compared with the current occlusion. This has the effect of remotivating the patient and reaffirming parental confidence in a clinician who takes an acute interest in the progress of the patient.

Mandibular incisor crowding

Creating space for the entire dentition is an ongoing problem in the treatment of malocclusion. Esthetic and periodontal considerations favor a result that will minimize rotated, overlapped, and blocked-out teeth. The overall arch length, however, will frequently not accommodate the total mesial-distal width of all the teeth. Any tooth, molars included, can be locked out of a normal occlusal position; but mandibular incisor teeth are the most often affected by crowding. The narrow mesial and distal contact area of the mandibular incisors predispose them to rotation. Incisors are also the focal points of mesial drift from the molars. A narrow mandible and lack of osseous development of the mental symphysis may exacerbate lower incisor crowding (Figs. 12-4a and b).

There is evidence that infant and childhood sleeping position can alter normal facial growth and cause dental crowding.

Mandibular Incisor Crowding

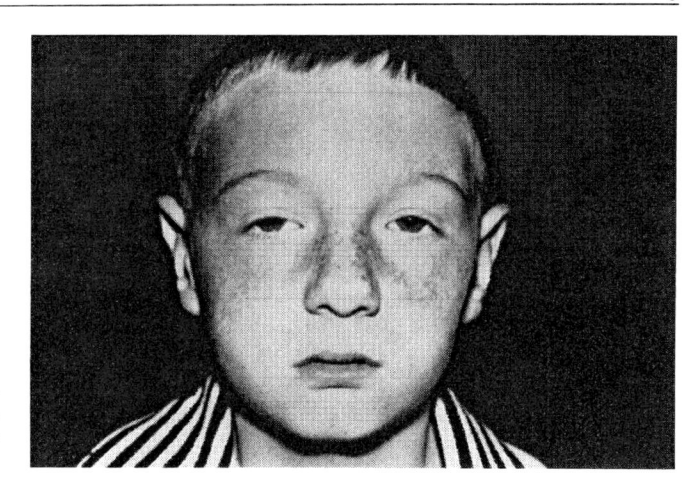

Figs. 12-4a and b A lack of facial fullness and skeletal development may lead to mandibular incisor crowding.

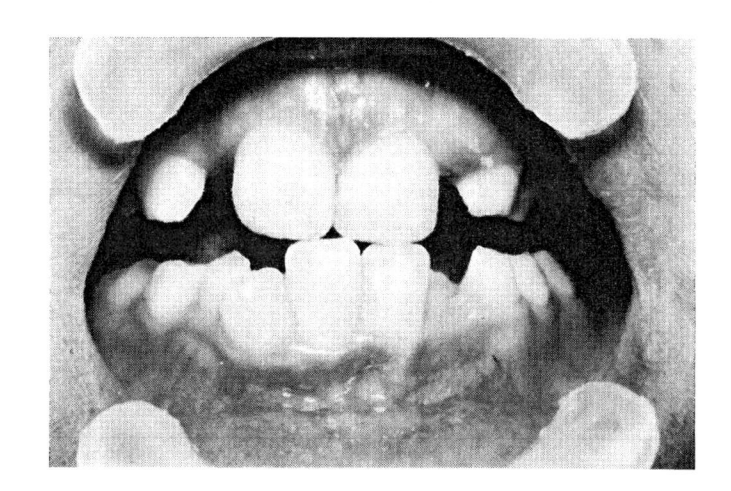

Fig. 12-4b

Stallard[1] and Huggins[2] suggest that an infant habitually sleeping on the stomach or side can develop orthopedic forces capable of changing the normal development of the craniofacial complex. These orthopedic forces can cause crossbite, dental crowding, and facial asymmetry (Fig. 12-5).

Incisor crowding has a tendency to recur after the completion of treatment (Figs. 12-6 and 12-7a and b). The mechanical correction and retention of lower anterior crowding frequently leads to relapse and consequential retreatment of the crowding after initial therapy. It has become evident that a more physiologically oriented and biologically stable solution to mandibular incisor crowding is required. Chapter 11 discusses the advantage of incisor, premolar, and molar extraction for minimizing anterior crowding. Peck and Peck[3] have studied the morphology of lower incisors and the relationship of tooth shape to dental stability. They contend that a large faciolingual incisor dimension and a smaller mesiodistal dimension will enhance lower incisor stability. Tooth shape helps determine the presence or absence of mandibular incisor crowding. Naturally, well-aligned mandibular incisor teeth have distinctive dimensional characteristics: mesiodistal di-

Special Problems in Treatment of Malocclusion

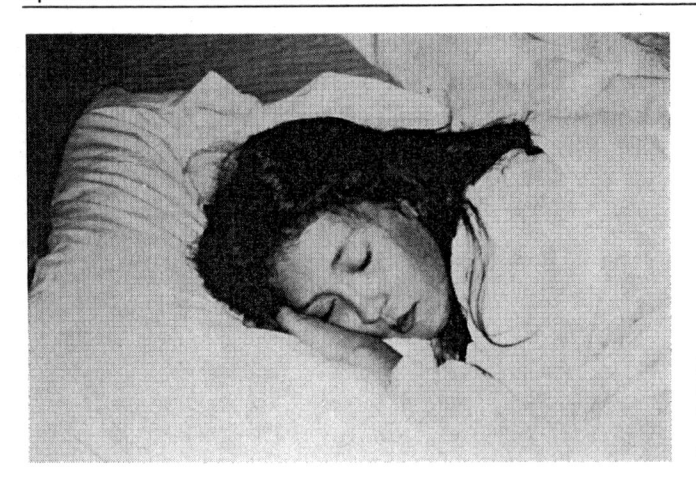

Fig. 12-5 This sleeping position should be discouraged. Osseous development of the face or temporomandibular joint may be adversely affected.

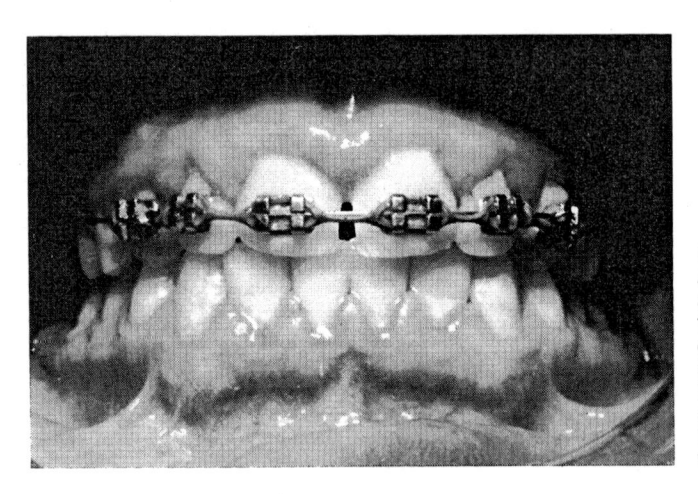

Fig. 12-6 The decalcified areas and relapse are evident shortly after removal of the mandibular fixed appliance. Generalized gingival inflammation is also present, especially in the maxillary arch where the fixed appliance is still in place. The patient has been treated for three years with a full-banded regime.

mensions are reduced and faciolingual dimensions are significantly greater than those found throughout the average population.[4,5] The concept of specific incisor shape adding to dental stability enhances the theory that interproximal stripping or narrowing of the mesiodistal incisor dimension will result in a more favorable, uncrowded, and stable incisor position.

Ballard[6] and Lavelle[7] have attempted to correlate tooth size with skull size. Ballard contended that mandibular incisor stability required an interproximal reduction to achieve optimal tooth-bone harmony where large mesiodistal dimensions existed. Lavelle considered facial pattern of prime importance when trying to identify potential relapse in a patient. Most of the population utilized, however, was of low-order statistical significance and should not be used for making clinical decisions for treatment. Nordeval et al.[8] have related mandibular anterior crowding to tooth size and craniofacial morphology. The study attempted to demonstrate a cephalometric propensity for mandibular incisor crowding. The cephalometric comparison of craniofacial morphology in a population with crowded mandibular incisors and a population with uncrowded mandibular incisors revealed

Mandibular Incisor Crowding

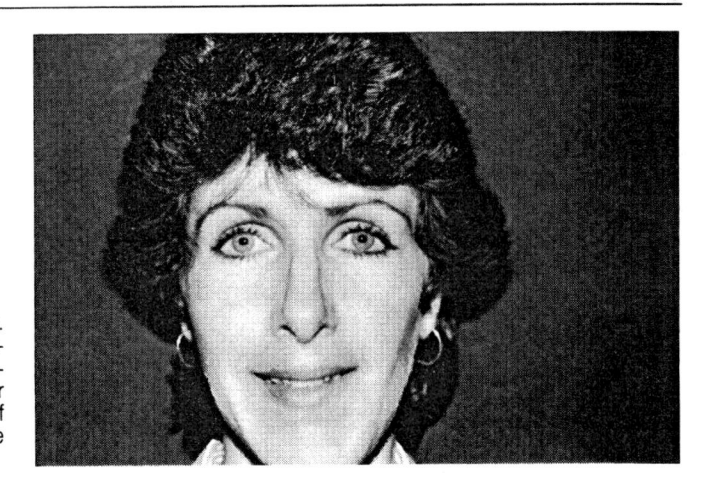

Figs. 12-7a and b Patient S. G. 24 years posttreatment. The facial skeletal features are harmonious as a result of four premolar extractions and three years of fixed appliance treatment at age 14 years.

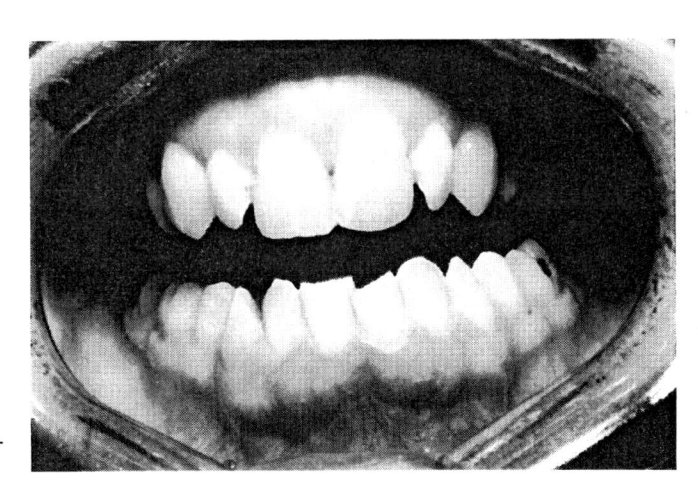

Fig. 12-7b The dental component shows complete relapse.

no significant correlations between the space available for the mandibular incisors and the craniofacial morphology of the two groups.

Baumrind et al.[9] have shown that residual errors in film tracing can be a source of cephalometric discrepancy. The clinician is encouraged not to make irreversible treatment decisions (e.g., interproximal stripping or extraction) based on "small differences in any set of magic numbers."

Treatment timing

Treatment timing is important in solving the problem of mandibular incisor crowding. The earlier the diagnosis of the cause for incisor crowding is made, the better the chance for a long-term esthetic result. Each patient requires an individual assessment of the probable level of his or her cooperation,[10] but early treatment planning and treatment for incisor crowding helps minimize the undesirable alternative of premolar extraction (see Chapter 11).

If the mandibular incisor crowding is a result of a maxillary malocclusion (e.g.,

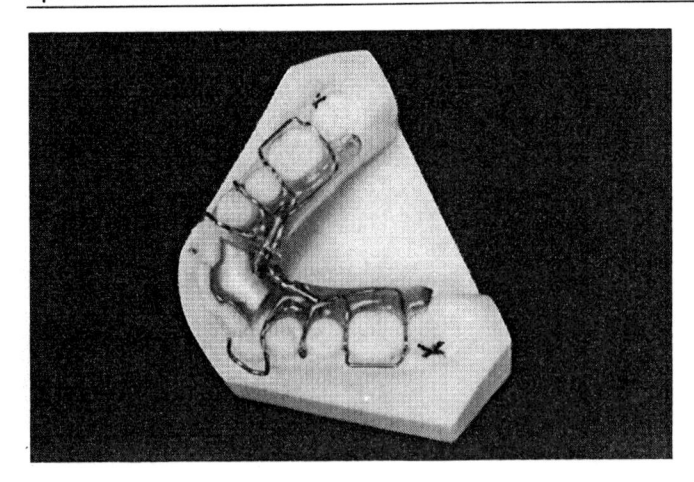

Fig. 12-8 The mandibular sagittal appliance is effective for correction of mandibular crowding when second molars are removed. (Courtesy of Dyna-Flex Orthodontic Laboratory, St. Louis, Mo.)

constricted arch from a thumb or facial sleeping habit), then correction of the habit and the maxillary malocclusion may allow spontaneous partial correction of the mandibular crowding.

Deep overbite malocclusion (as in Class II, Division 2 patients) may restrict osseous development of the mandible. The resulting mandibular incisal crowding may partially resolve on correction of the mandibular position. Pressure from the tongue, as the orthopedic appliance forces it to assume a more inferior position in the mouth, may account for a partial correction of mandibular incisal crowding.

Early treatment of mandibular incisor crowding also takes advantage of both the rapid growth and the greater potential for growth in the younger patient. Enlow[11] has shown that as the mandible develops, it takes on a three-dimensional growth characteristic (see Fig. 2-21 in Chapter 2).

Proper timing of appliance insertion will take advantage of bony remodeling in the mandibular incisor area. As the mandible is forced by an orthopedic appliance into a more protrusive position, several changes are taking place in the condyle[12] and in the mandibular anterior segment. The pressure exerted by the appliance on the lingual segment of the mandible may cause some slight lingual resorption and labial deposition to take place. As the labial plate undergoes remodeling, the incisors are able to upright and move into a more favorable and stable position in the arch (Fig. 12-8).

Spring retainer

After every conceivable precaution has been taken and assuming early biological treatment, occasionally the mandibular incisors are still not perfectly aligned. Barrer[13] has developed a combination treatment involving interproximal stripping and use of a spring retainer (Figs. 12-9a to c). This method takes advantage of mechanically aligning the incisors by creating broad, flat contact areas and applying contant rotational forces via a spring retainer. This technique should not be relied upon for gaining more than 3 to 4 mm of interproximal space. Care must be taken so that not more than one-half of the enamel is removed from the interproximal surfaces of the mandibular incisors. Too much enamel reduction could lead to increased susceptibility to dental caries, or to pulpal sensitivity to thermal changes or refined sugar in the diet. In addition, excessive reproximation of mandibular incisors followed by relapse

Mandibular Incisor Crowding

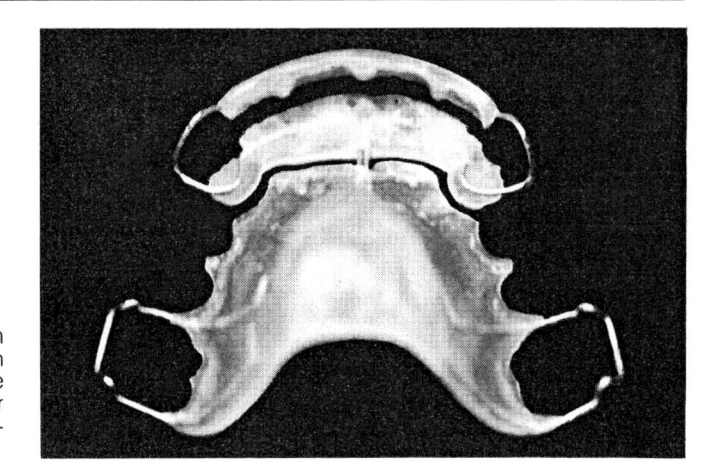

Fig. 12-9a Maxillary arch spring retainer for final correction of dental rotation. An appliance of this type is effective for anterior maxillary or mandibular correction of minor dental rotation.

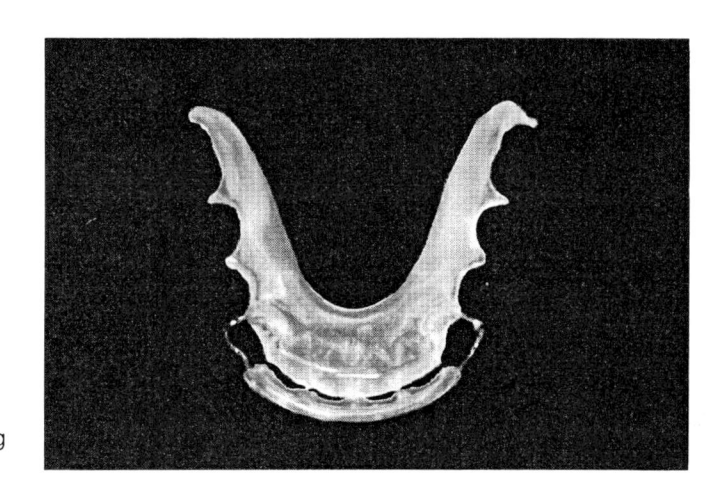

Fig. 12-9b Mandibular spring arch removable retainer.

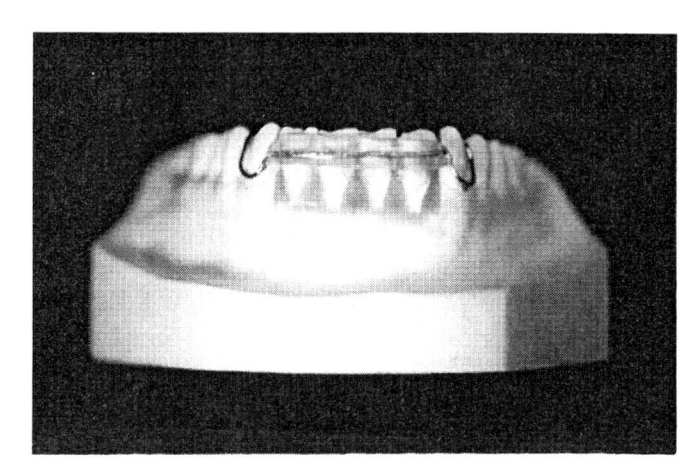

Fig. 12-9c Mandibular spring arch retainer in place, with the teeth realigned in wax. (Courtesy of New England Orthodontic Laboratory, Winchester, Mass.)

may shorten the mandibular arch length and deepen the anterior overbite.[14] The deepened overbite could lead to an unfavorable condylar-disc-fossa relationship (see Chapter 11).

The primary benefits of reproximation or "stripping" of the mandibular incisors are reviewed by Boese:[14] the reduction of enamel provides broader contact point areas and promotes stability and the amount of available space in the mandibular incisor area is increased. Treatment benefits outweigh the minimal risks.[15]

Reproximation is more effective if accomplished as necessary during various stages of treatment, rather than all at once. Although self-alignment may follow reproximation,[16] the best results are obtained by enamel removal after the mandibular incisors are aligned or after bracket removal. Several authors[13-22] have studied the problem of incisor uprighting and secondary crowding after treatment. Occasionally, additional reproximation may be necessary to compensate for this mandibular incisor crowding.

Dependence on mandibular incisor retention can be further reduced with the use of circumferential supracrestal fiberotomy. Boese[23] found that fiberotomy combined with reproximation had no significant impact on periodontal health. In addition, by recognizing the influence of displaced supra-alveolar connective tissue fibers associated with dental crowding, more effective long-term stability can be predicted.

Several studies[24-30] propose methods for assessing the severity and predicting the optimal treatment for dental crowding. There is considerable variation in the computation and correlation of reliable data used in these studies. Examiner treatment priority and variations in technique can lead to subjective assessments of crowding that can vary widely among clinicians.[31-35] Little[36] has minimized the subjective variable when assessing pretreatment and posttreatment status and posttreatment change in the mandibular incisors. He has developed an Irregularity Index, determined for each patient by the linear displacement of the adjacent anatomic contact points of the mandibular incisors. Although measurements were made from plaster casts, a predictable linear trend between clinical assessment and the proposed Irregularity Index was reported.

Schulhof et al.[37] have demonstrated no significant correlation between labiolingual incisor position and the propensity for relapse. Little difference was found in relapse potential after mandibular incisors were moved labially, lingually, or held in the same relative position during treatment. This finding is significant. Mechanotherapy with bands-brackets and straight-wire technique is used worldwide to attempt to correct spacing discrepancies and rotations. Without a correct diagnosis of the cause of the original malocclusion, much mechanotherapy is subject to relapse.

Some ethnic populations experience a higher degree of dental crowding than others. Hioki[38] has reported finding a significant frequency of bimaxillary crowding in the Oriental dentition. Likewise, the British orthodontic community shows more dental crowding than orthodontic populations from Mediterranean and Eastern European countries.[39-42] The frequency of dental extraction to improve orthodontic crowding can be directly related to ethnic biological differences throughout the world.[43]

If there is slight relapse after treatment, or incomplete resolution of mandibular incisor crowding after bracket removal and biological and mechanical therapy, then it is best to accept a small degree of mandibular incisor crowding. Little et al.[44] have noted that patients treated with premolar extraction have variable and unpredictable incisor alignment. Arch length and width were found to decrease after retention; crowding usually increased. This study found that less than 30% of patients that had undergone premolar extraction with routine edge-

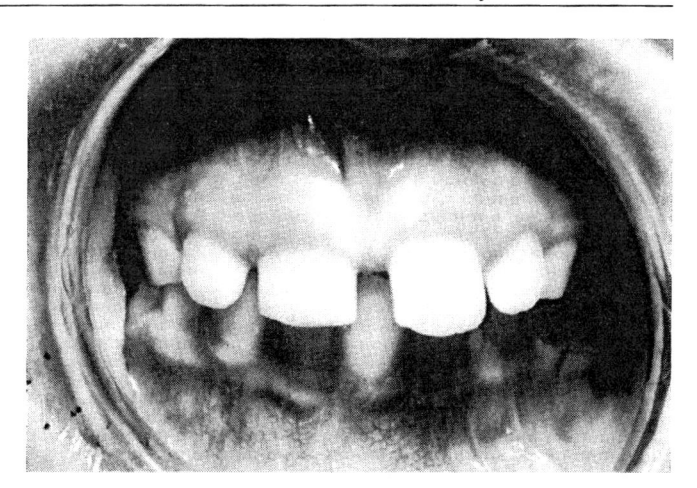

Fig. 12-10 Cosmetic correction of the diastema at an early age may stop unkind remarks from classmates.

wise mechanics maintained satisfactory mandibular anterior alignment after removal of retainers. Howe et al.[45] have demonstrated that dental crowding is associated with small dental arches, rather than with large teeth. Their study suggests treatment plans other than extraction that would increase dental arch length in patients with crowded dentitions.

In the case of a very crowded dentition, it would be wise to inform the parent or patient that slight crowding or rotations may remain after treatment. A slight degree of mandibular incisor crowding would be preferable to deepening the bite through premolar extraction and risking an unfavorable condylar-disc-fossa relationship.

The teeth comprise an important part of overall facial esthetics. In addition to facial fullness and uncrowded mandibular incisors, three additional tooth-related discrepancies require special consideration: the maxillary median diastema, the congenitally missing lateral incisor, and the impacted maxillary canine.

Maxillary median diastema

The maxillary median diastema is frequently the reason for initial patient contact. The parent of an 8- to 11-year-old patient may have a question about an extra wide space between the maxillary incisors (Fig. 12-10). Occasionally, parental desire for space closure will prompt the clinician to construct an appliance to close the diastema. Early treatment of the maxillary median diastema is often discouraged because, frequently, space closure is spontaneous with eruption of the maxillary permanent canines. Record gathering will differentiate the cause of the diastema: mesiodens, congenitally missing lateral incisor, thickened labial frenum, cyst, digit habit, or tooth size discrepancy.

Popovich et al.[46] contend that the labial frenum and the intermaxillary suture make only a minor contribution to the maxillary midline diastema. The primary factor contributing to maxillary diastema is the degree of maxillary dental crowding. Edwards[47] has shown, however, that there is a strong correlation between a clinically thickened maxillary midline frenum and a maxillary midline diastema. Edwards contends that patients with a maxillary midline diastema and a low, thickened labial frenum tend to undergo relapse after orthodontic closure of the diastema. Surgical removal of the labial frenal tissue is suggested, along with

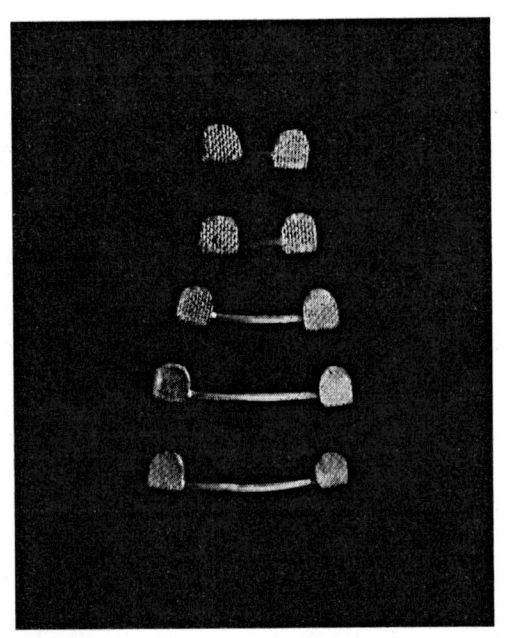

Special Problems in Treatment of Malocclusion

Fig. 12-11 The bondable lingual retainer will help to keep the diastema from reopening. The top two lingual retainers are for maxillary central incisors. The bottom three lingual retainers are for the mandibular arch.

removal of elastic fibers in the underlying periosteum. The transseptal fibers should also be surgically eliminated after orthodontic closure of a diastema. If these fibers are not destroyed, the orthodontic result may relapse and the diastema reappear. Campbell and his co-workers[48] have shown a very abnormal histological pattern to transseptal fibers after maxillary midline diastema correction. Once the transseptal fibers are dissected, a new and functionally adapted ligament forms within 30 days.[49]

Since the possibility exists for spontaneous diastema closure without orthodontic or surgical intervention, treatment for maxillary median diastema is best accomplished after eruption of the maxillary permanent canines, as long as no pathology is present (Fig. 12-11).

The congenitally missing lateral incisor

The congenitally missing lateral incisor can be a particularly vexing problem for the clinician. The two most common choices of treatment are: to mesialize the canine on the affected side and reshape it to resemble a lateral incisor,[50] or to distalize the canine and place a fixed prosthesis. If the arch exhibits dental crowding, then mesializing and reshaping the canine is readily accomplished with esthetic results. However, if the arch is not crowded, the dental and facial esthetics may be compromised by orthodontic closure of space: the smile may not look full; the face may have a concave appearance. In addition, when the maxillary arch length is reduced, the mandibular arch may be directed to a more retruded condylar relationship. A distal force vector on the condyle is not compatible with a healthy, full-functioning temporomandibular joint.

Mesializing and reshaping the canine to resemble a lateral incisor negates the possibility of a cuspid-protected occlusion: the maxillary canine occludes with the mandibular lateral incisor. Nordquist and McNeill[51] contend that establishment of a Class I cuspid-protected occlusion is not essential for a functional occlusion and that proper functional balance can be established by posttreatment occlusal equilibration. Emphasis is placed on gingival and periodontal health; fixed or removable replacement of lateral incisors is discouraged in this study. Carlson[52] encourages orthodontically closing the lateral incisor space and recontouring the canine so long as natural facial contours are not damaged. He expressed dissatisfaction with esthetic prosthodontic replacement. Tuverson[53] has described a method of recontouring the maxillary canine on the mesial, distal, labial, and lingual surfaces, and on the incisal edge in order to make it closely resemble the lateral incisor (Fig. 12-12).

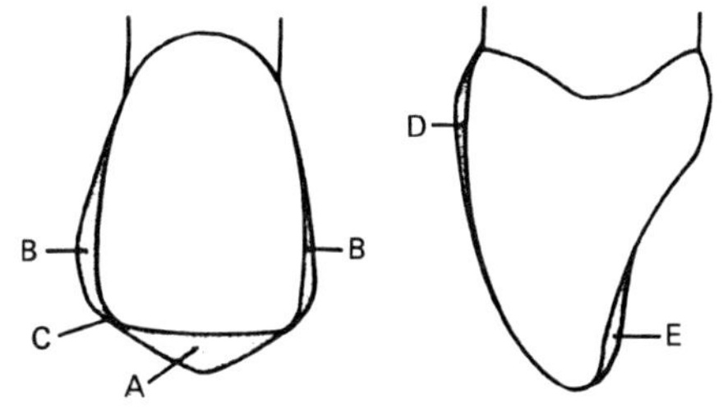

Fig. 12-12 A method of recontouring maxillary canines to resemble and function as lateral incisors. (From Dr. D. L. Tuverson, with permission. Courtesy of The C. V. Mosby Co., St. Louis, Mo.) (Enamel bonding can further aid the esthetic contouring of the canine.)

A Tip of canine flattened to produce an incisal edge. B Mesiodistal reduction. C Distal incisal angle is slightly rounded. D Reduction of canine eminence on labial surface. E Lingual surface is reduced at incisal area to enable adequate overbite and overjet to be established.

Senty[54] claims that there is no apparent change in facial contour when canines are moved mesially but that shade imbalance between the canine and the central incisor should be expected.

When presented with the problem of a missing lateral incisor, the clinician must make a treatment decision based on the data available: which compromise is best for the patient. Dental crowding would dictate consideration of mesialization of the canine. An excess of space would make distalization of the canine and prosthetic replacement more esthetically and functionally desirable. Strang[55] has indicated that facial and dental esthetics are enhanced when space is created for a prosthetic replacement. Wheeler[56] has commented on the cosmetic value of the position of the canine and the canine eminence. Dewel[57] has referred to the esthetic value of the canine and its strategic position at the angle of the arch. He contends that canine location is significant for determining occlusal symmetry and contour. Henns,[58] however, has shown that only minor changes in arch form are detected when canine position is altered mesially.

Zachrisson[50] has summarized details of treatment planning for missing maxillary incisors. He emphasizes clinical procedures that improve final results after orthodontic space closure: contouring of adjacent teeth, fiberotomy, and composite additions to incisal angles. Schwaninger and Shay[59] have also suggested careful management of patients with missing maxillary lateral incisors. If the canine is mesialized and recontoured, premature contact with the opposing teeth should be avoided.

The contention that canines can be mesialized and reshaped is well-represented in the literature. The procedure of reshaping or replacement requires individual consideration for each patient. None of the studies reviewed expressed concern about reduction in maxillary arch length or possible effect on the temporomandibular joint. Enhancing facial and dental esthetics and reducing plaque accumulations are important, but treatment planning should include consideration for a healthy temporomandibular joint. Joint noises (clicking or cracking) or headache as a posttreatment result would indicate inadequate treatment planning.

The impacted maxillary canine

The impacted maxillary canine can also

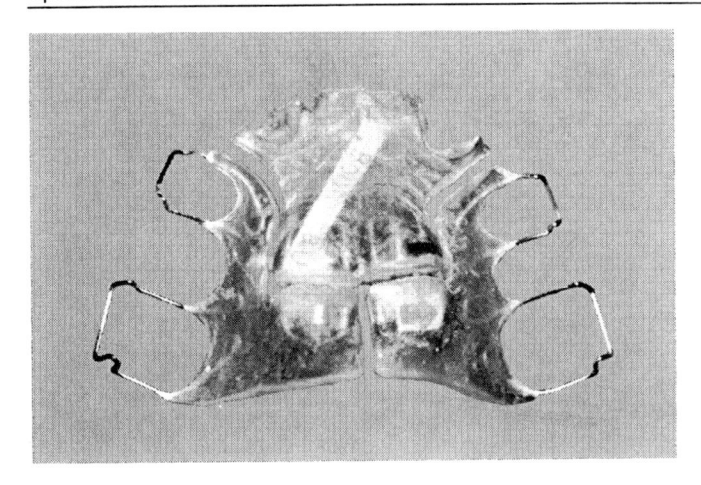

Special Problems in Treatment of Malocclusion

Fig. 12-13 The two-way sagittal appliance can effectively create arch length in the maxillary canine area.

create a perplexing situation for the clinician: should space be created and the canine surgically exposed and orthodontically guided into the arch; or should it be surgically extracted and the first premolar recontoured to resemble the canine? There are valid reasons for employing each procedure. The key to treatment lies in prevention, early diagnosis, and treatment planning.

The maxillary permanent canine is the most-often impacted tooth (excluding third molars) in the adult dentition.[60] Thilander and Myrberg[61] found permanent tooth impaction common in Swedish schoolchildren. Several authors have reported on the frequency of maxillary impacted cuspids.[62-64] Several causes of canine impaction have been suggested: long path of eruption (Broadbent[65]; Bass[60]), nonresorption of primary canine root (Lappin[66]), and a narrow maxilla in combination with retroclined incisors, dentigerous cysts, or congenitally missing lateral incisors (Kettle).[63] Becker et al.[67] have suggested that patients with anomalous lateral incisors (missing, peg-shaped, or smaller or larger than the mandibular counterpart) be evaluated for the possibility of palatally displaced canines. This study agreed with others[64,68] that found a relatively high incidence of palatally displaced canines in females.

Diagnosis of maxillary canine impaction should begin as early as the dental age of 8 years.[69] Screening would consist of palpating for a canine bulge and checking the intraoral radiograph for pathology or abnormal lateral incisor development. Once it has been determined that the maxillary permanent canine is at risk of being impacted, the extraction of the maxillary primary canine and location of the position of the permanent canine may aid in prevention of impaction. The relative location of a lingually positioned maxillary permanent canine can be determined by the Clark technique.[70] Two intraoral radiographs are exposed with the film in the same position and the radiographic source moved to a different horizontal angle. Comparing the two radiographs will help assess location of the maxillary canine in that the object closest to the film will shift to the same direction as the radiographic source in relation to another object closer to the source.

Once it is determined that a canine is impacted, surgical or fixed treatment techniques may be utilized to bring about eruption.[71,72] Elimination of severe dental crowding in the maxillary arch can make

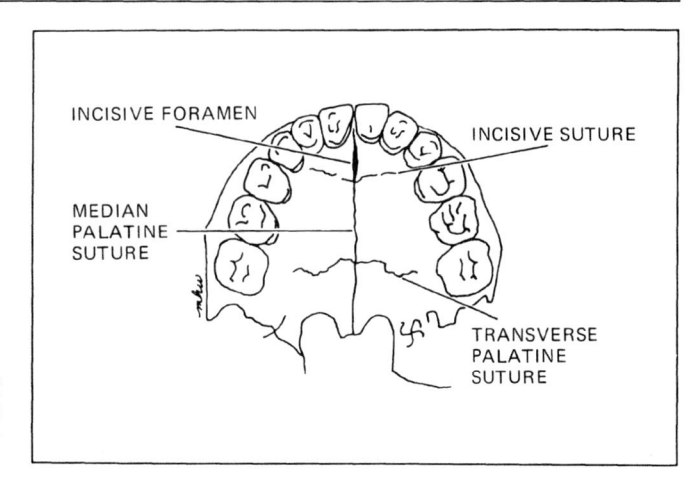

Fig. 12-14 The palatal view of the skeletal maxilla demonstrates the position of the incisive suture.

room for the impacted canine and possibly stimulate eruption. Since space is required in the crowded arch for this tooth, a sagittal appliance (Fig. 12-13) is used to enlarge the space at the incisive suture (Fig. 12-14).

Increasing arch length in the canine area is often accomplished in conjunction with the second molar extraction technique discussed in Chapter 11. Because of the value of premolar teeth in protecting the vertical dimension, it is rare that this tooth would ever be enucleated (as advocated by some)[73] in order to enhance canine eruption downward and backward into the premolar space. Early enucleation of premolar teeth usually is not beneficial with respect to either facial esthetics or health of the temporomandibular joint and has no place in standard maxillofacial orthopedic treatment of malocclusion.

An impacted canine that will erupt after space has been created may require surgical exposure, followed by orthodontic acceleration and guidance into occlusion. Shapira and Kuftinec have reviewed some of the complications and risks of repositioning impacted canines:[74] ankylosis of the canine prevents guided eruption and can cause discoloration or devitalization, root resorption, or loss of cervical bone with resulting long clinical crown and lack of attached gingival tissue. Caution is urged when wire ligation (lasso) is utilized to bring the impacted canine back into occlusion as suggested by Norton[75] and Ziegler[76] because of the chance that it will cause external root or enamel resorption.[77,78] A local inflammatory reaction may be responsible for enamel or cementum resorption of the impacted canine.[79]

Success resulting from exposing impacted canines, attaching a bonded bracket, and attempting orthodontic guidance is not always certain. Thoma[80] has described the impossibility of orthodontic treatment for certain horizontally impacted canines that may have their cusp tips against the root of the central or lateral incisor and the root apex distally approaching the first molar. Bishara et al.[81] have discussed the difficulties of surgical exposure and guidance of impacted maxillary canines and suggest a guarded prognosis.

Surgical treatment

The chance of untoward posttreatment sequelae, prolonged treatment time, and strain on the patient and clinician have prompted serious consideration before deciding on surgical removal of the impacted canine and reshaping and mesializing the first premolar to resemble the canine. Altman and his colleagues[82] have shown successful results when the maxillary permanent canine is surgically removed and the maxillary first premolar is used as a substitute canine. This procedure is advocated when the impacted canines are in an unfavorable (oblique or horizontal) position or when canine eruption would suggest premolar extraction.

When the first premolar is substituted for a canine, the lingual cusp is reduced to take it out of occlusion and prevent contact in lateral excursions. The best esthetic results dictate that the first premolar have the same axial position as the canine and that arch form be normal. Altman found that stability of the two-rooted premolar was not a problem and that, esthetically, the final results were very acceptable. No facial asymmetry could be detected even on unilateral extraction of an impacted canine.

Summary

Five special problems in treatment of malocclusion with orthopedic techniques have been reviewed: patient cooperation, lower incisor crowding, maxillary midline diastema, missing lateral incisor, and impacted maxillary canine. An orthopedic and biological approach to treatment has been stressed. Chapter 13 will focus on additional special situations and results of errors in diagnosis, treatment planning, and treatment of malocclusion with maxillofacial orthopedic appliance technique.

References

1. Stallard, H. A consideration of extraoral pressures in the etiology of malocclusions. Int. J. Orthodont. Oral Surg. Radiog. 16:5, 1930.
2. Huggins, H. A. Why Raise Ugly Kids? Westport, Conn.: Arlington House Publishers, 1981.
3. Peck, H., and Peck, S. An index for assessing tooth shape deviations as applied to the mandibular incisors. Am. J. Orthod. 61:384–400, 1972.
4. Peck, S., and Peck, H. Crown dimensions and mandibular incisor alignment. Angle Orthod. 42:2, 148–153, 1972.
5. Peck, S., and Peck, H. Orthodontic aspects of dental anthropology. Angle Orthod. 45:95–102, 1975.
6. Ballard, M. L. Asymmetry in tooth size; a factor in the etiology, diagnosis and treatment of malocclusion. Angle Orthod. 14:67–70, 1944.
7. Lavelle, C. L. The relationship between tooth and skull size. J. Dent. Res. 53:1301, 1974.
8. Nordeval, K., Wisth, P. J., and Böe, O. E. Mandibular anterior crowding in relation to tooth size and craniofacial morphology. Scand. J. Dent. Res. 83:267–273, 1975.
9. Baumrind, S., Miller, D., and Molthen, R. The reliability of head film measurements. Am. J. Orthod. 70:617–644, 1976.
10. Jacobson, A. Psychology and early orthodontic treatment. Am. J. Orthod. 76:511–529, 1979.
11. Enlow, P. Handbook of Facial Growth. Philadelphia: W. B. Saunders Co., 1975.
12. McNamara, J. A., Jr., and Carlson, D. S. Quantitative analysis of temporomandibular joint adaptations to protrusive function. Am. J. Orthod. 76:593–611, 1979.
13. Barrer, H. G. Protecting the integrity of mandibular incisor position through keystoning procedure and spring retainer appliance. J. Clin. Orthod. 9:486–494, 1975.
14. Boese, L. R. Fiberotomy and reproximation without lower retention, nine years in retrospect: part I. Angle Orthod. 50:88–97, 1980.
15. Paskew, H. Self-alignment following interproximal stripping. Am. J. Orthod. 58:240–249, 1970.
16. Betteridge, M. A. The effects of interdental stripping on the labial segments evaluated one year out of retention. Br. J. Orthod. 8:193–197, 1981.
17. DeKock, W. H. Dental arch depth and width studied longitudinally from 12 years of age to adulthood. Am. J. Orthod. 62:56–66, 1972.
18. Schudy, G. F. Posttreatment craniofacial growth, its implications in orthodontic treatment. Am. J. Orthod. 65:39–57, 1974.
19. Siatokowski, R. E. Incisor uprighting: mechanism for late secondary crowding in the anterior segments of the dental arches. Am. J. Orthod. 66:398–410, 1974.

References

20. Riedel, R. Retention and relapse. J. Clin. Orthod. 10:454–472, 1976.
21. Gardner, S., and Chaconas, S. Posttreatment and postretention changes following orthodontic therapy. Angle Orthod. 46:151–161, 1976.
22. Lombardi, A. Mandibular incisor crowding in completed cases. Am. J. Orthod. 61:374–383, 1972.
23. Boese, L. R. Fiberotomy and reproximation without lower retention nine years in retrospect: part II. Angle Orthod. 50:169–178, 1980.
24. Barrow, G., and White, J. Developmental changes of the maxillary and mandibular dental arches. Angle Orthod. 22:41–46, 1952.
25. Björk, A., Krebs, A., and Solow, B. A method for epidemiological registration of malocclusion. Acta Odontol. Scand. 22:27–41, 1964.
26. Carlos, J. Evaluation of indices of malocclusion. Int. Dent. J. 20:606–617, 1970.
27. Draker, H. Handicapping labio-lingual deviations: a proposed index for public health purposes. Am. J. Orthod. 46:295–305, 1960.
28. Moorrees, C., and Reed, B. Biometrics of crowding and spacing of the teeth of the mandible. Am. J. Phys. Anthropol. 12:77–88, 1954.
29. Proffit, W., and Ackerman, J. Rating the characteristics of malocclusion: a systemic approach for planning treatment. Am. J. Orthod. 64:258–269, 1973.
30. Salzmann, J. Handicapping malocclusion assessment to establish treatment priority. Am. J. Orthod. 54:749–765, 1968.
31. Summers, C. The occlusal index: a system for identifying and scoring occlusal disorder. Am. J. Orthod. 59:552–567, 1971.
32. Freer, T., Grewe, J., and Little, R. Agreement among the subjective severity assessment of ten orthodontists. Angle Orthod. 43:185–190, 1973.
33. Grewe, J., and Hagen, D. Malocclusion indices: a comparative evaluation. Am. J. Orthod. 61:286–294, 1972.
34. Hermanson, P., and Grewe, J. Examiner variability of several malocclusion indices. Angle Orthod. 40:219–222, 1970.
35. Popovich, F., and Thompson, G. A longitudinal comparison of the orthodontic treatment priority index and the appraisal of the orthodontist. J. Public Health Dent. 31:2–8, 1981.
36. Little, R. M. The irregularity index: a quantitative score of mandibular anterior alignment. Am. J. Orthod. 68:554–563, 1975.
37. Schulhof, R. J., et al. The mandibular dental arch: part I. Lower incisor position. Angle Orthod. 47:280–287, 1977.
38. Hioki, M. The attitude of Japanese orthodontists toward tooth extraction in orthodontic treatment. Int. Dent. J. 21:340–345, 1971.
39. Gardner, J. H. Malocclusion in Europe. Br. J. Orthod. 1:69–71, 1974.
40. Adam, M. Reflections on planning of orthodontic extractions. Cesk. Stomatol. 70:68–71, 1970.
41. Lavelle, C. L. B. A study of multiracial malocclusions. Comm. Dent. Oral Epidemiol. 4:38–41, 1976.
42. Van Kirk, L., and Pennel, E. Assessment of malocclusion in population groups. Am. J. Public Health 49:1157–1163, 1959.
43. Peck, S., and Peck, H. Frequency of tooth extraction in orthodontic treatment. Am. J. Orthod. 76:491–496, 1979.
44. Little, R. M., Wallen, T. R., and Riedel, R. A. Stability and relapse of mandibular anterior alignment: first premolar extraction cases treated by traditional edgewise orthodontics. Am. J. Orthod. 80:349–365, 1981.
45. Howe, R. P., McNamara, J. A., Jr., and O'Connor, K. A. An examination of dental crowding and its relationship to tooth size and arch dimension. Am. J. Orthod. 83:363–373, 1983.
46. Popovich, F., Thompson, G. W., and Main, P. A. The maxillary interincisal diastema and its relationship to the superior labial frenum and intermaxillary suture. Angle Orthod. 47:265–271, 1977.
47. Edwards, J. G. The diastema, the frenum, the frenectomy: a clinical study. Am. J. Orthod. 71:489–508, 1977.
48. Campbell, P. N., Moore, J. W., and Matthews, J. L. Orthodontically corrected midline diastemas. Am. J. Orthod. 67:139–158, 1975.
49. Parker, G. R. Transseptal fibers and relapse following bodily retraction of teeth; a histologic study. Am. J. Orthod. 61:331–334, 1972.
50. Zachrisson, B. U. Improving orthodontic results in cases with maxillary incisors missing. Am. J. Orthod. 73:274–289, 1978.
51. Nordquist, G. G., and McNeill, R. W. Orthodontic vs. restorative treatment of the congenitally absent lateral incisor, long-term periodontal and occlusal evaluation. J. Periodontol. 46:139–143, 1975.
52. Carlson, H. Suggested treatment for missing lateral incisor cases. Angle Orthod. 22:205–216, 1952.
53. Tuverson, D. L. Orthodontic treatment using canines in place of missing lateral incisors. Am. J. Orthod. 58:109–127, 1970.
54. Senty, E. L. The maxillary cuspid and missing lateral incisors: esthetics and occlusion. Angle Orthod. 46:365–371, 1976.
55. Strang, R. H. W. Textbook of Orthodontia. 2nd ed. Philadelphia: Lea & Febiger, 1943.
56. Wheeler, R. C. Textbook of Dental Anatomy. Philadelphia: W. B. Saunders Co., 1940.
57. Dewel, B. F. The upper cuspid: its development and impaction. Angle Orthod. 19:79–90, 1949.
58. Henns, R. J. The canine eminence. Angle Orthod. 44:326–328, 1974.
59. Schwaninger, B., and Shay, R. Management of cases with upper incisors missing. Am. J. Orthod. 71:396–405, 1977.
60. Bass, T. B. Observations on the misplaced upper canine tooth. Dent. Practit. 18:25–32, 1967.
61. Thilander, B., and Myrberg, N. The prevalence of malocclusion in Swedish school children. Scand. J. Dent. Res. 81:12–21, 1973.
62. Mead, S. V. Incidence of impacted teeth. Orthodont. Oral Surg. Rad. Int. J. 16:885–890, 1930.
63. Kettle, M. A. Treatment of the unerupted maxillary

canine. Dent. Practit. Dent. Res. 8:245–255, 1958.
64. Dachi, S. F., and Howell, F. V. A study of impacted teeth. Oral Surg. 14:1165–1169, 1961.
65. Broadbent, B. H. Ontogenic development of occlusion. Angle Orthod. 11:223–241, 1941.
66. Lappin, M. M. Practical management of the impacted maxillary cuspid. Am. J. Orthod. 37:769–778, 1951.
67. Becker, A., Smith, P., and Behar, R. The incidence of anomalous maxillary lateral incisors in relation to palatally-displaced cuspids. Angle Orthod. 51:24–29, 1981.
68. Howard, R. D. The displaced maxillary canine: positional variations associated with incisor resorption. Trans. Br. Soc. Study Orthodont. 57:149–157, 1970–1971.
69. Williams, B. H. Diagnosis and prevention of maxillary cuspid impaction. Angle Orthod. 51:30–40, 1981.
70. Langlais, R. P., Langland, O. F., and Morris, C. R. Radiographic localization techniques. Dent. Radiogr. Photogr. 52:69–77, 1979.
71. Becker, A., and Zilberman, Y. A combined fixed-removable approach to the treatment of impacted maxillary canines. J. Clin. Orthod. 9:162–169, 1975.
72. Becker, A., and Zilberman, Y. The palatally impacted canine: a new approach to treatment. Am. J. Orthod. 74:422–429, 1978.
73. Mayne, W. R. Serial extraction. In T. M. Graber (ed.) Current Orthodontic Concepts and Techniques. Philadelphia: W. B. Saunders Co., 1969.
74. Shapira, Y., and Kuftinec, M. Treatment of impacted cuspids: the hazard lasso. Angle Orthod. 51:203–207, 1981.
75. Norton, L. A. Treatment of impacted canines. J. Clin. Orthod. 5:454–455, 1971.
76. Ziegler, T. F. A modified technique for ligating impacted canines. Am. J. Orthod. 72:665–670, 1977.
77. Stafne, E. C., and Austin, L. T. Resorption of embedded teeth. J. Am. Dent. Assoc. 32:1003–1009, 1945.
78. Blackwood, H. J. Resorption of enamel and dentin in the unerupted tooth. Oral Surg. 11:79–85, 1958.
79. Azaz, B., and Shteyer, A. Resorption of the crown in impacted maxillary canine. Int. J. Oral Surg. 7:167–171, 1978.
80. Thoma, K. H. Oral Pathology. 2nd ed. St. Louis: The C. V. Mosby Co., 1944.
81. Bishara, S. E., et al. Management of impacted canines. Am. J. Orthod. 69:371–387, 1976.
82. Altman, J. A., Arnold, H., and Spector, P. Substituting maxillary first premolars for maxillary impacted canines in cases requiring the extraction of dental units as part of orthodontic correction. Am. J. Orthod. 75:618–629, 1979.

Chapter 13

Critical Errors in Diagnosis and Treatment of Malocclusion

Correction of malocclusion is gratifying for the patient, parent, and clinician. The changes brought about in the individual are not always confined to the dentition. Maxillofacial orthopedic appliances encourage facial growth and the results of treatment can greatly improve facial esthetics. Often a distinct behavioral change from an introverted personality to an extroverted personality will be evident posttreatment. As an individual becomes comfortable with a full, wide smile, an improved sense of well-being becomes pervasive. However, poor facial esthetics is not the usual motivation for a patient to seek help (Fig. 13-1).

Stricter[1] has reviewed the psychological issues pertaining to malocclusion and has consistently found certain patient motivations in seeking treatment: degree of malocclusion, parental influence, gender, and age. In many cases, it was found that the parents rather than the child wanted the treatment for the child.

Diagnostic and clinical errors

Following are some selected diagnostic and clinical errors that can short-circuit the best efforts of the clinician and transform routine treatment of a malocclusion into a thoroughly unpleasant and difficult experience: root resorption, premature decision to extract premolars, incisors chipped from appliance wear, utilization of a bulky appliance for an uncooperative patient, headgear treatment when it is not necessary or well-accepted by the individual, miscalculation of patient or parent commitment, the attempt to orthopedically correct gross skeletal deformities when surgical correction is necessary, late diagnosis of an existing etiology, and poor communication with the patient or parent.

Root resorption

Root resorption is deleterious to the oral health of the patient for at least two reasons: discoloration or devitalization of the tooth may result and mobility and periodontal pathology can occur. Ketcham[2,3] discussed the problem of root resorption as early as 1927. It was noted that appliances that encouraged bodily tooth movement caused a greater number of root resorptions than appliances that only tipped the teeth. Rudolph, in 1936,[4] demonstrated a higher degree of root resorption in older patients and less resorption in younger patients. It is evident from studies in 1954 by Massler and Malone[5] and in 1955 by Philips[6] that root resorption is prevalent when teeth are bodily moved through bone. In the Massler study, 93.3% of all teeth examined had at least 1 mm of resorption; in the Philips study, 84.0% of maxillary central incisors evidenced root resorption. DeShields,[7] in

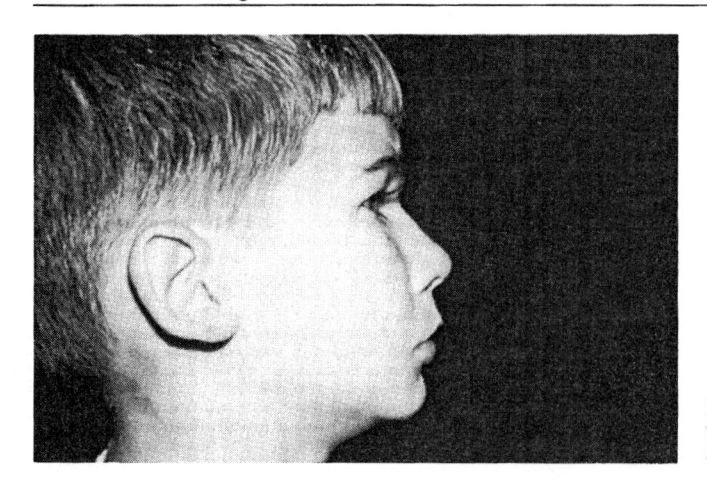

Fig. 13-1a This patient sought treatment for persistent headache.

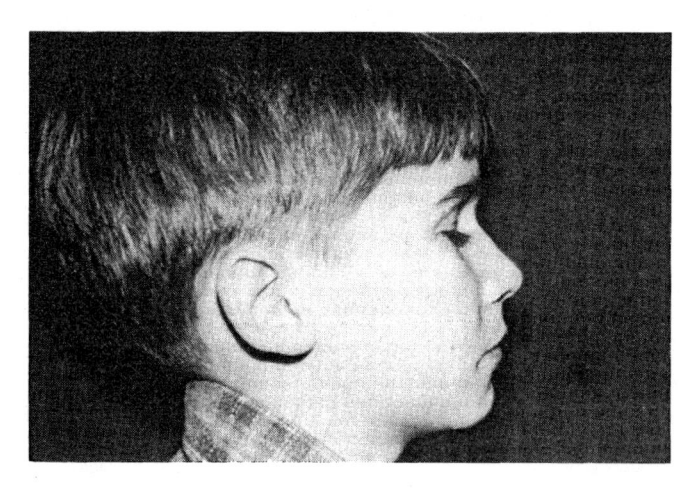

Fig. 13-1b An improvement in facial esthetics was of psychological benefit. Note the increase in lower face height and the improved chin profile. The patient and parent noted a cessation of headache approximately ten days after bionator appliance insertion.

1969, found that in a sample of nonextraction cases, 81.73% of maxillary central incisors underwent definite root resorption. The gender of the patient did not affect the amount or prevalence of root resorption. Since it was suspected that apical root movement could be a cause of root resorption, DeShields recommended that "unnecessary tooth movements should be avoided."

Most investigation of root resorption indicates that the more a tooth is moved mechanically (bodily or by tipping, torque, intrusion, or extrusion), the greater the chance for resorption of the roots. Since extraction of premolars requires relatively extensive tooth movements, this form of therapy for malocclusion could be expected to cause more frequent root resorption. Goldson and Henrikson[8] found root resorption especially prevalent in maxillary central incisors that underwent root torque when treated by the Begg technique. Hall[9] found severe root resorption during Stage II of the Begg technique and suggested that the resorption might be caused by movement of the incisor apices against the labial cortical plate (Figs. 13-2a to c).

Harry and Sims[10] have shown that root resorption is dependent on duration of

Diagnostic and Clinical Errors

Figs. 13-2a to c This patient had the maxillary incisors retruded to help the esthetic replacement of the congenitally missing lateral incisors.

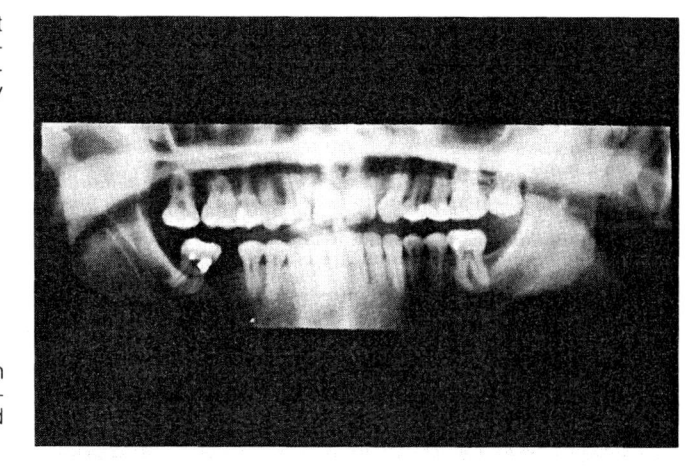

Fig. 13-2a No consideration was given to the possible untoward sequelae of resorbed roots.

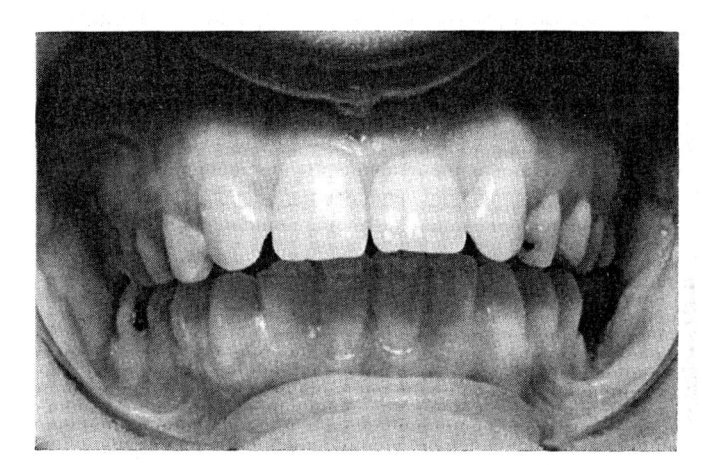

Fig. 13-2b Note the poor dental esthetics.

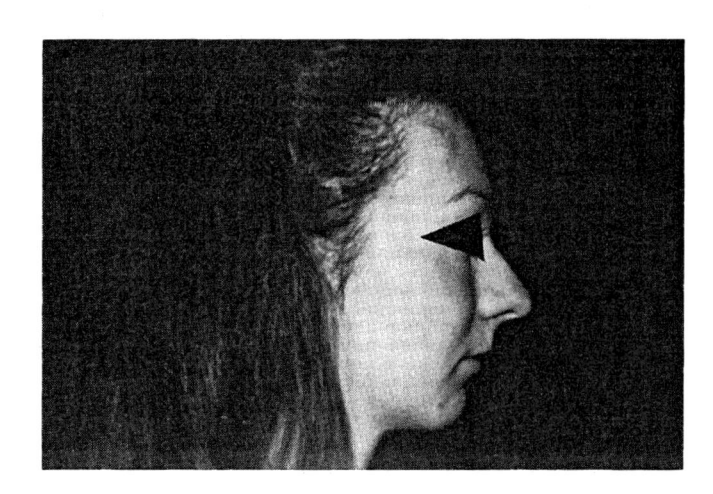

Fig. 13-2c Facial profile.

force but not necessarily on the magnitude of force. The lightest force in this study (50 g) produced some resorption in all experimental teeth.

For reasons other than root resorption, the regime of treatment that retracts maxillary incisors may be detrimental to the patient. The retracted maxillary incisors may guide the mandibular component to a retruded position on maximum intercuspation and hence affect adversely the condyle-disc-fossa relationship. In a study of components of Class II malocclusion in children, McNamara[11] demonstrated that mandibular skeletal retrusion was a much more common characteristic of Class II malocclusion than was maxillary protrusion. Indeed, it is suggested that a treatment plan that stimulates and directs mandibular growth would be more appropriate than a treatment plan that restricts maxillary growth. In light of the McNamara study, it appears that inhibiting maxillary growth via extraction of premolars and external anchorage retraction should be pursued very cautiously.

Premature decision to extract premolars

Extraction of any tooth for improvement of occlusion requires careful diagnosis and treatment planning (see Chapter 11). Baumrind et al.[12] caution against placing too much emphasis on cephalometric requirements for extraction. Peck and Peck[13] have stressed a need for a fuller facial profile than is commonly thought acceptable by cephalometric norms. Eirew[14] has shown pictorally the structural changes that can occur if premolars are removed without regard for long-term facial esthetics.

A premature decision to remove premolar teeth may jeopardize the long-term stability of the esthetic, the temporomandibular joint, and/or the dental component of the occlusion (Figs. 13-3a and b). If premolar teeth are to be extracted, it is wise to utilize as little mechanical therapy as possible in guiding the teeth into occlusion. Larsson and Ronnerman[15] have shown a high incidence of mandibular dysfunction symptoms in patients that have been treated with fixed appliances in the maxillary arch only. Janson and Hasund[16] found that, in a sample of 90 randomly selected patients from Bergen, Norway, nonextraction of premolars demonstrated excellent functional adaptation and was suggested wherever possible.

If early removal of primary first molars and enucleation of permanent first premolar teeth is undertaken, then the chance for an occlusion with a full complement of teeth is lost. This violates a fundamental and desirable goal established by Tweed[17] in 1945: "There must be a full complement of teeth, and each tooth must be made to occupy its normal position."

Wilson[18] questions the value of serial extraction, particularly in Class II, Division 2 (deep bite) patients, because it eliminates other choices, such as extraction of first or second molars.

Chipped incisal edge from appliance wear

Several types of orthopedic appliances are constructed to reposition the mandible in a more forward position. The goal, as outlined in Chapters 3 and 8, is to stimulate and direct mandibular growth. When the appliance is initially placed in a prepubertal individual and worn as directed, the mandible will reposition anteriorly quite rapidly. Prepubertal patients should be cautioned about chewing hard on their teeth during meals. Particular care should be given to chewing food at breakfast. After a full night of wear, the mandibular musculature is well-redirected for a more forward positioning of the mandible and the mandibular teeth. Closing hard on the incisors may

Diagnostic and Clinical Errors

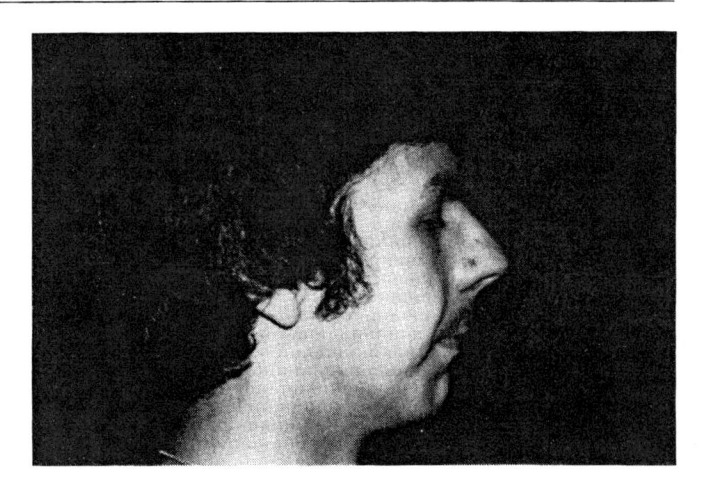

Figs. 13-3a and b This patient must struggle to keep his lips together. Nasal breathing is almost impossible. The facial profile esthetics have not improved after three years of edgewise full-banded treatment. Premolar extraction and incisor retraction have "dished in" the lower face.

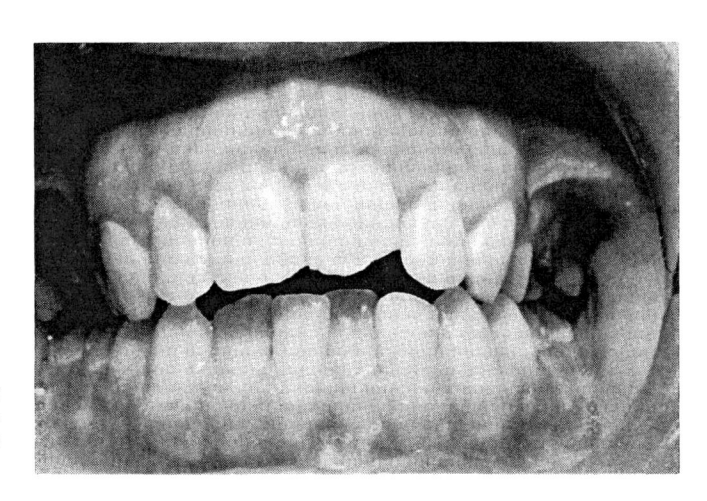

Fig. 13-3b The patient's mother is concerned about the red gingival tissue and crowded teeth two years after treatment.

cause chipping or abrading of the central or lateral incisors (Figs. 13-4a and b). Instructions to the patient to avoid hard chewing when the appliance is out of the mouth will avoid this treatment error.

Bulky appliances for uncooperative patients

Utilization of a bulky appliance for an uncooperative child may lead to incompletion of a treatment plan. However, many special-needs children that have a variety of handicapping disorders can be very adequately treated with removable orthopedic appliances. The value and appreciation of the result to parent and patient makes this treatment especially gratifying. Although cooperation can vary from marginal to 100%, the special-needs patient usually requires more in-office chair time for treatment. The extra effort required to take impressions, radiographs, and photographs and to accomplish treatment is well worthwhile for the special-needs patient (Figs. 13-5a and b).

Children that do not have special needs may require extra time for instructions and familiarization with orthopedic appliances.

305

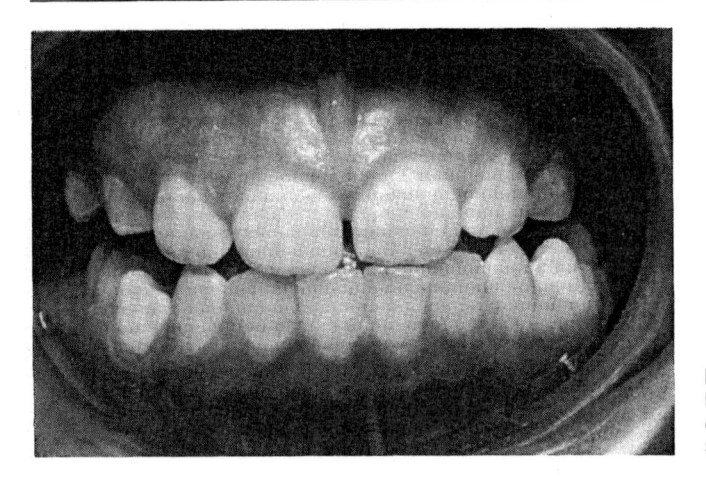

Figs. 13-4a and b Care must be taken to avoid incisal edge damage during orthopedic repositioning of the mandible.

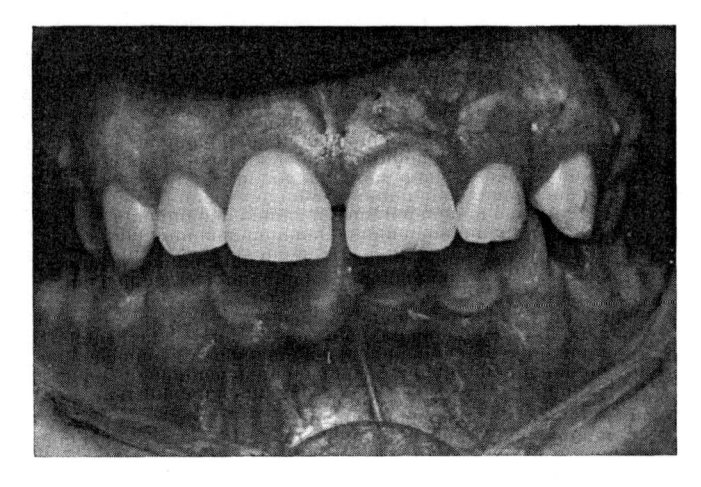

Fig. 13-4b

Observation and discussion with other children that already wear orthopedic appliances can do much to ameliorate the fears and anxieties that most children (and parents) harbor concerning appliance wear. Maj et al.,[19] in 1967, found that 75% out of a sample of 100 children regarded removable appliances as "troublesome" and 50% had fears of being excluded from the social group because of appliance wear. Lewis and Brown,[20] in 1973, showed a lower overall anxiety level than that of Maj et al. The most prevalent worry (37%) was of forgetting to wear the appliance, followed by those of being noticed by other people (36%), interference and embarrassment with speaking (36%), and worry about pain (23%). Careful patient selection and evaluation for treatment with maxillofacial orthopedic appliances will minimize noncompliance with the treatment plan.

Difficulties of headgear treatment

The problem of maxillary dental overjet (Class II, Division 1 malocclusion) has been considered by some investigators to be a growth discrepancy within the maxilla.

Diagnostic and Clinical Errors

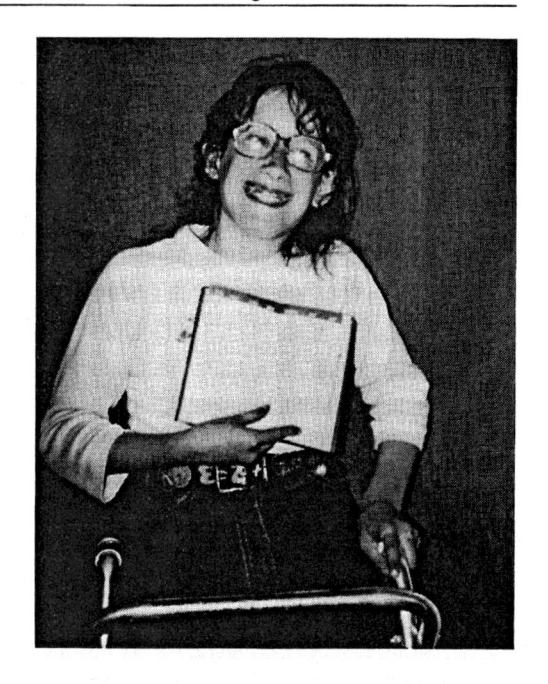

Figs. 13-5a and b Many special-needs patients accept removable appliance treatment with enthusiasm.

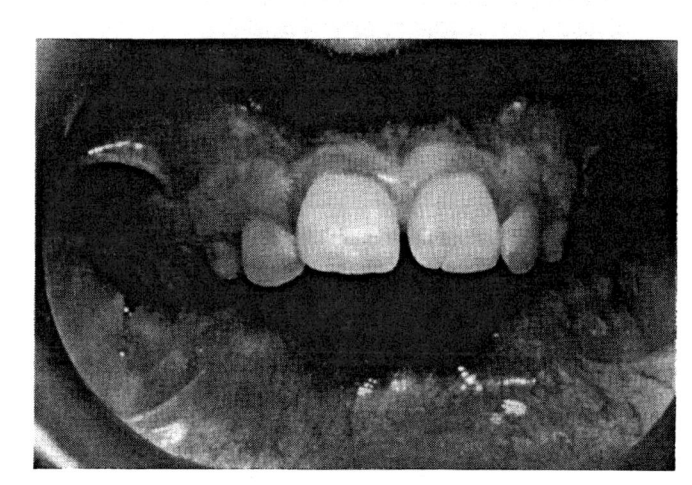

Fig. 13-5b The 12 mm overjet would not easily be treated with headgear and fixed-appliance therapy.

Tweed, in 1936[21] and 1941,[22] suggested that the treatment plan of Class II, Division 1 malocclusion be first directed toward "the most efficient manner possible for distal movement *en masse* of the maxillary teeth." Concern was also expressed that many Class II, Division 1 patients "never seem to develop much chin." Fischer, in 1948,[23] discussed the limitations of moving the mandibular teeth forward and stated that "anteroposterior malrelationship of the dental arches in maxillary protrusions and structural mandibular retrusions must be corrected by a posterior movement of the maxillary dental arch." Margolis, in 1953,[24] suggested that the clinician improve the contour of the lower third of the face by "reducing a bimaxillary dento-alveolar prognathism."

Dougherty,[25] in 1973, indicated that in Class II growth patterns the "maxilla proportionately outgrows the mandible." Baumrind et al., in 1979,[26] found that it was possible to "produce absolute distal displacement of the maxilla by the clinical use of distally directed forces to the maxilla."

Others have indicated that the Class II dental discrepancy was a hypoplastic growth problem of the mandible. Holdaway, in 1956, stated:[27]

> The treatment response most desired in most Class II cases is one of forward mandibular positioning due to alteration in the amount and direction of growth, primarily in the growth site at the head of the condyles.

Maxillofacial orthopedic appliances can be constructed (Chapter 8) to encourage the mandibular growth sought by Holdaway. If mandibular growth can be obtained to eliminate dental overjet, many patients that would otherwise object to wearing a headgear may receive treatment. Maxillary crowding is resolved first; then the maxilla serves as a skeletal guide for mandibular correction. The bionator appliance provides a reciprocal distal force to the maxilla as the mandible is repositioned forward (Chapters 3 and 8).

Patient cooperation for headgear wear can be difficult to obtain. Clemmer and Hayes[28] found that patients who most required headgear treatment had the greatest potential for a negative attitude toward orthodontics. Gabriel[29] suggests that the clinician can program and influence treatment results if there is good communication with the patient. The Clemmer and Hayes study indicated that females were more sensitive to dentofacial attractiveness and would cooperate with headgear wear more frequently than would males. Although an appeal to dental and facial esthetics was effective for motivating females, males required a goal and a sense of accomplishment. Fitch and Moxley[30] indicate that specific measures of accomplishment help reinforce cooperation.

The orthodontic progress report (Chapter 12) provides a method of continually reinforcing cooperation by giving measurable goals. A diary of appliance wear that demonstrates minimization or elimination of conspicuous headgear treatment will provide positive motivation for the patient.

Miscalculation of patient or parent commitment

It is important to know the patient before expecting total commitment and cooperation for the duration of a treatment plan. Some clinicians expect full cooperation after a 10- or 15-minute discussion of the treatment plan with the parent. Removable orthopedic appliances require excellent patient cooperation if treatment is to be successful. The clinician who knows the patient well has an improved chance of minimizing the risk of failure through poor cooperation. Slakter et al.[31] recognized patient cooperation as an important factor in the outcome of orthodontic treatment. Many clinicians in the Slakter study felt that two months was too soon to fully evaluate patient cooperation. It was also noted that early patient acceptance and cooperative compliance with the treatment plan was evidence of probable continued cooperation. Similarly, early noncompliance with instructions was indicative of probable continuing difficulty with patient cooperation.

Since patient cooperation is necessary for optimal results in the correction of malocclusion, it would be helpful to predict before treatment commenced which types of patients were likely to be the most cooperative. With complicated malocclusions, a high degree of patient assistance can determine the difference between average results and truly successful resolution.

Starnbach and Kaplan,[32] in a sample of 362 patients evaluated, found that the best orthodontic patients tended to be Protestant or Catholic females from rural industrial neighborhoods with fathers that were from farm, benchworker, or blue collar backgrounds. Croxton[33] found parental overpermissiveness to be a primary factor in dental management problems for children.

Maxillofacial orthopedic appliances are particularly effective when initiated during a growth period between the early mixed dentition stage and the pubertal stage of patient development. Stöckli[34] suggests that ages 8 to 11 coincide with responsiveness to parental authority and rapid growth so that conditions for patient cooperation with appliances is optimal. In a personality study of 30 12- to 18-year-old patients who were undergoing treatment for malocclusion, Allen and Hodgson[35] found younger patients more cooperative than older patients. They found no difference in cooperation on the basis of gender. They also found that personality profiles show the most cooperative patients to be those younger than 14 and "enthusiastic, outgoing, energetic, wholesome, self-controlled, responsible, trusting, determined to do well, hardworking, forthright, and obliging." The patient least likely to be cooperative is more than 14 years of age and is "of superior intelligence, hardheaded, independent, aloof, often nervous, temperamental, impatient, individualistic, easygoing, self-sufficient, intolerant of prolonged effort or attention, and tends to disregard the wishes of others when his own desires are involved."

Parental commitment is also necessary for the best occlusal and functional results. If the young patient cannot keep the adjustment appointments, progress may be thwarted. A miscalculation of parental commitment will bring about failure of the treatment plan.

Surgical consideration of skeletal deformities

Surgical treatment for correction of dentofacial deformities in the growing child is controversial. If the procedure is accomplished too early, without attempting correction via maxillofacial orthopedic technique, then the patient may be unnecessarily exposed to surgical risk. Also, early surgical treatment may relapse. However, some facial deformities are not readily corrected without surgical intervention. In addition, many children with facial deformities have difficulties with peer acceptance. Unintentional cruelty from friends and schoolmates can damage the developing psyche of the child.

Vertical maxillary deficiency

No attempt should be made to correct gross skeletal deformities without a previous surgical consultation (Chapter 3, Fig. 3-4). An example is vertical maxillary deficiency. When visualizing the patient with the lip in the postural position, no maxillary incisor teeth are visible. Orthopedic correction is all but impossible, and orthodontic correction would require excess extrusion of the incisors. Bell and Scheideman[36] describe the surgical technique (basically a LeFort I osteotomy) and the strategy for avoiding relapse with surgical treatment. Autogenous interpositional bone grafts are used to increase and stabilize facial height.

Vertical maxillary excess

Vertical dentofacial discrepancies have been studied by Sassouni and Nanda.[37] Eight patients with vertical maxillary excess and open bite from birth to adulthood were studied by superimposing cephalometric films. As compared with patients with nor-

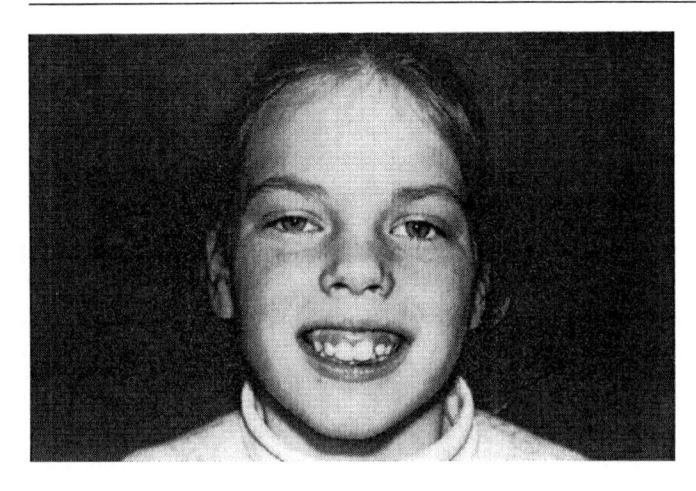

Fig. 13-6 The decision to correct vertical maxillary excess surgically may be given impetus by patients themselves if unkind remarks are making life difficult for them. Some authors feel that stable surgical results can be achieved during growth.[39] Final condylar position must be considered when choosing a surgical procedure that will alter vertical dimension.

mal dentofacial proportions (Fig. 13-6), the total maxillary dental height was greater in the incisor and molar area. Dentofacial relationships in the adults studied were present at about 6 years of age. Bell et al.[38] recommend careful use of cephalometric tracings in attempting to predict the long-term stability of surgical correction of vertical maxillary excess. Washburn et al.[39] have shown that surgical correction of vertical maxillary excess is successful in patients who are still growing. Early surgical intervention (in this study, between ages 10 and 16) favorably affected the disproportionate growth that is characteristic of vertical maxillary excess. The occlusal, skeletal, and esthetic results were stable after an average follow-up period of three years.

Primary failure of eruption

An attempt to treat a posterior open bite that is a result of primary failure of eruption is extremely frustrating. Since the etiology is not distinct, treatment modalities are not specific. If the teeth are not ankylosed, an orthodontic force tends to cause ankylosis. Fixed appliance therapy tends to intrude surrounding normal teeth rather than extrude the unerupted tooth (Figs. 13-7a to c and 13-8a to c). Proffit and Vig[40] suggest that the only reasonable method of managing primary failure of eruption is to surgically reposition the tooth or teeth by way of alveolar osteotomy without disturbing the periodontal ligament. A bone graft is positioned beneath the repositioned osseous segment and the repositioned tooth is held tightly in occlusion until healing is complete.

Mandibular prognathism

Severe mandibular prognathism that has been untreated by age 12 or that has not responded to early (ages 5 to 10) chin-cap treatment or maxillary sagittal appliance therapy should be considered for later surgical correction. Epker and Wolford[41] have described the surgical correction of mandibular excess deformities. Good communication between clinicians is stressed for optimal patient care. Wisth,[42] in a postoperative survey 10 years posttreatment, found that the surgical results of vertical ramus osteotomy were relatively stable. Most patients were generally satisfied with the surgical correction.

Surgical Consideration of Skeletal Deformities

Figs. 13-7a to c This patient has worn fixed appliances for five years. Two surgical procedures and lengthy mechanical extrusion have failed to bring about eruption of the permanent left maxillary canine. In place of canine eruption, the surrounding teeth have intruded.

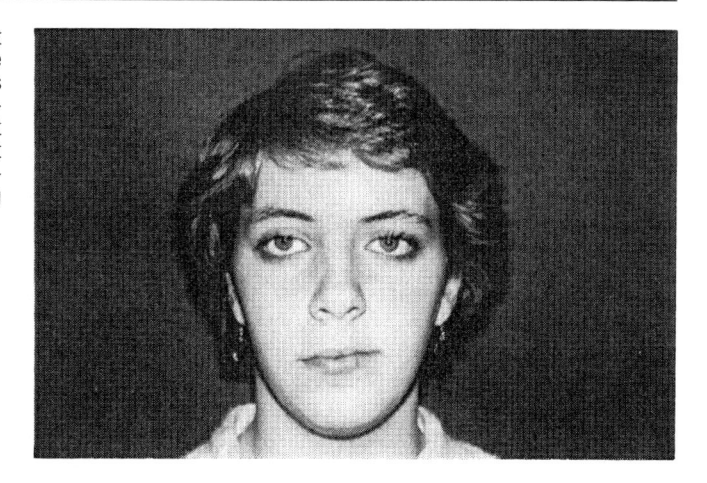

Fig. 13-7a Facial asymmetry.

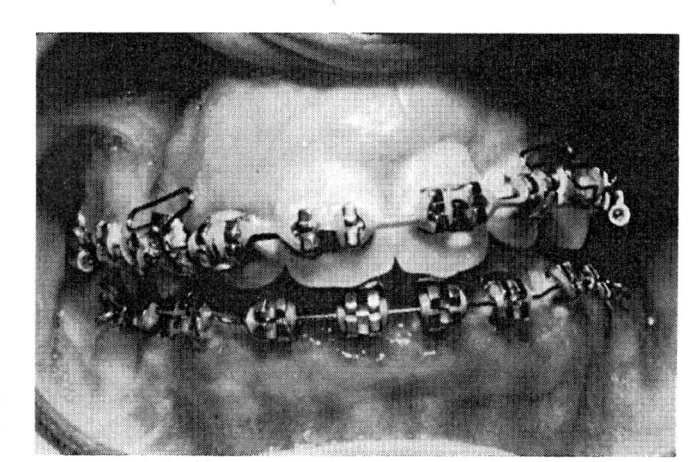

Figs. 13-7b and c Dental asymmetry and intrusion are evident.

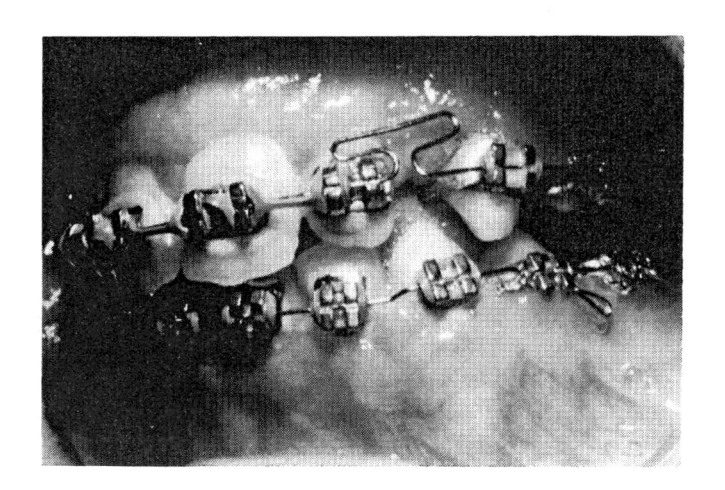

Fig. 13-7c

311

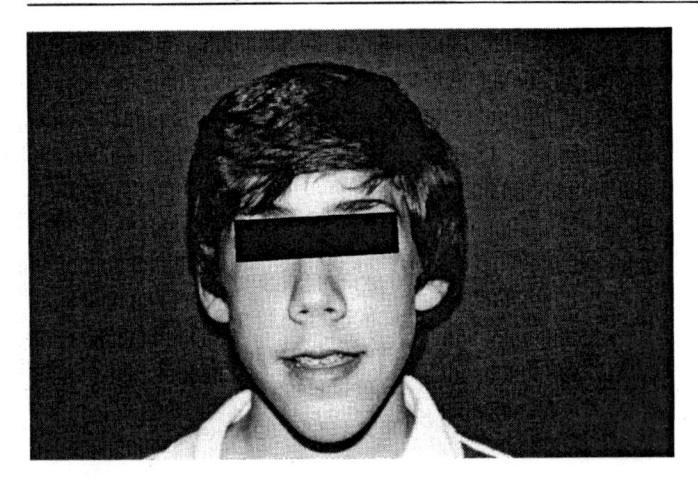

Critical Errors in Diagnosis and Treatment of Malocclusion

Figs. 13-8a to c At this stage of development (age 12 years), surgical correction is the best alternative for this patient. The patient presents with a mandibular skeletal protrusion, increased lower facial height, and a left deviation of the lower face.

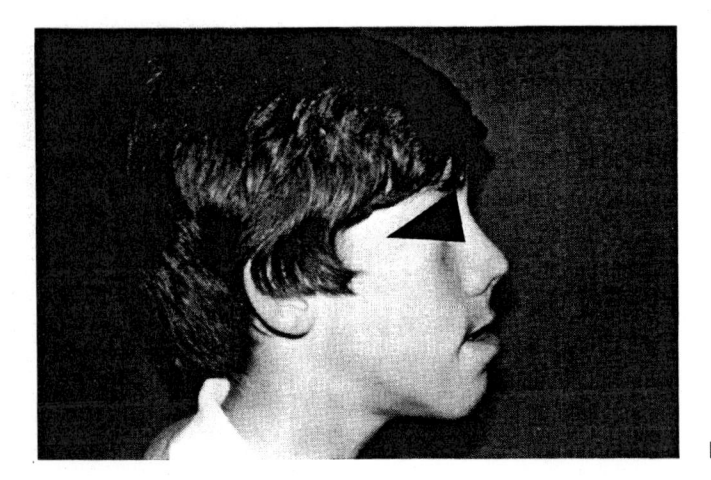

Fig. 13-8b

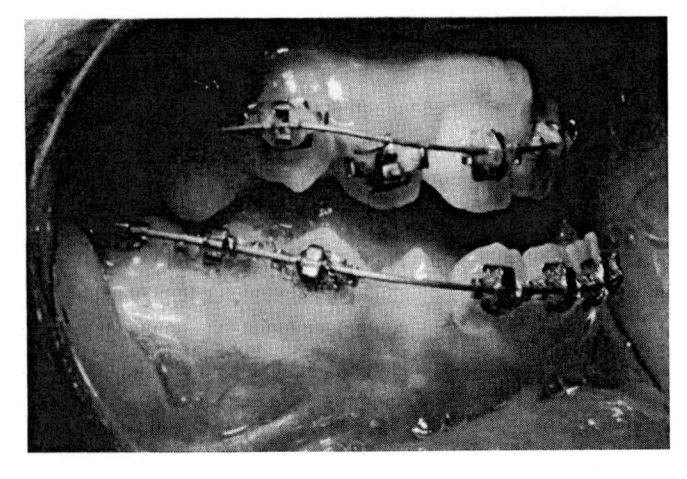

Fig. 13-8c

312

Late diagnosis of existing etiology

Nasal airway obstruction

Elimination of adenotonsillar tissue has been suggested[43-46] as a prophylactic method of treating potentially excessive mandibular growth. Rubin[47] has recommended early (prenatal) interest in malocclusion. Allergic nasal obstruction in an infant or growing child may alter the rest position and subsequent growth of the mandible (see Chapter 2). The introduction of adult foods (orange juice, eggs, and cereal) before the age of 6 months can cause allergic reactions in children.[48] Prospective mothers and parents of neonates should be counseled to breast-feed children in order to help avoid allergic reactions during the first year of life. If breast-feeding is impossible, a hypoallergenic soybean milk would be less allergenic than cows' milk.[49] There is evidence in primitive societies of excellent nutritional results from using breast milk as the sole food source for more than one year.[50] By avoiding allergies early in life, the allergic response mechanism may become quiescent[47-49]; hence one cause of nasal airway obstruction (allergic rhinitis) may be avoided.

Although the prevention of nasal airway obstruction (via nutritional considerations) and the elimination of adenoidal and tonsillar obstruction (via surgical intervention) have been discussed in the literature, neither technique has proved to reduce the potential for long-face syndrome or excessive mandibular growth. Howard in 1932,[51] Humphreys and Leighton in 1950,[52] and Leech in 1958[53] could not establish a direct relationship between mouth breathing and dentofacial form. Bushey,[54] in a 1979 study of adenoid obstruction in the nasopharynx, could not definitely establish the extent to which craniofacial morphology was influenced by the type of respiration. Morag and Ogra,[55] Ogra,[56] and Surjan and Surjan[57] point out that tonsillectomy and adenoidectomy may compromise the microbial defense or local immunological functions of the host. Since the evidence is inconclusive that removal of tonsillar and adenoidal tissue will influence facial growth, Diamond[58] suggests a conservative approach to treatment.

Mitani[59] has studied mandibular prognathism in Japanese females. The fundamental growth pattern of mandibular prognathism seemed to be established early in life. Once established, the mandibular growth rate was similar to that in the normal face before puberty.

McNamara[60] found a direct relationship between upper airway obstruction and craniofacial growth. The clinical cases presented in this study illustrate the problem of mouth breathing, and the effects of nasal airway obstruction on mandibular posture and its possible undesirable effects on craniofacial growth.

Since there are two distinct points of view concerning upper airway obstruction and early treatment of mandibular prognathism, it is urged that each patient with this problem be evaluated very carefully. Medical and dental consultation will ensure an individualized treatment plan that is best suited to the particular patient (Figs. 13-8a to c). The relationship between nasal airway function and dentofacial morphogenesis has been reviewed by O'Ryan et al.[61] A consistent relationship between obstructed nasorespiratory function and long-face syndrome could not be found in the literature. The relationship between airway obstruction and untoward facial growth requires further study and documentation.

Poor communication with patient or parent

Most parents and patients prefer a conservative approach to treatment as long as the original pretreatment goals are met. Good communication during all stages of treatment will help minimize problems with patient treatment and cooperation.[62] The first evening of appliance insertion is an especially good time to telephone the patient or parent in order to be sure of patient comfort. The parent will have a feeling of involvement with the treatment plan as long as open communication is emphasized and the clinician demonstrates a sincere interest in patient progress.

Teamwork is important for efficient correction of malocclusion. The parent should be included as part of a three-member team for treatment: parent, child, and dental staff. If the parent is involved in a team approach to treatment, there is less likelihood of an adversary relationship developing or litigation for unforeseen circumstances during treatment. Good parental-patient-staff communication will be rewarded by shortened treatment time, happier patients, and additional referrals. Poor communication may lead to a prolonged treatment time and poor patient cooperation. If communication is poor and a treatment plan seems endless, the patient or parent may discontinue treatment.[63]

Poor communication may also lead to appliance breakage or abuse. Oliver[64] has studied the frequency of unscheduled visits for fixed and removable appliances. Unscheduled visits can reduce patient and parent confidence in the treatment plan and waste valuable time for the clinician. Careful instructions for appliance usage will minimize carelessness and abuse.

One particularly difficult area of parent-patient-staff communication is renumeration for services. Many clinicians consider discussion of fees beneath the dignity of the doctor. This attitude will discourage patient/parent acceptance of a treatment plan and misplace the emphasis on *cost for* treatment instead of on the *value of* treatment. The cost of treatment can be easily calculated in terms of monetary and time commitment. If the parent or patient perceives the value of treatment as worth many times the cost of treatment, then most treatment plans will be readily accepted.[65]

Patient communication and effective management of a clinical practice may be as important as clinical expertise. An effective blending of high-quality clinical care and astute practice management should result in optimal patient care. Callender and Barbour[66] have discussed the financial arrangements most preferred by parents of orthodontic patients in two representative offices in Denver, Colorado. The survey found that most parents preferred that the child patient be present during the discussion. Parents seemed to prefer an initial payment of 25% to 33% with regular monthly payments; larger initial payments or quarterly payments were not appreciated. If a loan was necessary, the Callender study pointed out that most parents preferred bank or credit union financing. There was much opposition to finance companies or in-family loans.

If a monthly payment was late, a written or telephoned reminder was preferable to a reminder during an appointment. If regular payments became impossible, most parents wanted treatment to continue, with any late charges added to the payments due.

Summary

A strong management approach to clinical practice will result in better staff-patient communication and in more patients being treated more effectively. Once the clinician can see himself or herself as a highly skilled manager, then delegation of responsibility and development of an effective team approach to treatment will come easily. The clinical errors in this chapter are never committed in some offices; some occur routinely. If errors can be minimized, the patient and the clinical staff will both benefit.

References

1. Stricter, G. Psychological issues pertaining to malocclusion. Am. J. Orthod. 58:276–283, 1970.
2. Ketcham, A. H. A radiographic study of orthodontic tooth movement: a preliminary report. J. Am. Dent. Assoc. 14:1577–1598, 1927.
3. Ketcham, A. H. A preliminary report of an investigation of apical root resorption of permanent teeth. Int. J. Orthod. O. Surg. Rad. 13:97–127, 1927.
4. Rudolph, C. E. A comparative study in root resorption in permanent teeth. Am. J. Orthod. 23:822–826, 1936.
5. Massler, M., and Malone, A. J. Root resorption in human permanent teeth. Am. J. Orthod. 40:619–633, 1954.
6. Philips, J. R. Apical root resorption under orthodontic therapy. Angle Orthod. 25:1–22, 1955.
7. DeShields, R. W. A study of root resorption in treated Class II, Division 1 malocclusion. Angle Orthod. 39:231–245, 1969.
8. Goldson, L., and Henrikson, C. O. Root resorption during Begg treatment: a longitudinal roentgenologic study. Am. J. Orthod. 68:55–66, 1975.
9. Hall, A. M. Upper incisor root resorption during stage II of the Begg technique: two case reports. Br. J. Orthod. 5:47–50, 1978.
10. Harry, M. R., and Sims, M. R. Root resorption in bicuspid intrusion. Angle Orthod. 52:235–258, 1982.
11. McNamara, J. A., Jr. Components of Class II malocclusion in children 8–10 years of age. Angle Orthod. 51:177–202, 1981.
12. Baumrind, S., Miller, D., and Molthen, R. The reliability of head film measurements. Am. J. Orthod. 70:617–644, 1976.
13. Peck, H., and Peck, S. A concept of facial esthetics. Angle Orthod. 40:284–318, 1970.
14. Eirew, H. L. An orthodontic challenge. Br. Dent. J. 140:96–99, 1976.
15. Larsson, E., and Ronnerman, A. Mandibular dysfunction symptoms in orthodontically treated patients ten years after the completion of treatment. Eur. J. Orthod. 3:89–94, 1981.
16. Janson, M., and Hasund, A. Functional problems in orthodontic patients out of retention. Eur. J. Orthod. 3:173–179, 1981.
17. Tweed, C. W. A philosophy of orthodontic treatment. Am. J. Orthod. Oral Surg. 31:74–103, 1945.
18. Wilson, W. L. Multidirectional orthodontic treatment. Trans. 49th Congress of the Eur. Orthod. Soc. 223–229, 1973.
19. Maj, G., Grilli, A. T. S., and Belletti, M. F. Psychologic appraisal of children facing orthodontic treatment. Am. J. Orthod. 53:849–857, 1967.
20. Lewis, H. G., and Brown, W. A. B. The attitude of patients to the wearing of a removable orthodontic appliance. Br. Dent. J. 134:87–90, 1973.
21. Tweed, C. H. The application of the principles of the edgewise arch in the treatment of Class II, Division 1 malocclusion. Angle Orthod. 6:198–208, 1936.
22. Tweed, C. H. The application of the principles of the edgewise arch in the treatment of malocclusion: part II. Angle Orthod. 11:12–67, 1941.
23. Fischer, B. Treatment of Class II, Division 1 (Angle): II. Differential diagnosis and an analysis of mandibular anchorage. Am. J. Orthod. 34:461–490, 1948.
24. Margolis, H. I. A basic facial pattern and its application in clinical orthodontics. Am. J. Orthod. 39:425–433, 1953.
25. Dougherty, H. Failures in orthodontics. Trans. 49th Congress Eur. Orthod Soc. 231–241, 1973.
26. Baumrind, S., et al. Distal displacement of the maxilla and upper first molar. Am. J. Orthod. 75:630–640, 1979.
27. Holdaway, R. A. Changes in relationship of points A and B during orthodontic treatment. Am. J. Orthod. 42:176–193, 1956.
28. Clemmer, E. J., and Hayes, E. W. Patient cooperation in wearing orthodontic headgear. Am. J. Orthod. 75:517–524, 1979.
29. Gabriel, H. F. Motivation of the headgear patient. Angle Orthod. 38:129–135, 1968.
30. Fitch, M., and Moxley, R., Jr. Preventive dentistry with behavior modification. J. Am. Soc. Prev. Dent. 2:45–46, 1972.
31. Slakter, M. J., et al. Reliability and stability of the orthodontic patient cooperation scale. Am. J. Orthod. 78:559–563, 1980.
32. Starnbach, H. K., and Kaplan, A. Profile of an excellent orthodontic patient. Angle Orthod. 45:141–145, 1975.
33. Croxton, W. Child behavior and the dental experience. J. Dent. Child. 34:212–217, 1967.
34. Stöckli, P. W. Treatment timing. Trans. Eur. Orthod. Soc. 61–65, 1975.
35. Allan, T. K., and Hodgson, E. W. The use of personality measurements as a determinant of patient cooperation in an orthodontic practice. Am. J. Orthod. 54:433–440, 1968.
36. Bell, W. H., and Scheideman, G. B. Correction of vertical maxillary deficiency: stability and soft tissue changes. J. Oral Surg. 39:666–670, 1981.
37. Sassouni, V., and Nanda, S. Analysis of dentofacial vertical proportions. Am. J. Orthod. 50:801–823, 1964.
38. Bell, W. H., Sinn, D. P., and Finn, R. A. Cephalometric treatment planning for superior repositioning of the maxilla and concomitant mandibular advancement. J. Maxillofac. Surg. 10:42–49, 1982.
39. Washburn, M. C., Schendel, S. A., and Epker, B. N. Superior repositioning of the maxilla during growth. J. Oral Maxilofac. Surg. 40:142–149, 1982.
40. Proffit, W. R., and Vig, K. W. L. Primary failure of eruption: a possible cause of posterior open bite. Am. J. Orthod. 80:173–190, 1981.
41. Epker, B. N., and Wolford, L. M. Dentofacial Deformities, Surgical-Orthodontic Correction. St. Louis: The C. V. Mosby Co., 1980.
42. Wisth, P. J. What happened to them? Postoperative survey of patients 10 years after surgical correction of mandibular prognathisms. Am. J.

Orthod. 80:525-535, 1981.
43. Ricketts, R. M. Respiratory obstruction syndrome. Am. J. Orthod. 54:495-514, 1968.
44. Subtelny, J. D. Workshop on tonsillectomy and adenoidectomy. Supplement 19, Am. Otol. Rhinol. Laryngol. 84:250-254, 1974.
45. Linder-Aronson, S. Effects of adenoidectomy on the dentition and facial skeleton over a period of five years. pp. 85-100. *In* Trans. 3rd. Int. Orthodontic Congress. St. Louis: The C. V. Mosby Co., 1975.
46. Quinn, G. W. Airway interference and its effect upon the growth and development of the face, jaws, dentition and associated parts. N.C. Dent. J. 60:28-31, 1978.
47. Rubin, R. M. Mode of respiration and facial growth. Am. J. Orthod. 78:504-510, 1980.
48. Glaser, J. The prophylaxis of allergic disease in infancy. Pediatrics 29:835-862, 1962.
49. Johnstone, D. E., and Dutton, A. M. Dietary management of allergic disease in children. N. Engl. J. Med. 274:715-719, 1966.
50. Marks, M. B. Allergy in relation to orofacial dental deformities in children: a review. J. Allergy 36:293-302, 1965.
51. Howard, C. C. Inherent growth and its influence on malocclusion. J. Am. Dent. Assoc. 19:642-651, 1932.
52. Humphreys, H. F., and Leighton, B. C. A survey of anteroposterior abnormalities of the jaws of children between the ages of two and five-and-a-half years of age. Br. Dent. J. 88:3-15, 1950.
53. Leech, H. L. A clinical analysis of orofacial morphology and behavior of 500 patients attending an upper respiratory clinic. Dent. Practit. 9:57-68, 1958.
54. Bushey, R. S. Adenoid obstruction of the nasopharynx. *In* J. A. McNamara, Jr. (ed.) Naso-respiratory Function and Craniofacial Growth. Monogr. no. 9, Craniofacial Growth Series. Ann Arbor: Center for Human Growth and Development, Univ. of Michigan, 1979.
55. Morag, A., and Ogra, P. L. Immunologic aspects of tonsils. Ann. Otol. Rhinol. Laryngol. 84(suppl. 19):37-42, 1975.
56. Ogra, P. L. Effect of tonsillectomy and adenoidectomy on nasopharyngeal antibody response to polio virus. N. Engl. J. Med. 284:59-61, 1971.
57. Surjan, L., and Surjan, M. Immunologic role of human tonsils. Acta Otolaryngol. 71:190-193, 1971.
58. Diamond, O. Tonsils and adenoids: Why the dilemma? Am. J. Orthod. 78:495-503, 1980.
59. Mitani, H. Prepubertal growth of mandibular prognathism. Am. J. Orthod. 80:546-553, 1981.
60. McNamara, J. A., Jr. Influence of respiratory pattern on craniofacial growth. Angle Orthod. 51:269-300, 1981.
61. O'Ryan, F. S., Gallagher, D. M., LaBanc, J. P., and Epker, B. N. The relation between nasorespiratory function and dentofacial morphology: a review. Am. J. Orthod. 82:403-410, 1982.
62. Coote, J. D. Removable appliance therapy: patient cooperation and its assessment. Br. Dent. J. 134:91-94, 1973.
63. Keltzy, B. A pedodontist looks at orthodontics. Am. J. Orthod. 54:612-616, 1968.
64. Oliver, R. G. The casual attender. Br. J. Orthod. 9:154-157, 1982.
65. Gottlieb, E. L. Managing for success in orthodontics. J. Clin. Orthod. 15:319-328, 1981.
66. Callender, R. S., and Barbour, A. Effective communication with clients: financial arrangements. J. Clin. Orthod. 15:497-500, 1981.

Chapter 14

The Future

Total-health dentistry

This text has reviewed the craniofacial development and treatment of the child patient. It has also shown how total-health-oriented dentistry is the most effective way to care for skeletal malocclusion. Total-health dentistry (Chapter 5) needs to be emphasized more in practice. A specialty that concentrates on straightening or restoring teeth while ignoring a vitamin deficiency, obesity, chronic smoking, alcoholism, or other health hazard will have little chance for success in the 21st century.

Differential facial esthetic concepts

Facial esthetic development based on cephalometric "standards" is no longer adequate. In the United States racial characteristics are not always considered in diagnosis and treatment planning. There is a tendency today to treat all malocclusion alike.[1] Yet different esthetic standards for maxillary protrusion exist for different racial backgrounds.[2] Age, gender, and genetic heritage need to be considered when making diagnostic and treatment decisions.[3]

Computerized growth prediction

Cephalometric analysis is changing from an error-prone, time-consuming task[4] to a computer-oriented science where the entire cranium is evaluated in a three-dimensional plane. Several mathematical models for shape transformation such as the symmetric axis developed by Blum have helped make computerized analysis possible.[5-12] In the future, accurate computerized three-dimensional craniofacial growth prediction will be commonplace, making correction of craniofacial deformity possible very early in the patient's facial development. Maxillofacial orthopedic appliance design will improve and new developments in care for patients with malocclusion may include appliances that electrically or sonically stimulate the oral tissues.

Malocclusion correction in the year 2065: A possible scenario

Guided by a dental assistant, the patient or a guardian gives the patient's medical and dental history and any pertinent parental history to the office computer. In the examination room a small, fiber-optic type beam is passed over all aspects of the patient's dentition and craniofacial features, "photographically" entering the existing malocclusion into the computer. A tiny ultrasonic beam "radiographically" records the hard and soft structures of the oral cavity.

Evaluation by the computer is instantaneous. It notes any pathology and correlates this information with diet, personality, and historical data. The treatment plan best suited for the individual is printed out.

The assistant takes from stock the computer-selected prefabricated "smart" appliance, switches on its microcomputer, and has the patient occlude into the flexible material as the material adjusts and sets to the malocclusion. The patient might feel a slight tingling or warmth as preset piezoelectrical forces begin the correction of the malocclusion. This sensation is not unpleasant, and the patient adapts to it in a few minutes. The result is a removable appliance that coordinates muscular function with the ideal skeletal facial form and condylar position for the patient.

The computer generates a set of instructions regarding patient nutrition and care and use of the appliance. An appointment is set for a posttreatment examination in eight to 12 months.

Maxmen[13] has demonstrated a very plausible result for the physician and computer-based medical care. He suggests that much of clinical medicine will be performed by highly skilled technicians or physician assistants by the year 2000, and that most diagnostic skills will be housed in a well-programmed, continually updated data-based computer. It is imperative in the 1980s that private dental practitioners integrate computer technology into an efficient clinical practice and that we recognize that education and retraining are lifelong.

Preparing for the future

Much needs to be done to achieve optimal treatment of malocclusion worldwide in the coming decades. First, it is important to move away from a mechanical concept of correction toward biologic, preventive, and growth-guidance treatment techniques that are integrated for the total health of the individual. If teeth are straightened only to relapse, or a malocclusion corrected but a TMJ disorder exacerbated, of what value is the treatment for the patient? Of what value is any treatment to the oral cavity without at least some consideration for adequate nutrition, dental stability, craniomandibular health, and ongoing prevention?

Second, a commitment must be made to making correction of facial disharmony available for everyone. The psychosocial importance of facial esthetics makes it essential that the clinician devote maximum effort to correction of malocclusion and associated facial imbalance.

Disadvantaged people worldwide approach correction of malocclusion with an innate fatalism. They often express the feeling that, despite the availability of "competent and conscientious personal and professional care, the ultimate loss of teeth is one of the natural vicissitudes of life."[14] Their views are often justified. Dentists tend not to practice in low-income areas. And since only a small percentage of clinicians treat malocclusion, the cost of treatment is often prohibitive. Many third-party payment plans for dental care do not include orthodontic benefits which makes obtaining treatment for malocclusion even more difficult for the disadvantaged. And even when treatment is available, the poor often avoid it because of fear of the unknown.

Third, clinicians in all geographic areas must become familiar with the growth and development of the craniofacial complex and how this structure can be altered with maxillofacial orthopedic techniques. Undergraduate dental curricula should be expanded to include diagnosis, treatment planning, and treatment of malocclusion. Technological advances such as the straight-wire fixed appliance technique should be thoroughly familiar to graduating generalists and specialists. These techniques minimize headgear, wire bending, and uncomfortable prolonged treatment plans and bring about esthetic and stable results. DiSalvo[15] projected a step in this direction with the restructuring and redefining of orthodontic education in some pedodontic programs.

Efforts should now be directed toward individualizing dental school curriculums and eliminating archaic courses that have little to do with current clinical practice.[16]

Finally, dentistry cannot allow itself to become so specialized that it becomes difficult to incorporate new methods into clinical practice. "We are moving from the specialist who is soon obsolete to the generalist who can adapt," wrote Naisbitt,[17] suggesting that changes in the marketplace will force industrial specialists to retrain and learn new techniques. The same concept applies to the correction of malocclusion. What competent practitioner would consider premolar extraction without contemplating its effects on the craniomandibular articulation?

Handy[18] noted that despite the old managerial theory that concentration plus specialization equals efficiency, too much specialization is not always beneficial:

Specialization produces specialists, and concentration gives them some essential part in a larger integrated process. The combination gives them unique power of a negative kind—the power to hold the organization for ransom by withdrawing their specialty.

The same concept was discussed by Davenport[19] in the opening remarks at the 1913 meeting of the European Orthodontic Society: "There is a tendency for all specialization to have a narrowing influence and it is important to guard against that."

Davenport's advice still applies today. When one considers the benefit for the patient, it is possible to see why all clinicians will want to provide a more complete dental health service for the child and adolescent patient in the 1980s.

Conclusion

Treatment for malocclusion in the next decade and beyond will be based on current treatment trends. It makes sense to recognize these trends and take full advantage of craniofacial growth potential in the prepubertal and adolescent patient.

References

1. Watson, W. G. Fifty years of concern. Am. J. Orthod. 80:561–563, 1981.
2. Alexander, T. L., and Hitchcock, H. P. Cephalometric standards for American Negro children. Am. J. Orthod. 74:298–304, 1978.
3. Nass, G. G. Age changes in incisal inclination of American black and white children. Angle Orthod. 51:227–240, 1981.
4. Moyers, R. E., and Bookstein, F. L. The inappropriateness of conventional cephalometrics. Am. J. Orthod. 75:599–617, 1979.
5. Blum, H. Biological shape and visual science. Part I. J. Theor. Biol. 38:205–287, 1973.
6. Blum, H., and Nagel, R. N. Shape description using weighted symmetric axis features. Pattern Recognition 10:167–180, 1978.
7. Blum, H. Discussion paper: geometry for biology. Ann. N.Y. Acad. Sci. 231:19–30, 1974.
8. Bookstein, F. L. The study of shape transformation after D'Arch Thompson. Math. Biosci. 34:177–219, 1977.
9. Bookstein, F. L. Linear machinery for morphological distortion. Comp. Biomed. Res. 11:435–458, 1978.
10. Bookstein, F. L. Looking at mandibular growth: some new geometric methods. pp. 83–103. In D. S. Carlson (ed.) Craniofacial Biology. Monogr. no. 10, Craniofacial Growth Series. Ann Arbor: Center for Human Growth and Development, Univ. of Michigan, 1981.
11. Moss, M. L., et al. Space, time, and space-time in craniofacial growth. Am. J. Orthod. 77:591–612, 1980.
12. Saadia, A. M., et al. Symmetric axis geometry vs. conventional cephalometrics in mandibular growth. J. Dent. Res. 62:284, 1983.
13. Maxmen, J. S. The Post-Physician Era. New York: John Wiley & Sons, 1976.
14. Dunning, J. M. Dental Care for Everyone. Cambridge, Mass.: Harvard University Press, pp. 49–50, 1976.
15. DiSalvo, N. A. Orthodontics 1985–90: a panel discussion. Am. J. Orthod. 74:305–309, 1978.
16. Cherrick, H. M. Dentistry—a changing profession. J. Nebr. Dent. Assoc. 59(2):9–14, 1982.
17. Naisbitt, J. Megatrends. New York: Warner Books, 1982.
18. Handy, D. Through the organizational looking glass. Harv. Bus. Rev. 58:115–121, 1980.
19. Davenport, K. A. Trans. Eur. Orthod. Soc. 3, 1913.

Index

A

Activator appliances,	18, 73, 74, 76, 211
and craniofacial growth	194
See also Andresen activator appliances.	
Adenoids	59, 60
Age, emotional	143
Ahlgren, J.	20
Allergy	58, 59, 60
Andresen, Viggo	16, 18, 21
Andresen activator appliances	18, 23
Andresen-Häupl activator appliances	19, 21, 23
Andresen retractor appliances	215
Angle, E. H.	16, 17
Angle orthodontic appliances	16
Articular disc displacement	242, 243, 244, 248, 249
Ascorbic acid	124
Asymmetry, left-right	140
Auriculotemporal nerve	228

B

Babcock, J. H.	17
Batters, Wilhelm	20, 23
Balters appliances	20, 23, 76
Basic Diet Experiment	129, 130
Bimler, H. P.	20, 21
Bimler oral adaptor	20, 21, 73, 77
Bionator,	20, 23, 74, 76, 77, 149
adjustment	189, 190, 191
changes from use	184, 286
for Class II, Division 1 malocclusion	188, 192, 196
for deep bite	189
for headache	302
for open bite	188
for temporomandibular joint disorders	259
mode of action	186
proper construction	184
treatment planning	187
Bite opening	159
Bite plane, Kingsley	16
Bite registration,	
construction bite	183, 185
procedure,	
activator	212
bionator	183, 185, 212
Fränkel appliance	213
sagittal appliance	159, 162
Blanket sucking	64, 84, 85
See also Digit sucking, Thumb sucking, and Pacifiers.	
Bonding, orthodontic brackets	172
Bone,	
alveolar	47
and muscle function	33
apposition	48, 50
calcifying matrix	36, 41, 42, 44
cascade	42
central canal	36, 39
collagen	36, 39, 40
connective tissue effects on	43
development, and muscle function	47, 48
electrical energy effects	43
endochondral development	40, 41, 42
epiphysis	42, 50
formation methods	40, 41, 42, 43
growth,	
and maxillofacial orthopedic appliances	189

Index

plates	42, 44, 50
intramembranous ossification	39, 40, 41, 43
lacunae	36, 39
lacunae, Howship's	40
mechanical energy effects	43
modeling	40, 41, 42, 48
morphology-reorganization relation	47
origin of bone cells	36
remodeling	40, 48
"streaming" potentials in	44
stress potentials in	44
sutures	41, 48
temporal, histology	232
Brachycephalia	63, 64
"Brush border"	40
Bruxism	242, 252

C

Canine,	
impacted	295, 297
primary, extraction	267, 268
recontouring	295
size prediction	108
Cartilage	36, 40, 41, 42, 44, 232
Case presentation	143, 152
Cephalogram	96
Cephalometry,	92
ANB angle assessment	104, 105
analysis	95, 100, 120
landmarks	93
Y-axis angle assessment	111
Cervical nerves	118, 120
Cervical spine	117, 118
Chondroblasts	42
Chondrocytes	42, 232
Clarkson, P.	21
Communication	83, 313
Condyle,	
growth,	51, 52, 53
age and	75
environmental stimuli	74
in mandibular growth	50, 79
orthopedic appliances and	74
relation to teeth	47
histology	232
physiologic position	251
relation to fossa	87, 88, 141, 224, 247, 285
relation to temporomandibular disorders	250, 283, 285
Connective tissue,	
bioelectrical potentials in	43
effect on bone	43
Cranial base,	
and mandibular growth	44
and maxillary growth	44, 46
effect on maxillomandibular complex	32, 46
Craniofacial complex,	
adaptive changes in growth	52, 56
and malocclusion	61, 65
biological shaping	29–72
mastication effects	58
respiration effects	58, 59, 60, 61
soft-hard tissue relation	36, 67, 76
tongue effects	56
Craniofacial growth,	
and activator appliances	194
and extraoral traction	194
and Fränkel appliances	194
and maxillofacial orthopedic therapy	191
computerized prediction	317
cranial base effects	32, 57
dentoalveolar changes and	73
environmental factors	31, 74
genetic factors	31
hard-soft tissue relation	76
heredity factors	31
neuromuscular factors	33, 57, 76, 77
normal biological	29–72
orthopedic appliances and	73, 180, 181
sleep position and	166, 287, 288
teeth and	57
Craniomandibular articulation	232
Craniomandibular disorders. See Temporomandibular joint disorders.	
Craniomandibular joint. See Temporomandibular joint.	
Craniomandibular pain syndrome	240
Crossbite,	63, 64, 66, 87
anterior	164, 210, 212
correction timing	142, 151, 167
posterior	166
Crowding,	142
and maxillofacial development	284
and maxillofacial orthopedic appliances	287

321

Index

and sagittal appliances 290
assessment 292
Class I, 156, 160, 161
treatment 162, 163, 164, 165
ethnic relation 292
from premolar extraction 305
from primary tooth extraction 265, 266, 267
molar extraction for 277
treatment timing 289
Crown torque,
edgewise bracket 169
for Class I 170
for Class II 170
for Class III 170
straight-wire bracket 169
Crozat, George 18
Crozat appliances 18
Curve of Spee 48, 190

D

Deep bite, 179, 285
bionator for 189
treatment timing 151
Dental arch,
age changes 54
and maxilla growth 44, 45, 46
and tooth eruption 44, 45
"ideal" 15
leveling 143
Pont index 109, 112
Schwarz analysis 110, 112, 113
tooth effects 65
Dental plaque control 124
Dental rotation 143
Dentist-patient relations, 83, 313
and case presentation 144, 152
Dentition,
mixed 54
Tanaka and Johnson analysis 107, 113
permanent 56
primary 52, 54, 56
relation to muscle function 35, 47, 67
Diagnosis, differential 88, 99
Diastema 293
Diet,
American 126
relation to mandible form 46, 47

Digit sucking 64, 85
See also Blanket sucking, Thumb sucking, and Pacifiers.

E

Ear 228
Edgewise arch 17
Enamel,
decalcification 272, 288
stripping 291, 292
Endosteum 41
Energy,
electrical, effect on bone 43
mechanical, effect on bone 43
Esthetics,
concepts 317
dental 303
facial and premolar extraction 269, 270, 271
facial and second molar extraction 276
goals 139
European Orthodontic Society 17, 20, 21
Expansion plate 21
Exteroception, neuromuscular 77

F

F-S Index 240
Facial angle 95
Facial form and body position 120, 133
Facial growth,
and malocclusion 62, 63, 64, 66, 67, 68
appliance force and 180, 181
factors 29, 30, 31, 56
mid-face 46, 57
nasal airway obstruction and 58, 59, 60, 61
patterns 122
prenatal 29, 31
tongue effects 57
Facial height 140, 207
Facial pain, diagnosis 117
Facial profile, 99, 140, 154, 176, 202, 303, 305
esthetics 179, 180, 284
Family and treatment planning 143

Index

Farrar, John Nutting 19
Fauchard, Pierre 15
Fauconnier 18
Fossa,
  glenoid 247
  infratemporal 224
  relation to condyle 87, 88, 141, 224, 247, 285
Fränkel, Rolf 22, 23
Fränkel appliances 194
Fränkel functional regulator 20, 22, 74, 76, 79, 211
French Society of Stomatology 18
Functional orthodontic appliances 17, 21
Future 317–319

G

Gebissregelung mit Platten 21
Genetics, craniofacial growth 31
Gingiva,
  bleeding 142, 273
  inflammation 305
  stripping 146
Goals,
  esthetic 139
  functional 140
  stability as 141
  treatment 139, 140, 141
Grossman, W. J. 21
Growth. See Craniofacial growth, Facial growth.

H

HVGS 253
Habits 64, 84, 85
Harvold, E. P. 20
Häupl, Karl 16, 18, 19, 21
Hawley, C. A. 18
Head, ideal position 121
Headache, iatrogenic 302
Health 124, 125, 128
Health Quiz 129, 130
Height-weight table 134, 135
Heredity, craniofacial growth 31
Herren, P. 20
High voltage electrogalvanic stimulation (HVGS) 253
Hoffer, Oscar 19
Holistic dentistry 317
Hunter, John 15
Hydrocephalus 32

I

Incisal edge chip 304
Incisor,
  congenitally missing lateral 294
  crowding 289
  extraction effects 274
  mesiodistal width 107

J

Jaw-to-jaw relationship 143
"Jumping the bite" 16

K

K-F-S Index 241
Kantorowicz, A. 18
Kinetor appliances 20, 21, 22, 76
Kingsley, Norman William 15
Kingsley appliances 16
Korkhaus, G. 18

L

Law, William G. 17
Lingual arch appliances 18
Lips, examination 88
Litigation, and temporomandibular joint treatment 261

M

Malocclusion,
  and craniofacial form 64, 66
  and sleep position 166, 287, 288
  and thumb sucking 62
  Angle classification 17
  correction in 21st century 317
  diagnosis 18, 83–115
  diagnosis errors 301–316
  dynamic muscle balance 38
  early prevention 137
  early treatment 178, 204
  examination for 83–115
  extraction therapy 265–282
  functional orthopedic correction 19
  habits and 64

in brachycephalia	63, 64
maxillofacial orthopedic therapy	73, 74
muscle function relation	34
Schwarz classification	18
tooth extraction for	159
treatment errors	301–316
treatment problems	283–300
Malocclusion, Class I,	155–175
appliance choice	155
goal achievement	157
sagittal appliances for	156
straight-wire appliances for	167
treatment objectives	157, 163
treatment timing	146, 147, 155, 167
treatment, with crossbite	164, 166
treatment, with crowding	162, 163, 164, 165
Malocclusion, Class II,	123, 177–201
cross section	186
maxillofacial orthopedic appliances for	178
treatment timing	178
Malocclusion, Class II, Division 1,	176, 177
bionator	188, 192, 196
facial structure	176
treatment timing	147, 151
Malocclusion, Class II, Division 2	177
Malocclusion, Class III,	203–216
activators for	211
Andresen retractor appliances for	215
chin cup for	206
crossbite	210, 212
early treatment	204
facial height	207
facial structure	202
fixed interarch appliances for	211
Fränkel appliances for	211
labiolingual appliances for	211
mandibular rotation in	209
open bite	209
sagittal appliances for	210, 213
skeletal, surgery	204
tongue and	208
treatment timing	149, 151, 204
types	203
Mandible,	
age changes	54
closure	285
condylar change	50

form-diet relation	46, 47
form-function relation	46, 47
form-muscle relation	46
form-stress relation	46
form-teeth relation	46, 47
function differences	47, 49
growth	15, 50, 120
growth changes	49, 79
growth process	46, 47
growth, relation to maxilla	46
growth, relation to tongue	58
growth, stimulation	188, 195
position changes	34, 47, 48, 50
remodeling	48, 49
Mandibular movement	234
Mandibular ramus	48
Mandibular retrusion	75
Mastication,	
craniofacial effects	58
muscle function effects	34, 47
Maxilla,	
age changes	54
growth, process	44, 45, 46
growth, relation to mandible	46
Maxillofacial development	284
Maxillofacial orthopedic appliances,	
and bone growth	189
clinical needs	15
craniofacial disorder treatment	217–263
crowding and	287
development of	15, 18, 21
for Class II malocclusion	178
Maxillofacial orthopedic therapy,	
and facial growth	180, 181, 191
ascorbic acid relation	124
challenges of	28
craniofacial response	73–81, 180
facial skeleton response	80
for malocclusion	73, 74
for mandibular retrusion	75
history of	15–26
muscular changes in	77
neuromuscular response	76, 80
strategies	77
success factors	80
timing of	75, 79
Maxillopalatine complex growth process	44, 45
Medical history	84
Medical history forms	235, 236, 237
Mershon, J. V.	18

Metabolism defects, sucrose	136	etiology	59, 60, 61
Midline alignment	265, 267	Nasal floor	46
Models, study	103, 111, 112	*Natural History of Human Teeth*	15
Molar, first, extraction	275	Neuromuscular feedback	36
Molar, second, extraction	275, 276, 277, 278, 279	Neuromuscular system	33, 76, 80
		Nord, C. F. L.	17, 21
Molar, third,		Nutrition,	117–138
enucleation	280	adequate	127
extraction	277, 280	American diet	126
migration	279	needs	129
pathology	280	optimal	127, 128, 133
tipping	278	super	128, 129
Monoblock appliances	18	sweetener consumption	126
Motivation	89, 178	treatment planning	122
Mouth breathing	58, 60	U.S. population	125
Mouth opening limits	86, 232		
Muscle function,			
abnormal	34, 55, 66	**O**	
and skeletal changes	36, 47		
effect on bone	33, 47, 48	Occlusion,	
effect on mastication	34, 47	Class I face	154, 186
effect on muscles	47	dynamic muscle balance	38
hypermentalis activity	37	examination of	87
in malocclusion	34, 55	factors in	65
maxillofacial orthopedic therapy changes	77	premolar extraction effects	269, 270, 271, 272
normal	33	Oligodontia	67
relation to bone development	47	Open bite,	
relation to dentition	35, 47, 67	bionator for	188
Muscles,		etiology	159
activity in normal occlusion and malocclusion	79	in Class III malocclusion	209
		thumb sucking and	85
dynamic balance	38	treatment timing	151
evaluation of	87	Oral hygiene evaluation	88
lateral pterygoid	221, 222, 223, 228, 229, 242	Orthodontic appliances,	
		arch wire placement	173
masseter	221, 225	bracket bonding	173
masticatory	242	bracket positioning	169, 171, 172
medial pterygoid	221, 222, 227, 242	chin cup	206
		edgewise	305
of temporomandibular joint	221	edgewise, brackets	169, 171
physiological adaptation	36, 47	enamel decalcification	288
relation to mandible form	46	expansion screw plates	17
sternocleidomastoid	224, 230	extraoral traction and growth	181, 194, 306
temporalis	221, 222, 226, 242	fixed	142, 211, 289
Myostatic reflex	78	fixed interarch	211
		incisal edge chip from	304, 306
N		labiolingual	165, 211
		regulating	16
Nasal airway obstruction,	58, 61, 122, 313	removable	182
		sagittal,	

Index

bite opening 159
contraindications 156
design 157
for Class III
  malocclusion 210, 212
indications 156, 290
mode of action 156
patient instructions 161
three-way 148, 158, 160, 161
two-way 158, 296
straight-wire 167, 214
straight-wire, brackets 168, 169, 171
tubes for 17
See also specific named devices.
Orthodontic retention 79
Orthopedic corrector appliances 24, 251, 252, 254, 257
Orthopedic maxillofacial
  appliances, 15, 149
  advantages 144, 182
  disadvantages 145, 183
Osteoblasts 36, 40, 41, 42, 43
Osteoclasis 36
Osteoclasts 36, 40, 43
Osteocytes 36, 39, 40
Osteogenesis 36
Overbite 87, 285
Overjet 87, 123, 285

P

Pacifiers 64
See also Digit sucking, Blanket sucking, and Thumb sucking.
Pain. *See* specific anatomical region.
Parotid gland 228
Patient cooperation, 144, 152, 286, 305
  bionator 184
  headgear 308
  maxillofacial orthopedic
    appliances 283
  miscalculation of 308
  sagittal appliances 161
Patients,
  feedback from 83, 84
  initial contact 83
  special needs of 307
Perichondrium 42
Periodontium 271, 273
Periosteum 41, 48
Petrovic, A. 23
Photography 98, 100, 102
Pierre Robin syndrome 76
Pont's analysis 109, 112
Posture, 117–138
  and treatment planning 120
  body, and facial form 120, 133
  effect on temporomandibular
    joint 219, 220
  head 118, 121, 122, 133
A Practical Treatise on the Diseases of the Teeth 15
Premolar,
  extraction effects 269, 270, 271, 272, 273, 289, 304, 305
  size prediction 108
Proprioception, neuromuscular 38, 77

Q

Questionnaire, temporomandibular
  joint screening 233

R

Radiography,
  cephalometric 92
  examination by 90
  panoramic 91, 245, 246
  tomographic 246, 249
  transcranial 245
  transmaxillary 246, 248
Recommended Dietary
  Allowance (RDA) 125, 129
Relapse 142, 289, 292
Remoldable craniomandibular
  appliance 251, 252
Reproximation 292
Respiration, effects on craniofacial
  complex 58, 59, 60, 61
Retainer,
  Hawley 18
  lingual 294
  spring 290, 291
Robin, Pierre 16, 18, 20
Rogers, Alfred P. 18
Root, resorption 142, 301, 303
Roux, R. 19

S

Schwarz, A. M.	17, 19, 21
Schwarz analysis	110, 112, 113
Selmer-Olsen, R.	20
Skeletal changes	36, 75
Skeletal relationships,	
anterior dental	106, 107, 108, 109, 110
mandibular prognathism	310
mandibular protrusion	103, 312
mandibular retrusion	102
mandibular sagittal	101
maxillary protrusion	98
maxillary retrusion	97, 99
maxillary sagittal	96
normal dentoalveolar	96
normal maxillary	96
vertical	104
vertical maxillary deficiency	309
vertical maxillary excess	309, 310
Skull size	288
Sleep, position and malocclusion	166, 287, 288
Soft tissue	84, 88
Space analysis	107, 109
Splints, occlusal	150
Stability	141
Stockfisch, H.	20, 21, 22
Stress, mandible forms	46
Sucrose, metabolism	136
Swallowing, infantile pattern	52
Sweeteners, consumption	126, 133
Synovial joint, histology	229

T

TENS	253
Temporomandibular joint,	
anatomy	50, 220, 221, 222, 223
evaluation	84
functions	55
growth	54
innervation	224
ligaments	228
mechanical stress and	232
musculature	221, 222
pain	117, 118, 240, 252, 253
pathology	247
premolar extraction effects	271, 272, 273
radiography,	89, 243, 250
panoramic	245, 246
tomographic	246, 249
transcranial	245
transmaxillary	246, 248
vascularity	224, 231
visual index	241
wide open mouth effects	232
Temporomandibular joint disorders,	
bionator treatment	259
closed lock	242, 243, 244
diagnosis	118, 217, 248
examination forms	238, 239
examination procedure	234, 242
F-S Index	240
K-F-S Index	241
litigation	261
mandibular movement	234
maxillofacial orthopedic appliances for	217
noise	229, 243, 244, 245
orthopedic corrector appliances for	254, 257
patient history	254, 257
patient profile	217
posture and	219
relation to condyle	250
screening questionnaire	233
surgery	260
symptoms	86, 88
therapy success	253
treatment modalities	248
treatment planning	248
Textbook of Functional Jaw Orthopaedics	21
Thumb sucking	62, 85
See also Blanket sucking, Digit sucking, and Pacifiers.	
Tongue,	
and Class III malocclusion	208
effect on craniofacial complex	56
effect on mandibular growth	58
examination	88
Tonsils	60
Tooth,	
anatomy	67
birth to primary dentition	52
effects on dental arch	65
examination	88
impacted, canine	295
overretention	265, 266
relation to condyle growth	47
relation to mandible form	46, 47

relation to muscle function	35, 66, 67
size	65, 107, 108, 288
spacing	88
Tooth crown,	
angulation	169
in/out relation	168
inclination	168
Tooth eruption,	
and dental arch growth	44, 45, 52
failure	310, 311
Tooth extraction,	
adverse effects	121
for malocclusion therapy	265–282
incisor	274
molar, first	275
molar, second	275, 276, 277, 278, 279
molar, third	277, 280
premature exfoliation	265
premolar	179, 269, 289, 304, 305
primary, canine	265, 267, 268
serial	265
Transcutaneous electric nerve stimulation (TENS)	253
Treatment goals	139
Treatment planning,	89, 120, 122, 132, 139–152
bionator	187
combined approach	182
early intervention	146, 147, 148, 149, 151, 178
emotional age and	143
family constellation and	143
in temporomandibular joint disorders	248
philosophy	182
presentation	143
sequence	141
timing,	142, 145, 148
crowding	289
Class I malocclusion	146, 147
Class II malocclusion	147, 178
Class III malocclusion	149
crossbite	151
deep bite	151
open bite	151

U

Ultrasound	253

V

Vertical dimension,	
development	120
early evaluation	151
lack of	123, 149
normal	104
re-establishment of	150, 151
Vitamin supplements	132

W

Watry, F. M.	18, 20
Wiebrecht, Albert	18
Witt, E.	23
Witzig, John W.	24
Wolff, J.	19
Wolff's law	47, 56